Eye Care
SOURCEBOOK

Fifth Edition

Health Reference Series

Fifth Edition

Eye Care
SOURCEBOOK

Basic Consumer Health Information about Vision and Disorders Affecting the Eyes and Surrounding Structures, Including Facts about Hyperopia, Myopia, Presbyopia, Astigmatism, Cataracts, Macular Degeneration, Glaucoma, and Other Disorders of the Cornea, Retina, Macula, Conjunctiva, and Optic Nerve

Along with Guidelines for Recognizing and Treating Eye Emergencies, Advice about Protecting the Eyes at Work, Home, and Play, Tips for Living with Low Vision, a Glossary of Terms Related to the Eyes and Eye Disorders, and a Directory of Resources for Further Information

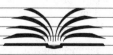

OMNIGRAPHICS

615 Griswold, Ste. 901, Detroit, MI 48226

Bibliographic Note
Because this page cannot legibly accommodate all the copyright notices, the Bibliographic
Note portion of the Preface constitutes an extension of the copyright notice.

* * *

Health Reference Series
Keith Jones, *Managing Editor*
***

OMNIGRAPHICS
A PART OF RELEVANT INFORMATION
***

Copyright © 2017 Omnigraphics
ISBN 978-0-7808-1532-2
E-ISBN 978-0-7808-1533-9

Library of Congress Cataloging-in-Publication Data

Names: Omnigraphics, Inc., issuing body.

Title: Eye care sourcebook: basic consumer health information about vision and
disorders affecting the eyes and surrounding structures, including facts about
hyperopia, myopia, presbyopia, astigmatism, cataracts, macular degeneration,
glaucoma, and other disorders of the cornea, retina, macula, conjunctiva, and optic
nerve; along with guidelines for recognizing and treating eye emergencies, advice
about protecting the eyes at work, home, and play, tips for living with low vision, a
glossary of terms related to the eyes and eye disorders, and a directory of resources
for further information. Other titles: Ophthalmic disorders sourcebook

Description: Fifth edition. | Detroit, MI: Omnigraphics, [2017] | Series: Health
reference series | Revision of: Ophthalmic disorders sourcebook. 2nd ed. c2003. |
Includes bibliographical references and index.

Identifiers: LCCN 2017004936 (print) | LCCN 2017006594 (ebook) | ISBN
9780780815322 (hardcover: alk. paper) | ISBN 9780780815339 (ebook) | ISBN
9780780815339 (eBook)

Subjects: LCSH: Eye--Diseases--Popular works. | Eye--Care and hygiene--Popular
works.

Classification: LCC RE51 .O64 2017 (print) | LCC RE51 (ebook) | DDC 617.7--
dc23

LC record available at https://lccn.loc.gov/2017004936

Table of Contents

Part Five: Eye Injuries and Disorders of the Surrounding Structures

Part Six: Congenital and Other Disorders That Affect Vision

Preface

About This Book

Recent statistics show that more than 39 million Americans have low vision or a disorder that can lead to it. Together these impairments cost $68 billion in annual direct healthcare costs, as well as lost productivity and diminished quality of life. These costs will continue to increase as the population increases. The most common causes of vision loss among adults in order of prevalence are cataracts, diabetic retinopathy, glaucoma, and age-related macular degeneration. Often these impairments can develop gradually and few are aware of the warning signs of serious eye disorders. Fewer still know that the effects of many of these disorders could be lessened or eliminated entirely with regular comprehensive eye exams and early detection which can help diagnose emerging vision problems before vision loss is noticeable.

Eye Care Sourcebook, Fifth Edition, provides information about common vision and eye-related problems and how they are diagnosed and treated. It includes facts about cataracts, corneal disorders, macular degeneration, glaucoma and other disorders of the optic nerve, retinal disorders, and refractive and eye movement disorders. It describes congenital and hereditary disorders that affect vision, and infectious diseases, traumatic injuries, and other disorders with eye-related complications. It also provides tips for recognizing and treating eye emergencies and suggestions to help prevent eye injuries. The book concludes with a summary of tips for living with low vision, a glossary of terms related to eye disorders, and a directory of resources for further help and information.

How to Use This Book

This book is divided into parts and chapters. Parts focus on broad areas of interest. Chapters are devoted to single topics within a part.

Part I: Eye and Eye Care Basics explains how the eyes work and describes the most common methods of diagnosing vision and other eye-related problems. It offers suggestions for maintaining healthy eyes and discusses common pediatric and age-related vision concerns. Finally, it describes ongoing research in the field of vision disorders.

Part II: Understanding and Treating Refractive, Eye Movement, and Alignment Disorders describes common disorders affecting the eyes' refractive ability, ability to move, and alignment, including astigmatism, hyperopia (farsightedness), myopia (nearsightedness), presbyopia, and strabismus. It provides details about the different types of eyeglasses and contact lenses used to treat refractive disorders and describes how to fit them and care for them properly. The section concludes with a discussion of the most common types of refractive surgery.

Part III: Understanding and Treating Disorders of the Cornea, Conjunctiva, Sclera, Iris, and Pupil discusses cataracts and other corneal disorders and provides a detailed description of treatments such as corneal transplant. It also discusses conjunctivitis, dry eye, and other common disorders of the conjunctiva and describes the methods used to diagnose and treat these disorders.

Part IV: Understanding and Treating Disorders of the Macula, Optic Nerve, Retina, Vitreous, and Uvea provides information about macular degeneration and other macular disorders, glaucoma, optic neuritis, and other disorders of the optic nerve, retinal detachment, retinopathy of prematurity, and other disorders of the retina, and disorders of the vitreous and uvea, including floaters, vitreous detachment, and uveitis. It details the signs and symptoms of these disorders and explains how they are diagnosed and treated.

Part V: Eye Injuries and Disorders of the Surrounding Structures discusses how to recognize and treat eye emergencies, including chemical burns, foreign objects in the eye, and blowout fractures, and how to prevent these injuries. It includes a description of recommended forms of workplace and sports eye protection. It also discusses the most common disorders of the eyelids and tear ducts, including blepharitis, and blocked tear ducts. The part concludes with a note on computer vision syndrome, which is a leading cause of eyestrain, and the methods to overcome it.

Part VI: Congenital and Other Disorders That Affect Vision describes the most common hereditary and other congenital disorders affecting vision, including color blindness, Down syndrome, and ocular albinism. It provides information about infectious diseases, such as herpes, toxoplasmosis, and trachoma, that affect the eyes, and describes diseases and injuries, including diabetes, multiple sclerosis, acquired immune deficiency syndrome (AIDS), strokes, and traumatic brain injury, that have eye-related complications.

Part VII: Living with Low Vision defines what is meant by the terms "low vision," and "legal blindness," and provides tips for coping with vision loss. It offers suggestions for home modification to improve safety and provides tips for independence and mobility for people with low vision. The section concludes with a discussion of social security for people who are blind or have low vision, and laws regarding employment of people with low vision.

Part VIII: Additional Help and Information discusses Centers for Disease Control and Prevention's (CDC's) Vision Health Initiative and its objectives, and also includes a glossary of terms related to eyes and eye disorders and a directory of resources for further help and support.

Bibliographic Note

This volume contains documents and excerpts from publications issued by the following U.S. government agencies: Centers for Disease Control and Prevention (CDC); *Eunice Kennedy Shriver* National Institute of Child Health and Human Development (NICHD); Federal Aviation Administration (FAA); Federal Occupational Health (FOH); Genetic and Rare Diseases Information Center (GARD); Genetics Home Reference (GHR); *Go4Life*; Military Health System (MHS); National Cancer Institute (NCI); National Eye Institute (NEI); National Human Genome Research Institute (NHGRI); National Institute of Arthritis and Musculoskeletal and Skin Diseases (NIAMS); National Institute of Diabetes and Digestive and Kidney Diseases (NIDDK); National Institute of Neurological Disorders and Stroke (NINDS); National Institute on Aging (NIA); National Institutes of Health (NIH); *NIH News in Health*; Occupational Safety and Health Administration (OSHA); Office of Disease Prevention and Health Promotion (ODPHP); Office on Women's Health (OWH); U.S. Agency for International Development (USAID); U.S. Department of Veterans Affairs (VA); U.S. Equal Employment Opportunity Commission (EEOC); U.S. Food and Drug Administration (FDA); U.S. Library of Congress (LOC); and U.S. Social Security Administration (SSA).

In addition, this volume contains copyrighted documents from the following organizations: American Association for Pediatric Ophthalmology and Strabismus (AAPOS); American Optometric Association; Boston Children's Hospital; The Gavin Herbert Eye Institute; National Stroke Association; and WebMD LLC.

It may also contain original material produced by Omnigraphics and reviewed by medical consultants.

About the Health Reference Series

The *Health Reference Series* is designed to provide basic medical information for patients, families, caregivers, and the general public. Each volume takes a particular topic and provides comprehensive coverage. This is especially important for people who may be dealing with a newly diagnosed disease or a chronic disorder in themselves or in a family member. People looking for preventive guidance, information about disease warning signs, medical statistics, and risk factors for health problems will also find answers to their questions in the *Health Reference Series*. The *Series*, however, is not intended to serve as a tool for diagnosing illness, in prescribing treatments, or as a substitute for the physician/patient relationship. All people concerned about medical symptoms or the possibility of disease are encouraged to seek professional care from an appropriate healthcare provider.

A Note about Spelling and Style

Health Reference Series editors use *Stedman's Medical Dictionary* as an authority for questions related to the spelling of medical terms and the *Chicago Manual of Style* for questions related to grammatical structures, punctuation, and other editorial concerns. Consistent adherence is not always possible, however, because the individual volumes within the *Series* include many documents from a wide variety of different producers, and the editor's primary goal is to present material from each source as accurately as is possible. This sometimes means that information in different chapters or sections may follow other guidelines and alternate spelling authorities.

Medical Review

Omnigraphics contracts with a team of qualified, senior medical professionals who serve as medical consultants for the *Health Reference Series*. As necessary, medical consultants review reprinted and originally written material for currency and accuracy. Citations including the phrase, "Reviewed (month, year)" indicate material reviewed by this team. Medical consultation services are provided to the *Health Reference Series* editors by:

Dr. Vijayalakshmi, MBBS, DGO, MD
Dr. Senthil Selvan, MBBS, DCH, MD
Dr. K. Sivanandham, MBBS, DCH, MS (Research), PhD

Our Advisory Board

We would like to thank the following board members for providing initial guidance on the development of this series:

- Dr. Lynda Baker, Associate Professor of Library and Information Science, Wayne State University, Detroit, MI

- Nancy Bulgarelli, William Beaumont Hospital Library, Royal Oak, MI

- Karen Imarisio, Bloomfield Township Public Library, Bloomfield Township, MI

- Karen Morgan, Mardigian Library, University of Michigan-Dearborn, Dearborn, MI

- Rosemary Orlando, St. Clair Shores Public Library, St. Clair Shores, MI

Health Reference Series *Update Policy*

The inaugural book in the *Health Reference Series* was the first edition of *Cancer Sourcebook* published in 1989. Since then, the *Series* has been enthusiastically received by librarians and in the medical community. In order to maintain the standard of providing high-quality health information for the layperson the editorial staff at Omnigraphics felt it was necessary to implement a policy of updating volumes when warranted.

Medical researchers have been making tremendous strides, and it is the purpose of the *Health Reference Series* to stay current with the most recent advances. Each decision to update a volume is made on an individual basis. Some of the considerations include how much new information is available and the feedback we receive from people who use the books. If there is a topic you would like to see added to the update list, or an area of medical concern you feel has not been adequately addressed, please write to:

Managing Editor
Health Reference Series
Omnigraphics
615 Griswold, Ste. 901
Detroit, MI 48226

Part One

Eye and Eye Care Basics

Chapter 1

How the Eyes Work

The human eye is a complex organ with more than two million working parts. Its main function is to take in the light that is reflected off objects in the environment and transfer an image to the human brain. The brain instantly interprets the information, which is what enables people to "see" objects. The eyes are responsible for 80 percent of the sensory information that is processed by an average person's brain.

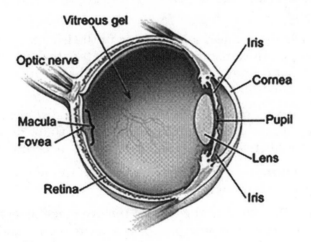

Figure 1.1. *The Human Eye*

(Source: "Diagram of the Eye," National Eye Institute (NEI).)

Structure of the Eye

The complex structure of the eye includes many specialized parts that work together to deliver light information to the brain for processing. Beginning at the front or exterior of the eye, the main parts include the following:

- **Eyelids:** thin folds of skin that help protect the eyes from damage and also keep them moist and clear of debris by blinking an average of 12,000 times per day.

- **Tear film:** a thin layer of moisture that carries oxygen to the cornea and helps keep the eyes healthy.

- **Sclera:** the protective outer membrane that is sometimes referred to as the "white" of the eye.

- **Cornea:** a clear layer that acts like a window and helps to focus light as it enters the eye. The cornea is unique because it is the only organ in the human body that does not have any blood vessels. It must be transparent in order to provide clear vision, so it receives oxygen from the air rather than from blood circulation.

- **Aqueous humor:** a liquid-filled chamber that helps maintain a constant pressure inside the eye.

- **Iris:** the circular, colored section of the eye that controls the size of the pupil.

- **Pupil:** a small, round, black opening in the iris that changes size to adjust the amount of light that enters the eye (getting larger in dark conditions to allow more light to enter, or smaller in bright conditions to allow less light to enter).

- **Lens:** a curved, transparent structure suspended by ligaments and muscles; it focuses light by adjusting its shape depending on the distance between the eye and the object reflecting the light.

- **Vitreous humor:** a clear, jelly-like substance that allows light to pass through the middle of the eye.

- **Retina:** a thin layer in the back of the eye made up of millions of light-sensitive photoreceptor cells known as rods and cones, which convert light into electrical signals or nerve impulses.

- **Rods:** the type of photoreceptor cells found around the edges of the retina, which are sensitive to light rather than color and allow the eye to see objects in dim light or in the periphery of the field of vision.

- **Cones:** the type of photoreceptor cells found near the center of the retina, which are sensitive to color and allow the eye to see in daylight and perceive color and fine details.

- **Macula:** the central focal point of the retina.

- **Fovea:** the bullseye in the center of the macula, which has more photoreceptors than any other part of the retina.

- **Optic nerve:** a bundle of thousands of nerve fibers that collects electrical signals from the photoreceptor cells in the retina and carries the information to the visual center in the brain for processing.

How Does the Light Pass through the Eye?

The eye basically works like a camera to capture light and create images. When light enters the eye, it passes through the cornea to the pupil. If the light is bright, the pupil will get smaller, or constrict, to reduce the amount of light that enters the eye. If the light is dim, the pupil will grow larger, or dilate, to increase the amount of light that enters the eye. Next, the light hits the lens, which adjusts automatically to focus the image on the retina. Since the lens is curved, it bends the light to create a reverse or upside-down image on the photoreceptor cells lining the back of the eye.

When the light energy that makes up the image reaches the retina, the photoreceptor cells turn it into electrical signals that travel to the optic nerve. The optic nerve carries these nerve impulses to the brain, which processes the information. Although the eyes can take in light and capture an image (like the lens of a camera), the visual center in the brain must interpret the image (like developing the film in a camera) for the person to be able to "see" it. As the brain processes the upside-down image, it automatically flips it over the right way again.

When the cornea, lens, and retina all work together perfectly, the result is clear vision. Unfortunately, a number of problems can occur to disrupt this complicated process. Two of the most common eyesight issues occur when the cornea and lens do not focus light on the retina properly. Myopia, or nearsightedness, occurs when the light is focused in front of the retina rather than directly on it. People with this condition have trouble seeing distant objects clearly. Hyperopia, or farsightedness, occurs when the light is focused behind the retina. People with this condition have trouble seeing close-up objects clearly. Both of these conditions can have a genetic component. Another common condition is presbyopia, in which the lens loses some of its ability to focus on close-up objects. Many people develop presbyopia in middle age as part of the natural aging process.

Testing and Correcting Vision

Doctors have developed tests to identify these common conditions affecting the quality of vision, which can often be corrected with prescription eyeglasses or contact lenses. The standard test of visual acuity used in eye examinations is called the Snellen system, after the Dutch ophthalmologist who developed it. It uses an eye chart with rows of letters that gradually decrease in size from top to bottom. The patient typically stands about 20 feet (6 meters) away from the chart and tries to read the letters on each line. The size of the letters on one of the lines corresponds to normal visual acuity, or what a person with normal eyesight can read from a distance of 20 feet.

Using the Snellen measurement system, a person with normal visual acuity is said to have 20/20 vision. The numerator of the Snellen fraction refers to the patient's distance from the eye chart, while the bottom number refers to the distance at which a person with normal visual acuity can read that line. About 35 percent of adults have 20/20 vision without corrective lenses. The goal of corrective measures like eyeglasses, contact lenses, and laser surgery is to bring a patient's vision to 20/20, and about 75 percent of adults can reach that goal.

People with 20/20 eyesight do not necessarily have perfect vision, however, because visual acuity is not the only factor determining the quality of vision. In real-life situations, the human eye is often called upon to distinguish between different colors, track moving objects, perceive depth of field, and see low-contrast objects that blend into the background. These tasks involve physical and neurological factors such as the sensitivity of the photoreceptive rods and cones in the retina, and the ability of the brain to process visual images received from the eyes. A more inclusive measurement of the quality of vision employs additional tests to assess these skills and abilities.

References

1. "The Eyes," Sightsavers, 2017.

2. Hellem, Amy, and Gary Heiting. "Is 20/20 Vision 'Perfect' Vision?" AllAboutVision, September 2016.

3. "How Do We See?" Coopervision, 2017.

4. "How We See," Bradbury Fields, 2017.

5. Vimont, Celia. "What Does 20/20 Vision Mean?" American Academy of Opthamology, November 30, 2016.

6. "Vision Basics: How Does Your Eye Work?" WebMD, October 3, 2015.

Chapter 2

Maintaining Eye Health

Chapter Contents

9

Section 2.1

Simple Tips for Healthy Eyes

This section includes text excerpted from "Simple Tips for Healthy Eyes," National Eye Institute (NEI), January 5, 2017.

Your eyes are an important part of your health. There are many things you can do to keep them healthy and make sure you are seeing your best. Follow these simple steps for maintaining healthy eyes well into your golden years.

Have a comprehensive dilated eye exam. You might think your vision is fine or that your eyes are healthy, but visiting your eye care professional for a comprehensive dilated eye exam is the only way to really be sure. When it comes to common vision problems, some people don't realize they could see better with glasses or contact lenses. In addition, many common eye diseases such as glaucoma, diabetic eye disease and age-related macular degeneration often have no warning signs. A dilated eye exam is the only way to detect these diseases in their early stages.

During a comprehensive dilated eye exam, your eye care professional places drops in your eyes to dilate, or widen, the pupil to allow more light to enter the eye the same way an open door lets more light into a dark room. This enables your eye care professional to get a good look at the back of the eyes and examine them for any signs of damage or disease. Your eye care professional is the only one who can determine if your eyes are healthy and if you're seeing your best.

Know your family's eye health history. Talk to your family members about their eye health history. It's important to know if anyone has been diagnosed with a disease or condition since many are hereditary. This will help to determine if you are at higher risk for developing an eye disease or condition.

Eat right to protect your sight. You've heard carrots are good for your eyes. But eating a diet rich in fruits and vegetables, particularly dark leafy greens such as spinach, kale, or collard greens is important for keeping your eyes healthy, too. Research has also shown there are eye health benefits from eating fish high in omega-3 fatty acids, such as salmon, tuna, and halibut.

Maintain a healthy weight. Being overweight or obese increases your risk of developing diabetes and other systemic conditions, which can lead to vision loss, such as diabetic eye disease or glaucoma. If you are having trouble maintaining a healthy weight, talk to your doctor.

Wear protective eyewear. Wear protective eyewear when playing sports or doing activities around the home. Protective eyewear includes safety glasses and goggles, safety shields, and eye guards specially designed to provide the correct protection for a certain activity. Most protective eyewear lenses are made of polycarbonate, which is 10 times stronger than other plastics. Many eye care providers sell protective eyewear, as do some sporting goods stores.

Quit smoking or never start. Smoking is as bad for your eyes as it is for the rest of your body. Research has linked smoking to an increased risk of developing age-related macular degeneration, cataract, and optic nerve damage, all of which can lead to blindness.

Be cool and wear your shades. Sunglasses are a great fashion accessory, but their most important job is to protect your eyes from the sun's ultraviolet rays. When purchasing sunglasses, look for ones that block out 99 to 100 percent of both UVA and UVB radiation.

Give your eyes a rest. If you spend a lot of time at the computer or focusing on any one thing, you sometimes forget to blink and your eyes can get fatigued. Try the 20-20-20 rule: Every 20 minutes, look away about 20 feet in front of you for 20 seconds. This can help reduce eyestrain.

Clean your hands and your contact lenses properly. To avoid the risk of infection, always wash your hands thoroughly before putting in or taking out your contact lenses. Make sure to disinfect contact lenses as instructed and replace them as appropriate.

Practice workplace eye safety. Employers are required to provide a safe work environment. When protective eyewear is required as a part of your job, make a habit of wearing the appropriate type at all times and encourage your coworkers to do the same.

Section 2.2

Supplements and Protection against Eye Diseases

This section includes text excerpted from "For the Public: What
the AREDS Means for You," National Eye Institute (NEI),
May 2013. Reviewed March 2017.

The Age-Related Eye Disease Study

Researchers with the Age-Related Eye Disease Study (AREDS)
reported in 2001 that a nutritional supplement called the AREDS
formulation can reduce the risk of developing advanced age-related
macular degeneration (AMD). The original AREDS formulation contains vitamin C, vitamin E, beta-carotene, zinc and copper.

In 2006, the same research group, which is based at National Institutes of Health's (NIH) National Eye Institute (NEI), began a second
study called AREDS2 to determine if they could improve the AREDS
formulation. They tested:

- adding the antioxidants lutein and zeaxanthin

- adding omega-3 fatty acids

- removing beta-carotene

- lowering the dose of zinc

This section provides information about the results and implications
of AREDS2. If you are at risk for advanced AMD or have a family
member who is at risk, the questions and answers below may help
you discuss using AREDS and related nutritional supplements with
a healthcare professional.

What Is the Original AREDS Formulation?

- 500 milligrams (mg) of vitamin C
- 400 international units of vitamin E
- 15 mg beta-carotene

- 80 mg zinc as zinc oxide
- 2 mg copper as cupric oxide

What Modifications Were Tested in AREDS2?

- 10 mg lutein and 2 mg zeaxanthin
- 1000 mg of omega-3 fatty acids (350 mg docosahexaenoic acid (DHA) and 650 mg eicosapentaenoic acid(EPA))
- No beta-carotene
- 25 mg zinc

Why Change the Formulation?

Why add lutein/zeaxanthin and omega-3 fatty acids? Previous studies had found that dietary intake of lutein/zeaxanthin and omega-3 fatty acids is associated with a lower risk of developing advanced AMD.

Why eliminate beta-carotene? During the AREDS trial, two large trials funded by the National Cancer Institute (NCI) found that beta-carotene may increase lung cancer risk among people who smoke. Lutein and zeaxanthin are in the same family of nutrients as beta-carotene and are believed to have important functions in the retina. Therefore, the researchers theorized that lutein/zeaxanthin might be a safer and possibly more effective alternative than beta-carotene.

Why reduce zinc? Although zinc was found to be an essential component of the AREDS formulation in the original trial, some nutritional experts recommended a lower dose.

What Are Lutein, Zeaxanthin and Beta-Carotene?

Lutein, zeaxanthin, and beta-carotene belong to a family of nutrients known as carotenoids. Carotenoids are made by plants and are especially enriched in green leafy vegetables. They can be stored in animal tissues and are found at relatively low levels in animal food products. In the body, beta-carotene is used to make Vitamin A, which is required by the retina to detect light and convert it into electrical signals. Beta-carotene itself is not found in the eye. In contrast, lutein and zeaxanthin are found in the retina and lens, where they may act as natural antioxidants and help absorb damaging, high-energy blue and ultraviolet light.

What Are Omega-3 Fatty Acids?

Omega-3 fatty acids are made by marine algae and enriched in fish oils; they are believed to be responsible for the health benefits associated with regularly eating fish, including lower rates of cardiovascular disease. The AREDS2 study focused on the omega-3 fatty acids DHA and its precursor EPA. DHA is needed for the integrity of the retinal cells, and has been shown to promote retinal development and repair in prior studies.

What Were the Effects of Changing the Original AREDS Formulation?

In the first AREDS trial, taking the original formulation reduced the risk of advanced AMD by about 25 percent over a five-year period. In the AREDS2 trial, adding DHA/EPA or lutein/zeaxanthin to the original formulation (containing beta-carotene) had no additional overall effect on the risk of advanced AMD. However, trial participants who took AREDS containing lutein/zeaxanthin and no beta-carotene had a slight reduction in risk of advanced AMD, compared with those who took AREDS with beta-carotene. Also, for participants with very low levels of lutein/zeaxanthin in their diet, adding these supplements to the AREDS formulation helped lower their risk of advanced AMD. Finally, former smokers who took AREDS with beta-carotene had a higher incidence of lung cancer. The investigators found no significant changes in the effectiveness of the formulation when they removed beta-carotene or lowered zinc.

Who Should Consider Taking a Combination of Antioxidants and Zinc Like Those Examined in AREDS and AREDS2?

People at high risk for developing advanced AMD should consider taking the antioxidant-zinc combinations examined in AREDS and AREDS2. These people are defined as having either:

1. **Intermediate AMD in one or both eyes.** Intermediate AMD can be detected by an eye care professional, but usually involves little or no vision loss.

2. **Advanced AMD in one eye, but not the other eye.** Advanced AMD involves either a breakdown of cells in the retina (called geographic atrophy or dry AMD), or the growth of

abnormal blood vessels under the retina (called neovascular or wet AMD). Either of these forms of advanced AMD can cause vision loss.

Will Taking an AREDS Formulation Prevent AMD?

There is no known treatment that can prevent the early stages of AMD. However, the AREDS formulations may delay progression of advanced AMD and help you keep your vision longer if you have intermediate AMD, or advanced AMD in one eye. The participants in the first AREDS trial have now been followed for 10 years, and the benefits of the AREDS formulation have persisted over this time.

Can I Take a Daily Multivitamin If I Am Taking One of the AREDS Formulations?

Yes. The AREDS formulation is not a substitute for a multivitamin. In the AREDS trial, two-thirds of the study participants took multivitamins along with the AREDS formulation. In AREDS2, almost nine of ten participants took multivitamins.

Can a Daily Multivitamin Alone Provide the Same Vision Benefits as an AREDS Formulation?

No. The vitamins and minerals tested in the AREDS and AREDS2 trials were provided in much higher doses than what is found in multivitamins. Also, it is important to remember that most of the trial participants took multivitamins. Taking an AREDS formulation clearly provided a benefit over and above multivitamins.

Can Diet Alone Provide the Same High Levels of Antioxidants and Zinc as the AREDS Formulations?

No. The high levels of vitamins and minerals are difficult to achieve from diet alone. However, previous studies have suggested that people who have diets rich in green, leafy vegetables—a good source of lutein/zeaxanthin—have a lower risk of developing AMD. In the AREDS2 trial, the people who seemed to benefit most from taking lutein/zeaxanthin were those who did not get much of these nutrients in their diet. Within this group, those who received lutein/zeaxanthin supplements had a 26 percent reduced risk of developing advanced AMD compared with those who did not receive the supplements.

What Is the Risk of Lung Cancer from Taking Beta-Carotene?

In the AREDS2 trial, current smokers or those who had quit smoking less than a year before enrollment were excluded from receiving beta-carotene. Despite this precaution, lung cancers were observed in 2 percent of participants who took an AREDS formulation with beta-carotene, compared with 0.9 percent of participants who took AREDS without beta-carotene. Across both groups, about 91 percent of participants who developed lung cancer were former smokers.

How Does Lutein/Zeaxanthin Compare to Beta-Carotene?

Lutein/zeaxanthin has not been associated with increased cancer risk. Moreover, analysis from the AREDS2 trial suggests that it offers similar or better protective benefits against advanced AMD, compared with beta-carotene. In the trial, participants who took an AREDS formulation containing lutein/zeaxanthin (no beta-carotene) had an 18 percent lower risk of progressing to advanced AMD compared with those who took AREDS containing beta-carotene (no lutein/zeaxanthin).

Does the High-Dose Vitamin E in the AREDS Formulations Affect the Risk of Prostate Cancer?

There have been conflicting data on the relationship between vitamin E and prostate cancer.

- In 1994, the Alpha-Tocopherol, Beta-Carotene (ATBC) trial found a 35 percent reduced risk of prostate cancer in men taking 50 mg of vitamin E daily for a follow-up of six years.

- In 2009, the Physicians Health Study II (PHS II) found that 400 IU of vitamin E every other day for a follow-up of eight years had no effect on the incidence of prostate cancer.

- In 2011, the Selenium and Vitamin E Cancer Prevention Trial (SELECT) found a 17 percent increase in the risk of prostate cancer among men taking 400 IU of vitamin E daily for a follow-up of seven years. That risk equates to 1–2 more prostate cancers per 1000 patients who took high-dose vitamin E for one year. For reasons that are unclear, men who took both vitamin E and selenium did not have an increased rate of prostate cancer.

In the AREDS trial, high-dose vitamin E had no effect on the risk of prostate cancer among male participants. The AREDS2 trial began in 2006 (before the SELECT trial was reported) and all study participants were offered an AREDS formulation containing vitamin E. A group of independent researchers monitoring the AREDS2 trial for safety noted no concerns about an increased risk prostate cancer. The final data from the study do not suggest a higher rate of prostate cancer among male participants than expected in an aging male population.

If you have concerns about vitamin E and prostate cancer, it is important to understand that many factors influence the risk of prostate cancer, including age, family history and race. Talk to your healthcare provider about the possible risks and benefits from taking vitamin E supplements.

Are There Any Other Side Effects or Risks from Taking the AREDS Formulations?

Many older Americans take prescription medications, and a considerable number use over-the-counter drugs, dietary supplements, and herbal medicines. High-dose supplemental nutrients can sometimes interfere with medications and compete with other vital nutrients for absorption into the body. Individuals who are considering taking an AREDS formulation should discuss this with their primary care doctors and/or eye care professionals.

Section 2.3

Smoking and Eye Health

This section includes text excerpted from "Vision Loss, Blindness, and Smoking," Centers for Disease Control and Prevention (CDC), January 10, 2017.

Overview of Smoking and Eyesight

Smoking is as bad for your eyes as it is for the rest of your body. If you smoke, you can develop serious eye conditions that can cause vision loss or blindness. Two of the greatest threats to your eyesight are:

- Macular degeneration

- Cataracts

Macular degeneration, also called age-related macular degeneration (AMD), is an eye disease that affects central vision. You need central vision to see objects clearly and for common tasks such as reading, recognizing faces, and driving.

There are two forms of AMD: dry AMD and wet AMD. Macular degeneration always begins in the dry form, and sometimes progresses to the more advanced wet form, where vision loss can be very rapid if untreated.

Cataracts cause blurry vision that worsens over time. Without surgery, cataracts can lead to serious vision loss. The best way to protect your sight from damage linked to smoking is to quit or never start smoking.

Symptoms of Eye Diseases Related to Smoking

You may think your eyes are fine, but the only way to know for sure is by getting a full eye exam. AMD often has no early symptoms, so an eye exam is the best way to spot this eye disease early. An eye specialist will place special drops in your eyes to widen your pupils. This offers a better view of the back of your eye, where a thin layer of tissue (the retina) changes light into signals that go to the brain. The macula is a small part of the retina that you need for sharp, central vision.

When symptoms of AMD do occur, they can include:

- blurred vision or a blurry spot in your central vision

- the need for more light to read or do other tasks

- straight lines that look wavy

- trouble recognizing faces

Eye injections are often the preferred treatment for wet AMD. Your doctor can inject a drug to stop the growth of these blood vessels and stop further damage to your eyes. You may need injections on a regular basis to save your vision.

How Does Smoking Affect Your Eyes?

Smoking causes changes in the eyes that can lead to vision loss. If you smoke:

- You are twice as likely to develop AMD compared with a nonsmoker.

- You are two to three times more likely to develop cataracts compared with a nonsmoker.

How Can You Prevent Vision Loss Related to Smoking?

If you smoke, stop. Quitting may lower your risk for both AMD and cataracts.

If you already have AMD, quitting smoking may slow the disease. AMD tends to get worse over time. Quitting smoking is something within your control that may help save your sight. Other healthy habits may also help protect your eyes from cataracts and AMD:

- Exercise regularly.
- Maintain normal blood pressure and cholesterol levels.
- Eat a healthy diet rich in green, leafy vegetables and fish.
- Wear sunglasses and a hat with a brim to protect your eyes from sunlight.

How Is a Cataract Treated?

The symptoms of an early cataract may improve with new eyeglasses, brighter lighting, anti-glare sunglasses, or magnifying lenses.

When glasses and brighter lighting don't help, you may need surgery. A doctor will remove the cloudy lens and replace it with an artificial lens. This clear, plastic lens becomes a permanent part of your eye.

Help for Vision Loss

Coping with vision loss can be frightening, but there is help to make the most of the vision you have left and to continue enjoying your friends, family, and special interests. If you've already lost some sight, ask your healthcare professional about low-vision counseling and devices such as high-powered lenses, magnifiers, and talking computers.

Section 2.4

Safe Use of Cosmetics

This section includes text excerpted from "Use Eye Cosmetics Safely,"
U.S. Food and Drug Administration (FDA), March 22, 2016.

The U.S. Food and Drug Administration (FDA) regulates all cosmetics marketed in the United States, including mascara, eye shadows, eye liner, concealers, and eyebrow pencils.

Safety experts within the Office of Cosmetics and Colors in FDA's Center for Food Safety and Applied Nutrition (CFSAN) offer consumers the following advice:

Keep everything clean. Dangerous bacteria or fungi can grow in some cosmetic products, as well as their containers. Cleanliness can help prevent eye infections.

Always wash your hands before applying eye cosmetics, and be sure that any instrument you place near your eyes is clean. Be especially careful not to contaminate cosmetics by introducing microorganisms. For example, don't lay an eyelash wand on a countertop where it can pick up bacteria. Keep containers clean, since these may also be a source of contamination.

Don't moisten cosmetic products. Don't add saliva or water to moisten eye cosmetics. Doing so can introduce bacteria. Problems can arise if you overpower a product's preservative capability.

Don't share or swap. People can be harmed by others' germs when they share eye makeup. Keep this in mind when you come across "testers" at retail stores. If you do sample cosmetics at a store, be sure to use single-use applicators, such as clean cotton swabs.

Don't apply or remove eye makeup in a moving vehicle. Any bump or sudden stop can cause injury to your eye with a mascara wand or other applicator.

Check ingredients, including color additives. As with any cosmetic product sold to consumers, eye cosmetics are required to have an ingredient declaration on the label. If they don't, they are considered misbranded and illegal.

In the United States, the use of color additives is strictly regulated. Some color additives approved for cosmetic use in general are not approved for areas near the eyes.

If the product is properly labeled, you can check to see whether the color additives declared on the label are in FDA's List of Color Additives Permitted for Use in Cosmetics.

Use only cosmetics intended for the eyes on the eyes. Don't use a lip liner as an eyeliner, for example. You may expose eyes either to contamination from your mouth or to color additives that are not approved for use near the eyes.

Say "no" to kohl! Also known as al-kahl, kajal, or surma, kohl is used in some parts of the world for enhancing the appearance of the eyes. But kohl is unapproved for cosmetic use in the United States.

Kohl contains salts of heavy metals such as antimony and lead. Reports have linked the use of kohl to lead poisoning in children.

Some eye cosmetics may be labeled with the word "kohl" only to indicate the shade, not because they contain true kohl.

A product's "ingredient statement" should not list kohl—this is not an FDA-approved color additive. Check the ingredient statement to make sure that kohl is not present.

Don't dye eyelashes and eyebrows. No color additives are approved by FDA for permanent dyeing or tinting of eyelashes and eyebrows. Permanent eyelash and eyebrow tints and dyes have been known to cause serious eye injuries.

Use care with false eyelashes or extensions. False eyelashes and extensions, as well as their adhesives, must meet the safety and labeling requirements for cosmetics. Since the eyelids are delicate, an allergic reaction, irritation, or injury in the eye area can occur. Check the ingredients to make sure you are not allergic to the adhesives.

Don't use eye cosmetics that cause irritation. Stop using a product immediately if irritation occurs. See a doctor if irritation persists.

Avoid using eye cosmetics if you have an eye infection. Discard any eye cosmetics you were using when you got the infection. Also, don't use eye cosmetics if the skin around the eye is inflamed.

21

Don't use old eye cosmetics. Manufacturers usually recommend discarding mascara two to four months after purchase. Discard dried-up mascara.

Don't store cosmetics at temperatures above 85°F. Preservatives that keep bacteria or fungi from growing can lose their effectiveness, for example, in cosmetics kept for long periods in hot cars.

Report Problems

If you need to contact FDA concerning an eye cosmetic product problem, go to FDA's MedWatch website (www.fda.gov/Safety/MedWatch/default.htm) and click on "Report a Problem," or fill in and send form FDA 3500B.

Chapter 3

Vision Disorders: A Statistical Picture

Chapter Contents

Section 3.1

Fast Facts about Vision Disorders

This section contains text excerpted from the following sources:
Text under the heading "Common Eye Disorders" is excerpted
from "Common Eye Disorders," Centers for Disease Control and
Prevention (CDC), September 29, 2015; Text under the heading
"Eye Disease Statistics" is excerpted from "Eye Disease Statistics,"
National Eye Institute (NEI), March 2014.

Common Eye Disorders

Approximately 11 million Americans aged 12 years and older
could improve their vision through proper refractive correction.
More than 3.3 million Americans aged 40 years and older are
either legally blind (having best-corrected visual acuity of 6/60
or worse (=20/200) in the better-seeing eye) or are with low vision
(having best-corrected visual acuity less than 6/12 (<20/40) in
the better-seeing eye, excluding those who were categorized as
being blind). The leading causes of blindness and low vision in
the United States are primarily age-related eye diseases such as
age-related macular degeneration, cataract, diabetic retinopathy,
and glaucoma. Other common eye disorders include amblyopia and
strabismus.

Refractive Errors

Refractive errors are the most frequent eye problems in the United
States. Refractive errors include myopia (nearsightedness), hyperopia
(farsightedness), astigmatism (distorted vision at all distances), and
presbyopia that occurs between age 40–50 years (loss of the ability to
focus up close, inability to read letters of the phone book, need to hold
newspaper farther away to see clearly) can be corrected by eyeglasses,
contact lenses, or in some cases surgery. Studies conducted by the
National Eye Institute (NEI) showed that proper refractive correction
could improve vision among 11 million Americans aged 12 years and
older.

Age-Related Macular Degeneration

Macular degeneration, often called age-related macular degeneration (AMD), is an eye disorder associated with aging and results in damaging sharp and central vision. Central vision is needed for seeing objects clearly and for common daily tasks such as reading and driving. AMD affects the macula, the central part the retina that allows the eye to see fine details. There are two forms of AMD—wet and dry.

The dry form is more common and accounts for 70–90 percent of cases of AMD and it progresses more slowly than the wet form. One of the most common early signs of dry AMD is drusen. Drusen are tiny yellow or white deposits under the retina. They often are found in people aged 60 years and older.

It is estimated that 1.8 million Americans aged 40 years and older are affected by AMD and an additional 7.3 million with large drusen are at substantial risk of developing AMD. The number of people with AMD is estimated to reach 2.95 million in 2020. AMD is the leading cause of permanent impairment of reading and fine or close-up vision among people aged 65 years and older.

Cataract

Cataract is a clouding of the eye's lens and is the leading cause of blindness worldwide, and the leading cause of vision loss in the United States. Cataracts can occur at any age because of a variety of causes, and can be present at birth. Although treatment for the removal of cataract is widely available, access barriers such as insurance coverage, treatment costs, patient choice, or lack of awareness prevent many people from receiving the proper treatment.

An estimated 20.5 million (17.2%) Americans aged 40 years and older have cataract in one or both eyes, and 6.1 million (5.1%) have had their lens removed operatively. The total number of people who have cataracts is estimated to increase to 30.1 million by 2020.

Diabetic Retinopathy

Diabetic retinopathy (DR) is a common complication of diabetes. It is the leading cause of blindness in American adults. It is characterized by progressive damage to the blood vessels of the retina, the light-sensitive tissue at the back of the eye that is necessary for good vision. DR usually affects both eyes.

It is the leading cause of blindness among U.S. working-aged adults aged 20–74 years. An estimated 4.1 million and 899,000 Americans are affected by retinopathy and vision-threatening retinopathy, respectively.

Glaucoma

Glaucoma is a group of diseases that can damage the eye's optic nerve and result in vision loss and blindness. Glaucoma occurs when the normal fluid pressure inside the eyes slowly rises. However, findings now show that glaucoma can occur with normal eye pressure. With early treatment, you can often protect your eyes against serious vision loss.

There are two major categories "open angle" and "closed angle" glaucoma. Open angle, is a chronic condition that progress slowly over long period of time without the person noticing vision loss until the disease is very advanced, that is why it is called "sneak thief of sight." Angle closure can appear suddenly and is painful. Visual loss can progress quickly; however, the pain and discomfort lead patients to seek medical attention before permanent damage occurs.

Amblyopia

Amblyopia, also referred to as "lazy eye," is the most common cause of vision impairment in children. Amblyopia is the medical term used when the vision in one of the eyes is reduced because the eye and the brain are not working together properly. The eye itself looks normal, but it is not being used normally because the brain is favoring the other eye. Conditions leading to amblyopia include strabismus, an imbalance in the positioning of the two eyes; more nearsighted, far-sighted, or astigmatic in one eye than the other eye, and rarely other eye conditions such as cataract.

Unless it is successfully treated in early childhood amblyopia usually persists into adulthood, and is the most common cause of permanent one-eye vision impairment among children and young and middle-aged adults. An estimated 2–3 percent of the population suffer from amblyopia.

Strabismus

Strabismus involves an imbalance in the positioning of the two eyes. Strabismus can cause the eyes to cross in (esotropia) or turn out (exotropia). Strabismus is caused by a lack of coordination between the eyes. As a result, the eyes look in different directions and do not focus simultaneously on a single point. In most cases of strabismus in children, the cause is unknown. In more than half of these cases, the problem is present at or shortly after birth (congenital strabismus). When the two eyes fail to focus on the same image, there is reduced or absent depth perception and the brain may learn to ignore the input from one eye, causing permanent vision loss in that eye (one type of amblyopia).

Eye Disease Statistics

Economic Burden[1]

$139 billion = estimated annual economic burden of vision loss and eye diseases and vision disorders in the United States.

Burden of Blindness and Low Vision[2]

- 1.3 million Americans are blind (≤20/200); an estimated 2.2 million Americans will be blind by 2030.

- 2.9 million Americans have low vision (<20/40); an estimated 5 million Americans will have low vision by 2030.

Major Eye Diseases[2]

Age-related Macular Degeneration (AMD)

- 2.1 million Americans have advanced AMD; an estimated 3.7 million will have advanced AMD by 2030.

Glaucoma

- 2.7 million Americans have glaucoma; an estimated 4.3 million will have glaucoma by 2030.

Diabetic Retinopathy

- 7.7 million Americans have diabetic retinopathy; an estimated 11.3 million will have diabetic retinopathy by 2030.

---

[1] *NORC and Prevent Blindness America.* Cost *of Vision Problems: The Economic Burden of Vision Loss and Eye Disorders in the United States. June 11, 2013.*
[2] *Prevent Blindness America and National Eye Institute. Vision Problems in the U.S. 2012.*

Cataract

- 24 million Americans are affected by cataract; an estimated 38.7 million will be affected by cataract by 2030.

Refractive Error

- 34.1 million Americans are nearsighted; an estimated 39 million will be nearsighted by 2030.

- 14.1 million Americans are farsighted; an estimated 20 million will be farsighted by 2030.

Section 3.2

Vision Loss: A Public Health Problem

This section contains text excerpted from the following sources: Text under the heading "Population Estimates" is excerpted from "The Burden of Vision Loss," Centers for Disease Control and Prevention (CDC), September 29, 2015; Text under the heading "Why Is Vision Loss a Public Health Problem?" is excerpted from "Why Is Vision Loss a Public Health Problem?" Centers for Disease Control and Prevention (CDC), September 28, 2015.

Population Estimates

More than 3.4 million (3%) Americans aged 40 years and older are either legally blind (having visual acuity [VA] of 20/200 or worse or a visual field of less than 20 degrees) or are visually impaired (having VA of 20/40 or less). The Federal Interagency Forum on Aging Related Statistics (2008) estimates that 17 percent of the age 65 and older population report "vision trouble." Twenty-one million Americans report functional vision problems or eye conditions that may compromise vision. Older people are more likely to experience vision loss because of age-related eye diseases. A Centers for Disease Control and Prevention (CDC) study revealed that self-reported vision loss (a little, moderate, or extreme difficulty) ranged from 14.3 percent to 20.5 percent among five states. Despite the magnitude of the population at risk for vision loss as well as the grave consequences of vision loss and blindness, many individuals do not benefit from available cost-effective early detection, timely treatments, and interventions to promote health.

Why Is Vision Loss a Public Health Problem?

A study had posed five criteria that define whether vision loss is a public health problem. They are:

1. Does vision loss affect a lot of people?

2. Does vision loss contribute a large burden in terms of morbidity, quality of life, and cost?

3. Has the problem recently increased and will it increase in the future?

4. Is vision loss perceived to be a threat by the public?

5. Is it feasible to act on the condition at a community or public health level?

The answer to each of these questions is "yes."

1. Does Vision Loss Affect a Lot of People?

Yes. More than 3.4 million Americans aged 40 years and older are blind (having a visual acuity of 20/200 or less or a visual field on 20 degrees or less) or visually impaired (having a visual acuity of 20/40 or less). Other estimates of "vision problems" range as high as 21 million, and a total of 80 million Americans have potentially blinding eye diseases. The major causes of vision loss are cataracts, age-related macular degeneration, diabetic retinopathy, and glaucoma.

2. Does Vision Loss Contribute a Large Burden in Terms of Morbidity, Quality of Life, and Cost?

Yes. People with vision loss are more likely to report depression, diabetes, hearing impairment, stroke, falls, cognitive decline, and premature death. Decreased ability to see often leads to the inability to drive, read, keep accounts, and travel in unfamiliar places, thus substantially compromising quality of life. The cost of vision loss, including direct costs and lost productivity, is estimated to exceed $35 billion.

29

3. Has Vision Loss Recently Increased and Will It Increase in the Future?

Yes. As the population of older people continues to accelerate, the number of people experiencing vision loss will continue to increase. And as the population of people experiencing diabetes increases, consequent increases will occur in diabetic retinopathy and other eye diseases. Prevent Blindness America estimates that the population of people experiencing blindness and visual impairment will double by 2030 unless corrective actions are taken.

4. Is Vision Loss Perceived to Be a Threat by the Public?

Yes. Vision loss ranks among the top ten causes of disability in the United States, and it is a condition feared by many.

5. Is It Feasible to Act on Vision Loss at a Community or Public Health Level?

Yes. Scientific evidence shows that early detection and treatment can prevent much blindness and vision impairment. Efficacious and cost-effective strategies to detect and treat diabetic retinopathy are available, but among people with diabetes, screening is received only by about two-thirds of persons for whom the exam is recommended and varies significantly across healthcare settings. Cataract removal surgery can restore vision, and this surgery is cost effective; however, among African Americans, unoperated senile cataracts remain a major cause of blindness. Glaucoma can be controlled, and vision loss stopped by early detection and treatment. Nevertheless, half the people with glaucoma are not diagnosed, and glaucoma is still the number one blinding disease among African Americans.

Public health serves to address each of these questions by conducting population-based investigations to determine the population, characteristics, circumstances, and trends of vision loss, as well as developing and implementing evidence-based, cost-effective interventions to assure access to vision care and health behaviors to prevent the onset of vision loss and to improve the health and quality of life for those who have lost vision.

Chapter 4

What You Need to Know about Eye Exams

Keep an Eye on Your Vision Health

Going to the doctor, going to the dentist—all part of taking care of your health. But going to the eye doctor? Also important! Eye exams at every age and life stage can help keep your vision strong.

Many people think their eyesight is just fine, but then they get that first pair of glasses or contact lenses and the world comes into clearer view—everything from fine print to street signs.

Improving your eyesight is important—about 11 million Americans over age 12 need vision correction—but it's just one of the reasons to get your eyes examined. Regular eye exams are also an important part of finding eye diseases early and preserving your vision.

Only Your Eye Doctor Knows for Sure

Eye diseases are common and can go unnoticed for a long time—some have no symptoms at first. A comprehensive dilated eye exam

This chapter contains text excerpted from the following sources: Text beginning with the heading "Keep an Eye on Your Vision Health" is excerpted from "Keep an Eye on Your Vision Health," Centers for Disease Control and Prevention (CDC), May 4, 2016; Text beginning with the heading "Eye Examination: The Basics" is excerpted from "Get Your Eyes Tested," Office of Disease Prevention and Health Promotion (ODPHP), U.S. Department of Health and Human Services (HHS), December 20, 2016.

by an optometrist or ophthalmologist (eye doctor) is necessary to find eye diseases in the early stages when treatment to prevent vision loss is most effective.

During the exam, visual acuity (sharpness), depth perception, eye alignment, and eye movement are tested. Eye drops are used to make your pupils larger so your eye doctor can see inside your eyes and check for signs of health problems. Your eye doctor may even spot other conditions such as high blood pressure or diabetes, sometimes before your primary care doctor does.

Vision Care Can Change Lives

Early treatment is critically important to prevent some common eye diseases from causing permanent vision loss or blindness:

- Cataracts (clouding of the lens), the leading cause of vision loss in the United States

- Diabetic retinopathy (causes damage to blood vessels in the back of the eye), the leading cause of blindness in American adults

- Glaucoma (a group of diseases that damages the optic nerve)

- Age-related macular degeneration (gradual breakdown of light-sensitive tissue in the eye)

Of the estimated 61 million U.S. adults at high risk for vision loss, only half visited an eye doctor in the past 12 months. Regular eye care can have a life-changing impact on preserving the vision of millions of people.

Start Early

Though people tend to have more vision problems as they get older, children need eye exams to ensure healthy vision, too. But less than 15 percent of preschool children get an eye exam and less than 22 percent receive vision screening. Vision screening can reveal a possible vision problem, but can't diagnose it. A comprehensive dilated eye exam is needed to diagnose eye diseases.

Amblyopia (reduced vision because the eye and brain aren't working together properly) is the most common cause of vision loss in children—2 to 3 out of 100 children. Amblyopia needs to be treated promptly to help avoid vision loss.

5 Ways to Protect Your Vision

1. Get regular eye exams.

2. Eat a healthy diet, including leafy greens such as spinach or kale, and maintain a healthy weight.

3. Know your family's eye health history.

4. Wear sunglasses that block out 99 percent to 100 percent of UVA and UVB radiation (the sun's rays).

5. Quit smoking or don't start.

Easy on the Eyes

If you spend a lot of time focusing on one thing, such as a computer screen, your eyes can get tired. Try the 20-20-20 rule to reduce eye-strain: every 20 minutes, look away about 20 feet in front of you for 20 seconds.

Eye Exams: How Often?

- Children's eyes should be checked regularly by an eye doctor or pediatrician. The U.S. Preventive Services Task Force (USPSTF) recommends vision screening for all children at least once between age 3 and 5 years to detect amblyopia or risk factors for the disease.

- People with diabetes should have a dilated eye exam every year.

- Some people are at higher risk for glaucoma and should have a dilated eye exam every 2 years:

  - African Americans aged 40 years and older

  - everyone older than age 60, especially Mexican Americans

  - people with a family history of glaucoma

Other Reasons to See Your Eye Doctor

If you have any of the following eye problems, don't wait for your next appointment—visit your eye doctor as soon as possible:

- Decreased vision

- Draining or redness of the eye

- Eye pain
- Double vision
- Diabetes
- Floaters (tiny specks that appear to float before your eyes)
- Circles (halos) around lights
- Flashes of light

Diabetes and Your Eyes

Diabetic retinopathy is a common complication of diabetes. High blood sugar damages the blood vessels in the retina (a light-sensitive part of the eye), where scarring can cause permanent vision loss.

Diabetic retinopathy is also one of the most preventable causes of vision loss and blindness. Early detection and treatment can prevent or delay blindness due to diabetic retinopathy in 90 percent of people with diabetes, but 50 percent or more of them don't get their eyes examined or are diagnosed too late for effective treatment.

People with diabetes are also at higher risk for other eye diseases, including glaucoma and cataracts. If you have diabetes, an eye exam every year is necessary to protect and preserve your eyesight and eye health.

Eye Examination: The Basics

Have your eyes tested (examined) regularly to help find problems early, when they may be easier to treat. The doctor will also do tests to make sure you are seeing as clearly as possible.

What Happens during an Eye Exam?

- The doctor will ask you questions about your health and vision.
- You will read charts with letters and numbers so the doctor can check your vision.
- The doctor will do tests to look for problems with your eyes, including glaucoma.
- The doctor will put drops in your eyes to dilate (enlarge) your pupils. A dilated eye exam is the only way to find some types of eye disease.

Am I at Risk for a Vision Problem?

As you get older, your eyes change. This increases your chance of developing a vision problem. You may be at higher risk if one of your parents had a vision problem, like needing to wear glasses.

Common vision problems are:

- **Nearsightedness**—when far away objects are blurry

- **Farsightedness**—when far away objects are easier to see than near ones

- **Astigmatism**—a condition that makes it hard to see fine details

- **Presbyopia**—a condition that older adults can get that makes it hard to see things up close

See an eye doctor right away if your vision or eyes suddenly change.

What's the Difference between a Vision Screening and an Eye Exam?

A vision screening is a short checkup for your eyes. It usually takes place during a regular doctor visit. Vision screenings can only find certain eye problems.

An eye exam takes more time than a vision screening, and it's the only way to find some types of eye disease.

These 2 kinds of doctors can perform eye exams:

- Optometrist

- Ophthalmologist

Take Action!

Protect your vision. Get regular eye exams so you can find problems early, when they may be easier to treat.

Schedule an Eye Exam

Ask your doctor or health center for the name of an eye care professional. Or use these tips for finding an eye doctor.

When you go for your exam, be sure to:

- Ask the doctor for a dilated eye exam.

- Tell the doctor if anyone in your family has eye problems or diabetes..

What about Cost?

Check with your insurance plan about costs and copayments. Medicare covers eye exams for:

- people with diabetes

- people who are at high risk for glaucoma

- some people who have age-related macular degeneration

If you don't have insurance, look for free or low-cost eye care programs where you live.

Get Regular Physical Exams

Get regular checkups to help you stay healthy. Ask your doctor or nurse how you can prevent type 2 diabetes and high blood pressure. These diseases can cause eye problems if they aren't treated.

Lower Your Risk of Falling

Poor vision or the wrong glasses can increase your risk of falling. One in 3 older adults will fall each year. Falling can cause serious injuries and health problems, especially for people over age 64.

Chapter 5

Screening and Diagnostic Tests for Vision and Other Eye-Related Problems

Chapter Contents

Section 5.1

Comprehensive Dilated Eye Exam

This section includes text excerpted from "What Is a
Comprehensive Dilated Eye Exam?" National Eye
Institute (NEI), December 23, 2014.

You may think your eyes are healthy, but visiting an eye care professional for a comprehensive dilated eye exam is the only way to really be sure. During the exam, each eye is closely inspected for signs of common vision problems and eye diseases, many of which have no early warning signs. Annual comprehensive dilated eye exams are generally recommended starting at age 60. However, African Americans are advised to start having comprehensive dilated eye exams starting at age 40 because of their higher risk of glaucoma. It's also especially important for people with diabetes to have a comprehensive dilated exam at least once a year.

Key elements of a comprehensive dilated eye examination include dilation, tonometry, visual field test and a visual acuity test.

Dilation is an important part of a comprehensive eye exam because it enables your eye care professional to view the inside of the eye. Drops placed in each eye widen the pupil, which is the opening in the center of the iris (the colored part of the eye). Dilating the pupil allows more light to enter the eye the same way opening a door allows light into a dark room. Once dilated, each eye is examined using a special magnifying lens that provides a clear view of important tissues at the back of the eye, including the retina, the macula, and the optic nerve.

In a person with **diabetic retinopathy**, the most common diabetic eye disease and a leading cause of blindness in the United States, the exam may show swelling or leaking of blood vessels in the retina, the light-sensitive layers of tissue at the back of the eye. The eye care professional may also see abnormal growth of blood vessels in the retina associated with diabetic retinopathy.

In **age-related macular degeneration (AMD)**, a common cause of vision loss and blindness in people over the age of 50, the exam may show yellow deposits called drusen or clumps of pigment beneath the retina. In some cases, the exam may also show abnormal growth of blood vessels beneath the retina. These AMD-related changes tend to cause deterioration of a small area of the retina called the macula, which is needed for sharp, central vision.

A comprehensive dilated eye exam is also critical for detecting **glaucoma**, a disease that damages the optic nerve, which carries information from the eyes to the brain. In a person with glaucoma, the dilated exam may show changes in the shape and color of the optic nerve fibers. The exam may also show excessive cupping of the optic disc, the place where the optic nerve fibers exit the eye and enter the brain.

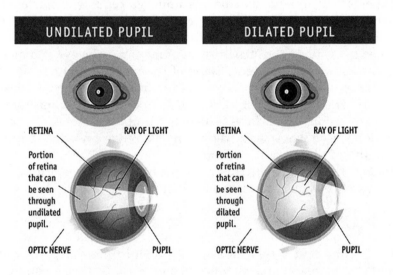

Figure 5.1. *Undilated and Dilated Pupil*

Tonometry is a test that helps detect glaucoma. By directing a quick puff of air onto the eye, or gently applying a pressure-sensitive tip near or against the eye, your eye care professional can detect elevated eye pressure, which can be a risk factor for glaucoma. Numbing drops may be applied to your eye for this test.

A **visual field test** measures your side (peripheral) vision. A loss of peripheral vision may be a sign of glaucoma.

A **visual acuity test** will require you to read an eye chart, which allows your eye care professional to gauge how well you see at various distances.

Section 5.2

Common Vision Tests

Experts recommend that people undergo regular, comprehensive eye examinations to check the clarity of their vision and the health of their eyes. A typical eye examination includes a number of tests designed to evaluate the structure and function of the eye and measure different aspects of eyesight. Some of the most common vision tests check the patient's ability to see details from a distance or close up, see colors, track moving objects, and see objects on the periphery of the field of vision. All of these tests help the ophthalmologist or optometrist determine whether corrective measures are needed to improve the quality of the patient's vision.

Some of the vision tests that are most likely to be performed during an eye examination include the following:

Visual Acuity Test

The visual acuity test measures the sharpness or clarity of the patient's near vision and distance vision. Both tests are usually conducted by asking the patient to read rows of letters on an eye chart. The test of distance vision, known as a Snellen test after the Dutch ophthalmologist who created it, uses a wall chart with rows of letters that gradually decrease in size from top to bottom. The patient typically stands about 20 feet (6 meters) away from the chart, covers one eye, and tries to read the letters on each line. The size of the letters on one of the lines corresponds to normal visual acuity, or what a person with normal eyesight can read from a distance of 20 feet.

Using the Snellen measurement system, a person with normal visual acuity is said to have 20/20 vision. The numerator (top number) of the Snellen fraction refers to the patient's distance from the eye chart, while the denominator (bottom number) refers to the distance at which a person with normal visual acuity can read that line. About 35 percent of adults have 20/20 vision without corrective lenses. A person with 20/40 vision would have visual acuity that is worse than normal, while a person with 20/10 vision would have visual acuity that is better than normal. The goal of corrective measures like eyeglasses, contact lenses, and laser surgery is to bring a patient's vision to 20/20, and about 75 percent of adults can reach that goal with correction.

Most states require people to demonstrate visual acuity of 20/40 or better in order to qualify for a driver's license. People whose visual acuity is measured at 20/200 or worse, even with corrective lenses, are considered legally blind.

The test of close-up vision is conducted using a Jaeger chart, which is a small card containing a few lines of printed text that get smaller moving from top to bottom. The patient holds the card about 14 inches from their face to determine the smallest print they can read comfortably. In the test of near vision, both eyes are tested at the same time. Many people experience a deterioration of their near vision as part of the normal aging process, so they require reading glasses or bifocals in middle age.

Refraction

The most common problems affecting visual acuity—nearsightedness (myopia) and farsightedness (hyperopia)—occur when the lens and cornea in the eye do not focus light on the retina accurately. Instead, the light is bent or refracted so that it is focused in front of or behind the retina, causing blurry vision when the patient looks at objects far away (myopia) or up close (hyperopia). The refraction test is used to determine the exact amount of the refraction error in each eye so that it can be corrected with an eyeglass prescription.

To perform a refraction, an eye doctor uses an instrument called a phoropter to show the patient a series of lenses. The patient must decide which lens option provides greater clarity in their vision. The lens power is fine-tuned through this interactive process until the eye doctor determines the final prescription for corrective lenses.

Retinoscopy

Retinoscopy is a test that can be used to approximate the results of a refraction. The patient looks through a series of lenses in a phoropter while the eye doctor shines a light into their eyes. When the light reflects onto the correct spot on the retina in the back of the patient's eye, the doctor can determine the lens power needed to correct the refraction error. This test can be used to speed up the refraction process or to determine the corrective lens prescription for young children and other people who may have trouble providing accurate feedback during other vision tests.

Machines called autorefractors and aberrometers can also be used to estimate the results of a refraction test. The autorefractor works the same way as a manual retinoscopy. The machine shines a light into the patient's eyes and determines the corrective lens power needed to focus the light accurately on the retina. An aberrometer is a sophisticated machine that uses wavefront technology to detect abnormalities in the way light travels through a patient's eye. It is usually used to determine the precise corrections to be made during surgical vision correction procedures.

Color Vision Test

Another test commonly performed in a comprehensive eye examination is designed to test the patient's ability to distinguish between colors. About 8 percent of men and 0.5 percent of women worldwide have a color vision deficiency or color blindness. Although most cases are hereditary, deficiencies in color vision can sometimes indicate problems with eye health. The typical color vision test asks patients to find colored numbers or symbols hidden within a pattern of different-colored dots. People with normal color vision are able to identify the numbers or symbols, while those with color vision deficiencies will have difficulty distinguishing one or more colors. Color vision tests are sometimes used to screen people for employment in jobs that require good color perception, such as electricians, pilots, and truck drivers.

Cover Test

A comprehensive eye examination also includes a simple test designed to check the patient's binocular vision, or how well their eyes work together. The cover test is performed by asking the patient to stare at an object while the doctor alternately covers one eye, then the other. The doctor watches to make sure that each eye is able to maintain its focus on the fixed object while it is covered and then uncovered.

Ocular Motility Test

Ocular motility is the eyes' ability to follow a moving object or shift focus quickly between two separate objects. To test ocular motility, an eye doctor will typically ask the patient to follow the movement of a small light with their eyes while keeping their head still. Ideally, the patient's eyes should move smoothly and in tandem. To test quick eye movements, an eye doctor may hold two objects some distance apart and ask the patient to move their eyes back and forth between them.

Stereopsis Test

Stereopsis, also known as depth perception, is the eyes' ability to discern the three-dimensional nature of objects. The two eyes must work together as a team to perceive depth. In the most common stereopsis test, the patient wears special 3D glasses while viewing a series of test patterns. For each pattern, the patient is asked to identify which letter or symbol appears closer.

Slit Lamp Exam

A slit lamp is a microscope that an eye doctor uses to examine the structures of the eye under magnification. This type of test can detect a variety of eye conditions and diseases, such as cataracts, macular degeneration, or corneal ulcers. It is often performed with the patient's pupils dilated in order to provide the best possible view of the internal structures of the eye. Pupil dilation is achieved by placing special drops in the patient's eyes. The effects can last for several hours, during which time the patient will likely be sensitive to light and have trouble focusing on close objects. If the patient will be exposed to bright light during this time, it is important for them to wear sunglasses to minimize glare and avoid damaging the eyes.

Glaucoma Test

Glaucoma is a serious eye condition caused by a buildup of pressure inside the eye when the fluid does not circulate properly. This interocular pressure can cause progressive damage to the optic nerve that carries visual signals to the brain, resulting in permanent, total blindness. Since people with glaucoma rarely experience any early symptoms or warning signs, it is important to get tested regularly. The most common glaucoma test, known as non-contact tonometry (NCT), involves a small puff of air being blown into the patient's open eye. The tonometer measures the eye's resistance to the puff of air in order to calculate its internal pressure. NCT is quick and painless, and the machine never touches the patient's eye.

Visual Field Test

A visual field test is used to detect gaps or blind spots in the patient's peripheral or side vision. Blind spots, known as scotomas, in the normal field of vision can indicate the presence of certain eye diseases or brain damage from a stroke or tumor. There are several different methods of testing a patient's field of vision. In a confrontation test, the patient covers one eye and stares at the doctor's eye or nose. The doctor slowly moves their hand from the edge of the patient's visual field toward the center, and the patient indicates the point at which they are able to see the hand. In a perimetry test, the patient stares at a dot inside a machine called a perimeter. The machine flashes lights at various points around the visual field, and the patient pushes a button each time they see a flash. At the end of the test, the machine prints a report showing any gaps or blind spots within the patient's field of vision.

If any of the above tests indicate problems with the patient's eye health or vision, the patient may be referred to a specialist for further testing.

References

1. Heiting, Gary, and Jennifer Palombi. "What to Expect during a Comprehensive Eye Exam," All About Vision, September 2016.

2. "Vision Tests," WebMD, 2017.

Chapter 6

Talking to Your Eye Care Doctor

Find an Eye Care Professional

There are several steps you can take to get in contact with an eye care professional.

- **Ask family members and friends** about eye care professionals they use.

- **Ask your family doctor** for the name of a local eye care professional.

- **Contact a state or county association** of ophthalmologists or optometrists. These groups, usually called academies or societies, may have lists of eye care professionals with specific information on specialty and experience.

- **Contact your insurance company or health plan** to learn whether it has a list of eye care professionals that are covered under your plan.

This chapter contains text excerpted from the following sources: Text beginning with the heading "Find an Eye Care Professional" is excerpted from "Healthy Eyes: Visiting Your Eye Care Professional," National Institute on Aging (NIA), National Institutes of Health (NIH), November 2015; Text under the heading "Tips for Talking to Your Doctor" is excerpted from "Tips for Talking to Your Doctor," National Eye Institute (NEI), February 8, 2017.

Prepare for Your Eye Care Visit

Today, patients take an active role in their healthcare. You and your eye care professional will work together to keep your eyes healthy. An important part of this relationship is good communication. To get the best out of your visit with your eye care professional, ask questions and continue to do so until you understand. It is also helpful to write down the questions before your visit, and write down what your eye care professional says.

Also, think about specific ways your vision has changed or specific times when you are aware of visual problems. For example, you may be more bothered by oncoming traffic lights when you are driving at night, or you may have trouble perceiving the depth of stairs or curbs. Sharing this information can help alert your eye care professional to any conditions you may have.

What to Bring to Your Visit

There are things you can bring to your visit that will help you to be more prepared. Remember to take along

- **A notebook and pen** to write down the responses to your questions.

- **A family member** or friend to take notes or for support.

- **Glasses or contacts**, if you use them.

- **An interpreter**, if you need of one.

- **Any medications** that you are currently taking.

Tips for Talking to Your Doctor

You should be active in the care of your eyes. You and your doctor can work together to keep your vision healthy. Good communication is the key to this relationship.

Ask questions. It's the best way to learn how to take care of your sight.

Questions about my eye disease or condition:

- What eye disease or condition do I have?

- What caused it?

- How will this affect my vision now and in the future?

Questions about contacting my doctor:

- Should I watch for any particular symptoms?
- When should I notify you if they occur?
- How can I take care of my eyes?
- Where should I go if I have an emergency?

Questions about my tests:

- What kinds of tests will I need?
- When should I have these tests done?
- Do I have to do anything special to prepare for any of the tests?
- What do you expect to find out from these tests?
- When will I know the results?
- Do these tests have any side effects or risks?
- Will I need more tests later?

Questions about treatment:

- What is the treatment for my condition?
- Are there other types of treatment?
- What is the best treatment and why?
- What are the benefits of this treatment, and how successful is it?
- What are the risks and side effects associated with this treatment?
- When will I start my treatment?
- How long will my treatment last?
- Should I follow a schedule for my treatment?
- Are there foods, drugs, or activities I should avoid while I'm on this treatment?
- If my treatment includes taking medication, what should I do if I miss a dose?

What else should I do?

Be sure you understand your doctor's answers. If you don't understand, ask questions until you do. Here are additional tips when talking with your doctor:

- Ask your doctor to write down all of your instructions. Repeat what your doctor said to make sure you understood everything.

- If you have an eye disease, ask for brochures to learn more about your condition.

- If you still have questions, ask where you can get more information.

- Remember you can also ask your nurse or pharmacist about your eye condition or treatment.

Chapter 7

Pediatric Vision Concerns

Vision Concerns in Children: The Basics

It's important for children to have their vision checked at least once before age 6, even if there aren't any signs of eye problems. Finding and treating eye problems early on can save a child's sight.

Healthy eyes and vision are very important to a child's development. Growing children constantly use their eyes, both at play and in the classroom.

What Are Common Eye Problems in Children?

These common eye problems can be treated if they are found early enough:

- Lazy eye (amblyopia)

- Crossed eyes (strabismus)

Other conditions—like being nearsighted or farsighted—can be corrected with glasses or contact lenses. Conditions like these are called refractive errors.

This chapter includes text excerpted from "Get Your Child's Vision Checked," Office of Disease Prevention and Health Promotion (ODPHP), U.S. Department of Health and Human Services (HHS), January 24, 2017.

Is My Child at Risk for Vision Problems?

If your family has a history of childhood vision problems, your child may be more likely to have eye problems. Talk to the doctor about eye problems in your family.

Eye Exams Are Part of Regular Checkups

The doctor will check your child's eyes during each checkup, beginning with your child's first well-baby visit.

Around age 3 or 4, the doctor will give your child a more complete eye exam to make sure her vision is developing normally. If there are any problems, the doctor may send your child to an eye doctor.

Take Action!

Follow these steps to protect your child's vision.

Talk to Your Child's Doctor

Ask the doctor or nurse if there are any problems with your child's vision.

If the doctor recommends a visit to an eye care professional:

- Ask your child's doctor for the name of an eye doctor who is good with kids.
- Write down any information about your child's vision problem.
- Plan your child's visit to the eye doctor.

What about Cost?

Under the Affordable Care Act (ACA), the healthcare reform law passed in 2010, health insurance plans must cover vision screening for kids.

- If you have private insurance, your child may be able to get screened at no cost to you. Check with your insurance provider.
- Medicaid and Children's Health Insurance Program (CHIP) also cover vision care for kids.

If you don't have health insurance, check these websites for free or low-cost eye care programs for children.

- Financial Aid for Eye Care
- Sight for Students

- VISION USA
- InfantSEE

Look out for Problems

Schedule an eye exam for your child if you see signs of an eye problem, like if your child's eyes:

- are crossed all the time
- turn out
- don't focus together
- are red, crusted, or swollen around the eyelids

Know the warning signs of vision problems in children.

Protect Your Child's Eyes

- Don't let your child play with toys that have sharp edges or points.
- Keep sharp or pointed objects, like knives and scissors, away from your child.
- Protect your child's eyes from the sun. Look for kids' sunglasses that block 100 percent of UVA and UVB rays.
- Keep chemicals and sprays (like cleaners and bug spray) where kids can't reach them.
- Make sure your child wears the right eye protection for sports.

Help Develop Your Child's Vision

It takes skill to match what we see with what we want to do—like when we want to bounce a ball or read a book.

Here are ways to help your child develop vision skills:

- Read to your child. As you read, let your child see what you are reading.
- Play with your child using a chalkboard, finger paints, or different shaped blocks.
- Take your child to the playground to climb the jungle gym and walk on the balance beam.
- Play catch with your child.

Chapter 8

Adult Vision Concerns

Chapter Contents

Section 8.1

Common Vision Problems in Adults

This section includes text excerpted from "Common Vision Problems,"
National Eye Institute (NEI), January 5, 2017.

The most common vision problems are refractive errors, more commonly known as nearsightedness, farsightedness, astigmatism and presbyopia. Refractive errors occur when the shape of the eye prevents light from focusing directly on the retina. The length of the eyeball (either longer or shorter), changes in the shape of the cornea, or aging of the lens can cause refractive errors. Most people have one or more of these conditions.

What Is Refraction?

Refraction is the bending of light as it passes through one object to another. Vision occurs when light rays are bent (refracted) as they pass through the cornea and the lens. The light is then focused on the retina. The retina converts the light-rays into messages that are sent through the optic nerve to the brain. The brain interprets these messages into the images we see.

What Are the Different Types of Refractive Errors?

The most common types of refractive errors are nearsightedness, farsightedness, astigmatism and presbyopia.

- **Nearsightedness** (also called myopia) is a condition where objects up close appear clearly, while objects far away appear blurry. With nearsightedness, light comes to focus in front of the retina instead of on the retina.

- **Farsightedness** (also called hyperopia) is a common type of refractive error where distant objects may be seen more clearly than objects that are near. However, people experience farsightedness differently. Some people may not notice any problems with their vision, especially when they are young. For people with significant farsightedness, vision can be blurry for objects at any distance, near or far.

- **Astigmatism** is a condition in which the eye does not focus light evenly onto the retina, the light-sensitive tissue at the back of the eye. This can cause images to appear blurry and stretched out.

- **Presbyopia** is an age-related condition in which the ability to focus up close becomes more difficult. As the eye ages, the lens can no longer change shape enough to allow the eye to focus close objects clearly.

Who Is at Risk for Refractive Errors?

Presbyopia affects most adults over age 35. Other refractive errors can affect both children and adults. Individuals that have parents with certain refractive errors may be more likely to get one or more refractive errors.

What Are the Signs and Symptoms of Refractive Errors?

Blurred vision is the most common symptom of refractive errors. Other symptoms may include:

- Double vision

- Haziness

- Glare or halos around bright lights

- Squinting

- Headaches

- Eye strain

How Are Refractive Errors Diagnosed?

An eye care professional can diagnose refractive errors during a comprehensive dilated eye examination. People with a refractive error often visit their eye care professional with complaints of visual discomfort or blurred vision. However, some people don't know they aren't seeing as clearly as they could.

How Are Refractive Errors Corrected?

Refractive errors can be corrected with eyeglasses, contact lenses, or surgery.

Section 8.2

Normal Changes in the Aging Eye and Their Symptoms

This section includes text excerpted from "Aging and Your Eyes," National Institute on Aging (NIA), National Institutes of Health (NIH), January 2017.

Are you holding the newspaper farther away from your eyes than you used to? Join the crowd—age can bring changes that affect your eyesight. Some changes are more serious than others, but for many problems, there are things you can do to protect your vision. The key is to have regular eye exams so you can spot problems early.

Steps to Protect Your Eyesight

Have your eyes checked regularly by an eye care professional— either an ophthalmologist or optometrist. People over age 65 should have yearly dilated eye exams. During this exam, the eye care professional should put drops in your eyes that will widen (dilate) your pupils so that he or she can look at the back of each eye. This is the only way to find some common eye diseases that have no early signs or symptoms. If you wear glasses, your prescription should be checked, too. See your doctor regularly to check for diseases like diabetes and high blood pressure. These diseases can cause eye problems if not controlled or treated.

See an eye care professional right away if you:

- suddenly cannot see or everything looks blurry

- see flashes of light

- have eye pain

- experience double vision

- have redness or swelling of your eye or eyelid

Protect your eyes from too much sunlight by wearing sunglasses that block ultraviolet (UV) radiation and a hat with a wide brim when you are outside. Healthy habits, like not smoking, making smart food choices, and maintaining a healthy weight can also help protect your vision.

Common Eye Problems

The following common eye problems can be easily treated. But, sometimes they can be signs of more serious issues.

- **Presbyopia** is a slow loss of ability to see close objects or small print. It is normal to have this problem as you get older. People with presbyopia often have headaches or strained, tired eyes. Reading glasses usually fix the problem.

- **Floaters** are tiny specks or "cobwebs" that seem to float across your vision. You might see them in well-lit rooms or outdoors on a bright day. Floaters can be a normal part of aging. But, sometimes they are a sign of a more serious eye problem such as retinal detachment. If you see many new floaters and/or flashes of light, see your eye care professional right away.

- **Tearing** (or having too many tears) can come from being sensitive to light, wind, or temperature changes, or having a condition called dry eye. Wearing sunglasses may help. So might eye drops. Sometimes tearing is a sign of a more serious eye problem, like an infection or a blocked tear duct. Your eye care professional can treat these problems.

- **Eyelid problems** can result from different diseases or conditions. Common eyelid problems include red and swollen eyelids, itching, tearing, and crusting of eyelashes during sleep. These problems may be caused by a condition called blepharitis and treated with warm compresses and gentle eyelid scrubs.

Eye Diseases and Disorders

The following eye conditions can lead to vision loss and blindness. They may have few or no early symptoms. Regular eye exams are your best protection. If your eye care professional finds a problem early, there are often things you can do to keep your eyesight.

- **Cataracts** are cloudy areas in the eye's lens causing blurred or hazy vision. Some cataracts stay small and don't change your eyesight a lot. Others become large and reduce vision. Cataract surgery can restore good vision. It is a safe and common treatment. If you have a cataract, your eye care professional will watch for changes over time to see if you would benefit from surgery.

- **Corneal diseases** and conditions can cause redness, watery eyes, pain, problems with vision, or a halo effect of the vision (things appear to have an aura of light around them). Infection and injury are some of the things that can hurt the cornea. Some problems with the cornea are more common in older people. Treatment may be simple—for example, changing your eyeglass prescription or using eye drops. In severe cases, surgery may be needed.

- **Dry eye** happens when tear glands don't work well. You may feel itching, burning, or other discomfort. Dry eye is more common as people get older, especially for women. Your eye care professional may tell you to use a home humidifier, special eye drops (artificial tears), or ointments to treat dry eye.

- **Glaucoma** often comes from too much fluid pressure inside the eye. If not treated, it can lead to vision loss and blindness. People with glaucoma often have no early symptoms or pain. You can protect yourself by having regular dilated eye exams. Glaucoma can be treated with prescription eye drops, lasers, or surgery.

- **Retinal disorders** are a leading cause of blindness in the United States. Retinal disorders that affect aging eyes include:

  - **Age-related macular degeneration (AMD).** AMD can harm the sharp vision needed to see objects clearly and to do common things like driving and reading. During a dilated eye exam, your eye care professional will look for signs of AMD. There are treatments for AMD. If you have AMD, ask if special dietary supplements could lower your chance of it getting worse.

  - **Diabetic retinopathy.** This problem may occur if you have diabetes. Diabetic retinopathy develops slowly and often has no early warning signs. If you have diabetes, be sure to have a dilated eye exam at least once a year. Keeping your blood sugar under control can prevent diabetic retinopathy or slow its progress. Laser surgery can sometimes prevent it from getting worse.

- **Retinal detachment.** THIS IS A MEDICAL EMERGENCY. When the retina separates from the back of the eye, it's called retinal detachment. If you see new floaters or light flashes, or if it seems like a curtain has been pulled over your eye, go to your eye care professional right away. With surgery or laser treatment, doctors often can prevent loss of vision.

Low Vision

Low vision means you cannot fix your eyesight with glasses, contact lenses, medicine, or surgery. Low vision affects some people as they age. You may have low vision if you:

- can't see well enough to do everyday tasks like reading, cooking, or sewing
- have difficulty recognizing the faces of your friends or family
- have trouble reading street signs
- find that lights don't seem as bright

If you have any of these problems, ask your eye care professional to test you for low vision. Special tools can help people with low vision to read, write, and manage daily tasks. These tools include large-print reading materials, magnifying aids, closed-circuit televisions, audio tapes, electronic reading machines, and computers with large print and a talking function.

Other things that may help:

- Change the type of lighting in your room.
- Write with bold, black felt-tip markers.
- Use paper with bold lines to help you write in a straight line.
- Put colored tape on the edge of your steps to help you see them and prevent you from falling.
- Install dark-colored light switches and electrical outlets that you can see easily against light-colored walls.
- Use motion lights that turn on when you enter a room. These may help you avoid accidents caused by poor lighting.

- Use telephones, clocks, and watches with large numbers; put large-print labels on the microwave and stove.

Remember to ask your eye doctor if your vision is okay for safe driving.

Section 8.3

Age-Related Eye Diseases and Conditions

This section includes text excerpted from "Helping Older Adults
See Well for a Lifetime," National Eye Health Education Program
(NEHEP), National Eye Institute (NEI), October 30, 2015.

With the aging of the population, vision loss from eye disease is becoming a major public health concern. More than 40 million people are age 65 or older, and that number is expected to grow to more than 88 million by 2050. By that same year, the number of Americans with age-related eye diseases is expected to double, and the number of people living with low vision is projected to triple.

Common Vision Problems as We Age

Some vision changes are common with the natural aging of the eye, including difficulty seeing close-up objects clearly; declining sensitivity; having trouble distinguishing colors, such as blue from black; and needing more light to see well. These changes often can be easily corrected with a new prescription for glasses or improved lighting. But it is important for older adults to know the difference between changes that are normal and those that are not.

What Are Age-Related Eye Diseases?

As people age, they are at higher risk for certain eye diseases and conditions, including age-related macular degeneration (AMD), cataract, diabetic retinopathy, glaucoma, and dry eye. Many of these diseases and conditions have no warning signs but can be detected in their early stages during a comprehensive dilated eye exam. Early detection and treatment are key to saving sight.

- AMD is the leading cause of vision loss and blindness among adults ages 50 and older. It gradually destroys the macula, which is the part of the eye that provides sharp, central vision. A variety of treatments are available to help reduce the risk of vision loss in people with this condition.

- Cataract is a clouding of the lens in the eye that causes loss of vision. Cataracts are very common in older people, and surgery is the only effective treatment. By age 80, more than half of all Americans either have cataracts or have had cataract surgery.

- Diabetic retinopathy (DR) is a complication of diabetes that damages blood vessels in the retina, which is the light-sensitive tissue at the back of the eye. Early detection, timely treatment, and appropriate follow-up care can reduce the risk of vision loss by 95 percent.

- Glaucoma is a group of diseases that can cause fluid and pressure to build up in the eye and damage the optic nerve. It first affects side, or peripheral, vision but can lead to total vision loss if left uncontrolled.

- Dry eye occurs when the eye does not produce tears properly or when tears evaporate too quickly. Left untreated, this condition can lead to pain, ulcers, or scars on the cornea, and some loss of vision. Dry eye can be treated with artificial tears, prescription eye drops, gels, gel inserts and ointments, and punctal or tear duct plugs.

What Is Low Vision?

Left untreated, many age-related eye diseases and conditions can lead to low vision. Low vision is a visual impairment that cannot be corrected with glasses, contact lenses, medication, or surgery. While vision that has been lost usually cannot be restored, people can learn to make the most of their remaining vision with vision rehabilitation.

What Are the Numbers?

Two million adults ages 40 and over have AMD, 24.4 million have cataract, 7.7 million have diabetic retinopathy, 2.7 million have glaucoma, and 3 million have low vision. These rates are expected to increase as the population of older adults grows.

Table 8.1. Prevalence of Eye Disease/Conditions and Their Projections (in Millions)

Eye Disease/Condition	Current Estimate	2030	2050
AMD	2.0	3.7	5.4
Cataract	24.4	38.7	50.2
Diabetic retinopathy	7.7	11.0	14.6
Glaucoma	2.7	4.3	6.3
Low vision	3.0	5.0	8.9

Ways to Prevent Vision Loss

Encouraging older adults to have regular comprehensive dilated eye exams is the most important thing you can to do help them protect their sight. Even if they haven't noticed any problems with their vision, it's still important to remind them that although many age-related eye diseases don't have any early symptoms, they can be detected and treated early before noticeable vision loss occurs. Many lifestyle factors can also play an important role in protecting vision as we age. It's important to remind older adults to take the following actions:

- Eat a balanced diet that includes dark, leafy greens and fish high in omega-3 fatty acids.
- Maintain a healthy weight.
- Do not smoke.
- Keep diabetes under control.
- Wear sunglasses and a brimmed hat outdoors.
- Wear protective eyewear.
- Know their family's eye health history and discuss it with their eye care professional.

Comprehensive Dilated Eye Exams—The Best Advice to Help Seniors Save Their Sight

The most important advice you can share with older adults to help them maintain good eye health is "Get a comprehensive dilated eye exam." During this exam, drops are placed in the eye to dilate or widen the pupils, and an eye care professional uses a special magnifying lens to examine the retina and optic nerve for signs of disease. Everyone age 50 should have a dilated eye exam. How often a person needs one depends on his or her individual risk factors.

Section 8.4

Vision Concerns in Pregnancy

During pregnancy, a woman's body undergoes many physical changes in order to support a growing baby. Natural fluctuations in hormone levels, metabolism, circulation, and fluid retention can affect the eyes just as they affect other organs. As a result, many pregnant women experience changes in their eyes or vision. Although most pregnancy-related eye issues are minor and disappear on their own after delivery, a few types of vision changes can indicate a health condition that requires medical attention. Experts recommend that expectant mothers check with their doctors if they experience any of the following symptoms:

- double vision;
- temporary loss of vision;
- sensitivity to light; or
- seeing spots, auras, or blinking lights.

Normal Vision Changes during Pregnancy

Most of the vision changes that occur during pregnancy are temporary. Although they can be annoying, they are usually not a cause for concern. They occur due to changing hormone levels and fluid retention, which are a normal part of pregnancy. Some of the common eye changes that occur during pregnancy include blurry vision, dry eyes, and puffy eyelids.

Blurry Vision

The fluid retention that most women experience during pregnancy can temporarily change the thickness and shape of the cornea, the transparent layer that helps focus light as it enters the eye. These changes can affect the power of corrective lenses the woman needs, resulting in blurry vision. Since the cornea will likely return to normal following delivery, experts generally recommend against getting a new prescription for corrective lenses during pregnancy. Many eye doctors can provide a temporary lens if the blurry vision makes it difficult to drive a car or perform other everyday tasks safely.

Dry Eyes

Many expectant mothers find that their eyes become dry and irritated during pregnancy and breastfeeding. This problem can be uncomfortable and make it difficult to wear contact lenses. Experts suggest using over-the-counter lubricating or rewetting eye drops to soothe dry eyes and relieve discomfort. Pregnant women may also be helpful to switch to glasses temporarily and take frequent breaks while working at a computer to avoid eyestrain.

Puffy Eyelids

Many women experience swollen ankles during pregnancy as a result of water retention. A lesser known effect of pregnancy hormones is swelling around the eyes and puffy eyelids, which can interfere with peripheral vision. To limit fluid retention, experts recommend drinking lots of water and eating a healthy diet low in sodium and caffeine.

Vision Changes of Concern during Pregnancy

A few vision changes that may occur during pregnancy can be symptoms of a serious medical condition, such as preeclampsia or gestational diabetes. Expectant mothers who experience sudden or severe vision disruptions should seek medical attention.

Preeclampsia

Preeclampsia is a complication that occurs in between 5 percent and 8 percent of all pregnancies. The main symptoms are high blood pressure, swelling of the hands and feet, and protein in the urine. Many women who develop preeclampsia experience vision problems, such as double vision, temporary loss of vision, sensitivity to light, or seeing spots, auras, or blinking lights. Preeclampsia can progress quickly to cause bleeding, organ damage, and detachment of the retinas in the eyes. Expectant mothers who experience symptoms of preeclampsia should seek medical attention and have their blood pressure checked immediately.

Diabetes and Gestational Diabetes

Diabetes is a disease that affects the body's ability to metabolize carbohydrates, resulting in high levels of sugar in the blood. High blood sugar can damage the blood vessels in the retina, causing a serious eye condition called diabetic retinopathy. Women who are diabetic need to monitor their blood sugar closely and get regular eye screenings to check for damage to the retina. This is especially important during pregnancy, which increases the risk of vision loss associated with diabetes.

Gestational diabetes is a form of diabetes that develops during pregnancy. Expectant mothers who develop the condition should be examined by an eye doctor for signs of retinopathy. Pregnant women with either form of diabetes should also seek medical attention if they experience blurry vision, which can be a sign of elevated blood sugar levels.

References

1. "Can Pregnancy Affect Your Eyes?" WebMD, 2017.

2. "How Pregnancy Affects Vision," Northwest Vision, August 30, 2015.

3. "Pregnancy and Your Vision," Prevent Blindness, 2017.

4. "Vision Changes during Pregnancy," BabyCenter, 2017.

Chapter 9

Current Vision Research

Chapter Contents

Section 9.1

Visual Impairment, Blindness Cases Expected to Double

This section includes text excerpted from "Visual Impairment, Blindness Cases in U.S. Expected to Double by 2050," National Institutes of Health (NIH), May 19, 2016.

With the youngest of the baby boomers hitting 65 by 2029, the number of people with visual impairment or blindness in the United States is expected to double to more than 8 million by 2050, according to projections based on the most recent census data and from studies funded by the National Eye Institute (NEI), part of the National Institutes of Health (NIH). Another 16.4 million Americans are expected to have difficulty seeing due to correctable refractive errors such as myopia (nearsightedness) or hyperopia (farsightedness) that can be fixed with glasses, contacts or surgery.

The researchers were led by Rohit Varma, M.D., director of the University of Southern California's Roski Eye Institute, Los Angeles, and published their analysis May 19, 2016 in JAMA Ophthalmology. They estimate that 1 million Americans were legally blind (20/200 vision or worse) in 2015. Having 20/200 vision means that for clear vision, you would have to be 20 feet or closer to an object that a person with normal vision could see from 200 feet away.

Meanwhile, 3.2 million Americans had visual impairment in 2015— meaning they had 20/40 or worse vision with best possible correction. Another 8.2 million had vision problems due to uncorrected refractive error.

"These findings are an important forewarning of the magnitude of vision loss to come. They suggest that there is a huge opportunity for screening efforts to identify people with correctable vision problems and early signs of eye diseases. Early detection and intervention—possibly as simple as prescribing corrective lenses—could go a long way toward preventing a significant proportion of avoidable vision loss," said NEI Director Paul A. Sieving, M.D., Ph.D.

Over the next 35 years, Varma and his colleagues project that the number of people with legal blindness will increase by 21 percent each decade to 2 million by 2050. Likewise, best-corrected visual impairment will grow by 25 percent each decade, doubling to 6.95 million. The greatest burden of visual impairment and blindness will affect those 80 years or older as advanced age is a key risk factor for diseases such as age-related macular degeneration and cataract.

The researchers analyzed data on visual impairment and blindness from six large studies: the Beaver Dam Eye Study (Beaver Dam, Wisconsin), Baltimore Eye Survey and Salisbury Eye Evaluation Study (Maryland), the Chinese American Eye Study (Monterey Park, California), Los Angeles Latino Eye Study, and Proyecto VER (Nogales and Tucson, Arizona). They used the 2014 census and population growth projections to estimate the nationwide prevalence of vision impairment and blindness now and in 2050.

In terms of absolute numbers, non-Hispanic whites, particularly white women, represent the largest proportion of people affected by visual impairment and blindness, and their numbers will nearly double. By 2050, 2.15 million non-Hispanic white women are expected to be visually impaired and 610,000 will be blind. "Based on these data, there is a need for increased screening and interventions across all population, and especially among non-Hispanic white women," Varma said.

African Americans currently account for the second highest proportion of visual impairment, but that is expected to shift to Hispanics around 2040, as the Hispanic population—and particularly the number of older Hispanics—continues to grow. Hispanics have particularly high rates of diabetes, which is associated with diabetic eye disease, a treatable cause of visual impairment.

African Americans, meanwhile, are expected to continue to account for the second highest proportion of blindness. "African Americans are at disproportionately high risk for developing glaucoma, a potentially blinding eye disease that typically causes the loss of peripheral, but not central vision, so people tend to not realize that they are losing their vision and do not seek treatment," he said.

Section 9.2

Use It or Lose It: Visual Activity Regenerates Neural Connections between Eye and Brain

This section includes text excerpted from "Use It or Lose It: Visual Activity Regenerates Neural Connections between Eye and Brain," National Eye Institute (NEI), July 11, 2016.

A study in mice funded by the National Institutes of Health (NIH) shows for the first time that high-contrast visual stimulation can help damaged retinal neurons regrow optic nerve fibers, otherwise known as retinal ganglion cell axons. In combination with chemically induced neural stimulation, axons grew further than in strategies tried previously. Treated mice partially regained visual function. The study also demonstrates that adult regenerated central nervous system (CNS) axons are capable of navigating to correct targets in the brain. The research was funded through the National Eye Institute (NEI), a part of NIH.

"Reconnecting neurons in the visual system is one of the biggest challenges to developing regenerative therapies for blinding eye diseases like glaucoma," said NEI Director Paul A. Sieving, M.D., Ph.D. "This research shows that mammals have a greater capacity for central nervous system regeneration than previously known."

The optic nerve is the eye's data cable, carrying visual information from the light-sensing neurons of the retina to the brain. Like a bundle of wires, it consists of about a million axons that each extend from an individual retinal ganglion cell. A variety of optic neuropathies, such as glaucoma, cause vision loss when they destroy or damage these axons. In adults, retinal ganglion cell axons fail to regrow on their own, which is why vision loss from optic neuropathies is usually permanent.

The researchers induced optic nerve damage in mice using forceps to crush the optic nerve of one eye just behind the eyeball. The mice were then placed in a chamber several hours a day for three weeks where they viewed high-contrast images—essentially changing patterns of black lines. The mice had modest but significant axonal regrowth compared to control mice that did not receive the high-contrast visual stimulation.

Prior work by the scientists showed that increasing activity of protein called mechanistic target of rapamycin (mTOR) promoted optic nerve regeneration. And so they wondered if combining visual stimulation with increased mTOR activity might have a synergistic effect. Two weeks prior to nerve crush, the scientists used gene therapy to cause the retinal ganglion cells to overexpress mTOR. Optic nerve crush was performed and mice were exposed to high-contrast visual stimulation daily. After three weeks, the scientists saw more extensive regeneration, with axons growing through the optic nerve as far as the optic chiasm, a distance from the eye of about 6 millimeters. Encouraged by these results, the researchers again increased mTOR activity but then forced mice to use the treated eye during visual stimulation by suturing shut the good eye. This combined approach of increasing mTOR activity with intense visual stimulation promoted regeneration down the full length of the optic nerve and into various visual centers of the brain.

"We saw the most remarkable growth when we closed the good eye, forcing the mice to look through the injured eye," said Andrew Huberman, Ph.D., associate professor, Stanford University School of Medicine's department of neurobiology, and lead author of the report, published online on July 11, 2016 in Nature Neuroscience. In three weeks, the axons grew as much as 12 millimeters, a rate about 500 times faster than untreated CNS axons.

The regenerating axons also navigated to the correct brain regions, a finding that Huberman said sheds light on a pivotal question in regenerative medicine: "If a nerve cell can regenerate, does it wander or does it recapitulate its developmental program and find its way back to the correct brain areas?"

Using transgenic mouse lines designed to express fluorescent proteins only in specific retinal ganglion cell subtypes (about 30 exist), the investigators traced where regenerating axons went. "The two types of retinal ganglion cells that we looked at—α-cells and melanopsin cells—seemed fully capable of navigating back to correct locations in the brain, plugging in and forming synapses," said Huberman. "And just as interesting, they didn't go to the wrong places." Fluorescent axons appeared in brain regions where α-cells and melanopsin cells would be expected but were absent in other regions.

Visual function was partially restored in animals that received visual/mTOR combination therapy. The investigators used four tests to assess four types of visual perception: ability to track moving objects, pupillary reflex, depth perception, and ability to detect an overhead predator—a stimulus that normally causes mice to freeze or flee for cover. Mice treated with combination therapy performed significantly better than untreated mice in two of the four tests.

"This study's striking finding that activity promotes nerve regrowth holds great promise for therapies aimed at degenerative retinal diseases," noted Thomas Greenwell, NEI program director for retinal neuroscience research. Greenwell said the research has great relevance to the NEI Audacious Goals Initiative (AGI), a sustained effort to develop regenerative medicine for retinal diseases.

For future therapies that preserve optic nerve axons, Huberman envisions the development of filters for virtual reality video games, television programs, or eyeglasses designed to deliver regeneration-inducing visual stimulation. A drawback of the optic nerve crush model is that it does not mimic typical blinding diseases or injuries. The investigators are therefore currently examining the effect of intense visual stimulation in a mouse glaucoma model. Going forward, they are homing in on the specific qualities of visual stimulation that drive retinal regeneration.

Part Two

Understanding and Treating Refractive, Eye Movement, and Alignment Disorders

Chapter 10

Refractive Disorders

Chapter Contents

Section 10.1

Facts about Refractive Errors

This section includes text excerpted from "Facts about
Refractive Errors," National Eye Institute (NEI),
October 2010. Reviewed March 2017.

Refractive Errors Basics

What Are Refractive Errors?

Refractive errors occur when the shape of the eye prevents light
from focusing directly on the retina. The length of the eyeball (longer
or shorter), changes in the shape of the cornea, or aging of the lens
can cause refractive errors.

What Is Refraction?

Refraction is the bending of light as it passes through one object
to another. Vision occurs when light rays are bent (refracted) as they
pass through the cornea and the lens. The light is then focused on
the retina. The retina converts the light rays into messages that are
sent through the optic nerve to the brain. The brain interprets these
messages into the images we see.

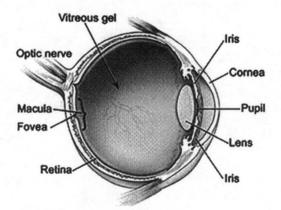

Figure 10.1. *Cross-Section of the Eye*

What Are the Different Types of Refractive Errors?

The most common types of refractive errors are myopia, hyperopia, presbyopia, and astigmatism.

Myopia (nearsightedness) is a condition where objects up close appear clearly, while objects far away appear blurry. With myopia, light comes to focus in front of the retina instead of on the retina.

Hyperopia (farsightedness) is a common type of refractive error where distant objects may be seen more clearly than objects that are near. However, people experience hyperopia differently. Some people may not notice any problems with their vision, especially when they are young. For people with significant hyperopia, vision can be blurry for objects at any distance, near or far.

Astigmatism is a condition in which the eye does not focus light evenly onto the retina, the light-sensitive tissue at the back of the eye. This can cause images to appear blurry and stretched out.

Presbyopia is an age-related condition in which the ability to focus up close becomes more difficult. As the eye ages, the lens can no longer change shape enough to allow the eye to focus close objects clearly.

Risk Factors

Presbyopia affects most adults over age 35. Other refractive errors can affect both children and adults. Individuals that have parents with certain refractive errors may be more likely to get one or more refractive errors.

Symptoms and Detection of Refractive Errors

What Are the Signs and Symptoms of Refractive Errors?

Blurred vision is the most common symptom of refractive errors. Other symptoms may include:

- double vision
- haziness
- glare or halos around bright lights
- squinting

- headaches

- eye strain

How Are Refractive Errors Diagnosed?

An eye care professional can diagnose refractive errors during a comprehensive dilated eye examination. People with a refractive error often visit their eye care professional with complaints of visual discomfort or blurred vision. However, some people don't know they aren't seeing as clearly as they could.

Treatment of Refractive Errors

Refractive errors can be corrected with eyeglasses, contact lenses, or surgery.

Eyeglasses are the simplest and safest way to correct refractive errors. Your eye care professional can prescribe appropriate lenses to correct your refractive error and give you optimal vision.

Contact Lenses work by becoming the first refractive surface for light rays entering the eye, causing a more precise refraction or focus. In many cases, contact lenses provide clearer vision, a wider field of vision, and greater comfort. They are a safe and effective option if fitted and used properly. It is very important to wash your hands and clean your lenses as instructed in order to reduce the risk of infection. If you have certain eye conditions you may not be able to wear contact lenses. Discuss this with your eye care professional.

Refractive Surgery aims to change the shape of the cornea permanently. This change in eye shape restores the focusing power of the eye by allowing the light rays to focus precisely on the retina for improved vision. There are many types of refractive surgeries. Your eye care professional can help you decide if surgery is an option for you.

Section 10.2

Astigmatism

This section includes text excerpted from "Facts about Astigmatism," National Eye Institute (NEI), October 2010. Reviewed March 2017.

Astigmatism Basics

What Is Astigmatism?

Astigmatism is a common type of refractive error. It is a condition in which the eye does not focus light evenly onto the retina, the light-sensitive tissue at the back of the eye.

Normal cornea   Cornea with astigmatism

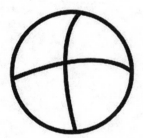 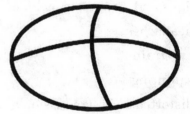

Figure 10.2. *Cornea with Astigmatism*

What Is Refraction?

Refraction is the bending of light as it passes through one object to another. Vision occurs when light rays are bent (refracted) as they pass through the cornea and the lens. The light is then focused on the retina. The retina converts the light rays into messages that are sent through the optic nerve to the brain. The brain interprets these messages into the images we see.

Causes and Risk Factors of Astigmatism

How Does Astigmatism Occur?

Astigmatism occurs when light is bent differently depending on where it strikes the cornea and passes through the eyeball. The cornea of a normal eye is curved like a basketball, with the same degree of roundness in all areas. An eye with astigmatism has a cornea that is curved more like a football, with some areas that are steeper or more rounded than others. This can cause images to appear blurry and stretched out.

Who Is at Risk for Astigmatism?

Astigmatism can affect both children and adults. Some patients with slight astigmatism will not notice much change in their vision. It is important to have eye examinations at regular intervals in order to detect any astigmatism early on for children.

Symptoms and Detection of Astigmatism

What Are the Signs and Symptoms of Astigmatism?

Signs and symptoms include:

- headaches
- eyestrain
- squinting
- distorted or blurred vision at all distances
- difficulty driving at night

If you experience any of these symptoms, visit your eye care professional. If you wear glasses or contact lenses and still have these issues, a new prescription might be needed.

How Is Astigmatism Diagnosed?

Astigmatism is usually found during a comprehensive dilated eye exam. Being aware of any changes in your vision is important. It can help in detecting any common vision problems. If you notice any changes in your vision, visit your eye care professional for a comprehensive eye dilated examination.

Can You Have Astigmatism and Not Know It?

It is possible to have mild astigmatism and not know about it. This is especially true for children, who are not aware of their vision being other than normal. Some adults may also have mild astigmatism without any symptoms. It's important to have comprehensive dilated eye exams to make sure you are seeing your best.

Treatment of Astigmatism

Astigmatism can be corrected with eyeglasses, contact lenses, or surgery. Individual lifestyles affect the way astigmatism is treated.

Eyeglasses are the simplest and safest way to correct astigmatism. Your eye care professional will prescribe appropriate lenses to help you see as clearly as possible.

Contact Lenses work by becoming the first refractive surface for light rays entering the eye, causing a more precise refraction or focus. In many cases, contact lenses provide clearer vision, a wider field of vision, and greater comfort. They are a safe and effective option if fitted and used properly. However, contact lenses are not right for everyone. Discuss this with your eye care professional.

Refractive Surgery aims to change the shape of the cornea permanently. This change in eye shape restores the focusing power of the eye by allowing the light rays to focus precisely on the retina for improved vision. There are many types of refractive surgeries. Your eye care professional can help you decide if surgery is an option for you.

Section 10.3

Hyperopia

This section includes text excerpted from "Facts about Hyperopia,"
National Eye Institute (NEI), July 2016.

Hyperopia Basics

What Is Hyperopia?

Hyperopia, also known as farsightedness, is a common type of
refractive error where distant objects may be seen more clearly than
objects that are near. However, people experience hyperopia differently. Some people may not notice any problems with their vision,
especially when they are young. For people with significant hyperopia,
vision can be blurry for objects at any distance, near or far.

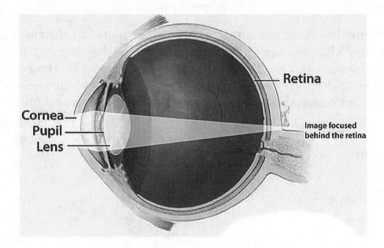

Figure 10.3. *Hyperopia*

What Is Refraction?

Refraction is the bending of light as it passes through one object
to another. Vision occurs when light rays are bent (refracted) as they

pass through the cornea and the lens. The light is then focused on the retina. The retina converts the light rays into messages that are sent through the optic nerve to the brain. The brain interprets these messages into the images we see.

What Are Refractive Errors?

In refractive errors, the shape of the eye prevents light from focusing on the retina. The length of the eyeball (longer or shorter), changes in the shape of the cornea, or aging of the lens can cause refractive errors.

Causes and Risk Factors

How Does Hyperopia Develop?

Hyperopia develops in eyes that focus images behind the retina instead of on the retina, which can result in blurred vision. This occurs when the eyeball is too short, which prevents incoming light from focusing directly on the retina. It may also be caused by an abnormal shape of the cornea or lens.

Who Is at Risk for Hyperopia?

Hyperopia can affect both children and adults. It affects about 5 to 10 percent of Americans. People whose parents have hyperopia may also be more likely to get the condition.

Symptoms and Detection

What Are the Signs and Symptoms of Hyperopia?

The symptoms of hyperopia vary from person to person. Your eye care professional can help you understand how the condition affects you.

Common signs and symptoms of hyperopia include:

- headaches
- eyestrain
- squinting
- blurry vision, especially for close objects

How Is Hyperopia Diagnosed?

An eye care professional can diagnose hyperopia and other refractive errors during a comprehensive dilated eye examination. People with this condition often visit their eye care professional with complaints of visual discomfort or blurred vision.

Treatment of Hyperopia

Hyperopia can be corrected with eyeglasses, contact lenses, or surgery.

Eyeglasses are the simplest and safest way to correct hyperopia. Your eye care professional can prescribe lenses that will help correct the problem and help you see your best.

Contact Lenses work by becoming the first refractive surface for light rays entering the eye, causing a more precise refraction or focus. In many cases, contact lenses provide clearer vision, a wider field of vision, and greater comfort. They are a safe and effective option if fitted and used properly. However, contact lenses are not right for everyone. Discuss this with your eye care professional.

Refractive Surgery aims to permanently change the shape of the cornea which will improve refractive vision. Surgery can decrease or eliminate dependency on wearing eyeglasses and contact lenses. There are many types of refractive surgeries and surgical options should be discussed with an eye care professional.

Section 10.4

Myopia

This section includes text excerpted from "Facts about Myopia,"
National Eye Institute (NEI), October 2016.

What Is Myopia?

Myopia, also known as nearsightedness, is a common type of refractive error where close objects appear clearly, but distant objects appear blurry.

When you look at an object, light rays reflect off that object and pass through the cornea and the lens of the eye, which bend (or refract) the light and focus it on the retina at the back of the eye. If you have perfect vision, the rays focus directly on the surface of the retina. But in a myopic eye, the eyeball is usually too long from front to back. This causes light rays to focus at a point in front of the retina, rather than directly on its surface. This makes distant objects blurry.

Myopia can also be the result of a cornea that is too curved for the length of the eyeball or a lens that is too thick. For some people, their myopia may be caused by a combination of problems in the cornea, lens, and length of the eyeball.

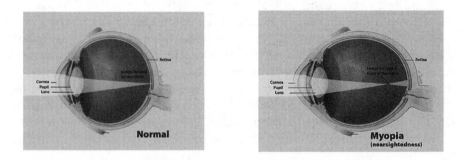

Figure 10.4. *Normal Vision and Myopic Vision*

What Are the Symptoms of Myopia?

If you have myopia, you have trouble seeing things far away, but you can see nearby things clearly. This is why myopia is commonly called nearsightedness.

If you can see well enough to read what's on your laptop or in a book, but you struggle to see what's on the television or a movie screen, you may be nearsighted. Sometimes people with undiagnosed myopia will have headaches and eyestrain from struggling to clearly see things in the distance.

Why Does the Eyeball Grow Too Long?

What causes the eyeball to grow too long isn't completely known, but researchers are exploring a number of factors. For many people, myopia appears to be an inherited condition—in other words, if you have a parent with myopia you are at higher risk for developing it. Researchers are also looking at the effects of sex, age, ethnicity, and environmental exposures—such as sunlight and the amount of time spent doing close-up work—on the development of myopia. More recently, scientists have been considering the influence of circadian rhythms (sometimes referred to as our biological or body clock), which regulate systems in the body according to the daily cycles of light and dark, as a factor in the development of myopia.

How Common Is Myopia?

Based on a study published in 2008, experts at National Institutes of Health (NIH) estimated that at least 33 percent of Americans are nearsighted. According to a 2009 study, the number of Americans with myopia has increased significantly from the 1970s to the early 2000s. The prevalence of myopia has also been increasing in many other countries around the world. It is particularly prominent among school-aged children living in urban areas in some Asian countries. In the past, people thought children might become myopic from spending too much time reading and writing, which require close-up vision, or from reading in poorly lit rooms. Studies suggest that the increase of myopia in children could be related to a decrease in the amount of time they spend outdoors.

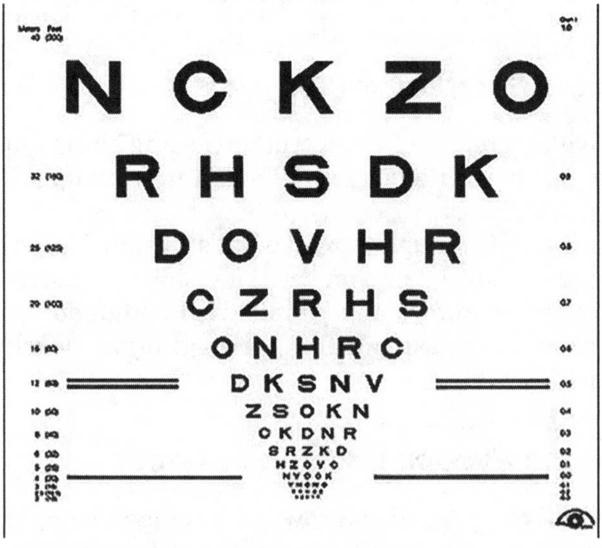

Figure 10.5. *EDTRS chart*

How Is Myopia Diagnosed?

An eye care professional can diagnose myopia during an eye exam, which usually begins with a visual acuity test. This test uses a standardized chart or card with rows of letters that decrease in size from top to bottom. Covering one eye, you will be asked to read out loud the smallest line of letters that you can see. When done, you will test the other eye. If the vision test shows that you are nearsighted, your doctor will use a retinoscope to shine light into your eyes and observe the reflection off the retina to determine the amount of refractive error you have.

What Kinds of Treatments Are Available for Myopia?

The most common way to treat myopia is to prescribe eyeglasses or contact lenses. Refractive surgery, once the eyes have stopped growing, has become another option for many people.

To find out the amount of myopia you have, an eye care professional uses a device called a phoropter to place a series of lenses in front of your eyes until you are seeing clearly. The combination of the results from both eyes is written as a prescription that will correct your vision to make it as normal as possible.

Eyeglasses use curved lenses to refocus light rays onto the retina, instead of in front of it.

Contact lenses correct vision in the same way as eyeglasses, except they rest directly on the eye.

Refractive surgery changes the shape of the cornea to correct myopia. There are different types of refractive surgery, but the most common are LASIK and PRK.

- LASIK removes tissue from the inner layers of the cornea. To do this, a section of the outer corneal surface is cut and folded back to expose the inner cornea. A laser removes a precise amount of tissue to reshape the cornea and then the flap of outer tissue is placed back in position to heal. The correction possible with LASIK is limited by the amount of corneal tissue that can be safely removed.

- PRK removes a thin layer of tissue from the surface of the cornea to change its shape. This allows light to focus more accurately on the retina. Like LASIK surgery, with PRK there is a limit to how much tissue can safely be removed and the amount of nearsightedness that can be corrected.

Many people will experience dry eye symptoms after refractive surgery and a small number may develop chronic dry eye syndrome. Some people may also develop vision symptoms such as double vision/ghosting, starbursts, glare, and halos, especially at night. Ask your eye doctor to discuss with you the risks and benefits of LASIK or PRK surgery before you undergo either procedure.

Phakic intraocular lenses (IOLs) are a new option for people who are very nearsighted or whose corneas are too thin to allow the use of laser procedures such as LASIK and PRK. Phakic lenses are surgically placed inside the eye.

What Is High Myopia?

High myopia is a severe form of myopia in which the eyeball continues to grow and becomes very long from front to back. It can increase the risk for retinal detachment, early development of cataracts and glaucoma.

What Is Degenerative Myopia?

Degenerative myopia (also called pathological or malignant myopia) is a rare and mostly inherited type of myopia that begins in early childhood. In degenerative myopia, the eyeball elongates rapidly and causes severe myopia, usually by the teenage or early adult years. Degenerative myopia may also progress far into the adult years. People with the condition have a significantly increased risk of retinal detachment and other degenerative changes in the back of the eye, including choroid neovascularization (abnormal blood vessel growth), and glaucoma.

What Research Is Being Done?

From 1996–2013 the COMET (Correction of Myopia Evaluation Trial) made many contributions to our understanding of why myopia develops and how it can be treated. One of the COMET reports, published in 2014, looked at seasonal differences in how quickly myopia progresses in young children.

The Pediatric Eye Disease (PED) Consortium is a project that brings together all existing population-based studies of eye diseases among preschool children around the world. It creates a repository of population-based survey data on vision health among more than 17,000 children between the ages of six and 72 months. PED Consortium researchers are using the data to look for demographic, behavioral, and clinical factors associated with the development of moderate to severe refractive errors.

A number of National Eye Institute (NEI)-funded studies are investigating how natural light exposure and daily circadian rhythm patterns influence the development of the eyeball. These studies are especially important since abnormal growth in the length of the eyeball is what causes myopia. Early studies with animal models have shown that environments that exclude natural daylight, or are solely lit by artificial light, or that switch day for night, influence how long the eyeball grows. Better understanding of the relationship between circadian rhythms and light exposure could provide new ways to decrease the risk for developing myopia.

NEI-supported researchers are also exploring the genetic causes of degenerative myopia. One study is working with members of a large, extended family, many of whom have degenerative myopia. The researchers are using genetic linkage analysis to identify possible causative genes, and then exploring what these genes do in eye tissue. Understanding the underlying mechanisms of degenerative myopia will help scientists work toward better treatments.

LASIK has become a popular surgical method to correct myopia in the United States, but not much is known about the long-term outcomes of LASIK surgery. In October 2009, the U.S. Food and Drug Administration (FDA), the National Eye Institute (NEI), and the Department of Defense (DOD) launched a collaborative study to look at how people fared after LASIK surgery. These studies—Patient Related Outcomes with LASIK (PROWL I and II)—laid the groundwork for a computer based questionnaire used to assess how many, of a select group of people who all received the same standardized LASIK treatment, experienced significant problems such as dry eye or vision irregularities (double vision, haloing, starbursts, or glare) over a period of 3 months following the procedure.

Section 10.5

Presbyopia

This section includes text excerpted from "Facts about Presbyopia," National Eye Institute (NEI), October 2010. Reviewed March 2017.

Presbyopia Basics

What Is Presbyopia?

Presbyopia is a common type of vision disorder that occurs as you age. It is often referred to as the aging eye condition. Presbyopia results in the inability to focus up close, a problem associated with refraction in the eye.

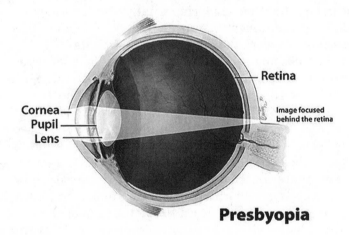

Figure 10.6. *Presbyopia*

Can I Have Presbyopia and Another Type of Refractive Error at the Same Time?

Yes. It is common to have presbyopia and another type of refractive error at the same time. There are several other types of refractive errors: myopia (nearsightedness), hyperopia (farsightedness), and astigmatism.

An individual may have one type of refractive error in one eye and a different type of refractive error in the other.

What Is Refraction?

Refraction is the bending of light as it passes through one object to another. Vision occurs when light rays are bent (refracted) by the cornea and lens. The light is then focused directly on the retina, which is a light-sensitive tissue at the back of the eye. The retina converts the light rays into messages that are sent through the optic nerve to the brain. The brain interprets these messages into the images we see.

Causes and Risk Factors

How Does Presbyopia Occur?

Presbyopia happens naturally in people as they age. The eye is not able to focus light directly onto the retina due to the hardening of the natural lens. Aging also affects muscle fibers around the lens making it harder for the eye to focus on up close objects. The ineffective lens causes light to focus behind the retina, causing poor vision for objects that are up close.

When you are younger, the lens of the eye is soft and flexible, allowing the tiny muscles inside the eye to easily reshape the lens to focus on close and distant objects.

Who Is at Risk for Presbyopia?

Anyone over the age of 35 is at risk for developing presbyopia. Everyone experiences some loss of focusing power for near objects as they age, but some will notice this more than others.

Symptoms and Detection

What Are the Signs and Symptoms of Presbyopia?

Some of the signs and symptoms of presbyopia include:

- hard time reading small print
- having to hold reading material farther than arm's distance
- problems seeing objects that are close to you
- headaches
- eyestrain

If you experience any of these symptoms you may want to visit an eye care professional for a comprehensive dilated eye examination. If you wear glasses or contact lenses and still have these issues, a new prescription might be needed.

How Is Presbyopia Diagnosed?

Presbyopia can be found during a comprehensive dilated eye exam. If you notice any changes in your vision, you should visit an eye care professional. Exams are recommended more often after the age 40 to check for age-related conditions.

Treatment of Presbyopia

Eyeglasses are the simplest and safest means of correcting presbyopia. Eyeglasses for presbyopia have higher focusing power in the lower portion of the lens. This allows you to read through the lower portion of the lens and see properly at distant through the upper portion of the lens. It is also possible to purchase reading eyeglasses. These types of glasses do not require a prescription and can help with reading vision.

Chapter 11

Eye Movement and Alignment Disorders

Chapter Contents

Section 11.1

Amblyopia

This section includes text excerpted from "Amblyopia,"
National Eye Institute (NEI), October 2, 2015.

What Is Amblyopia?

The brain and the eye work together to produce vision. Light enters
the eye and is changed into nerve signals that travel along the optic
nerve to the brain. Amblyopia is the medical term used when the vision
in one of the eyes is reduced because the eye and the brain are not
working together properly. The eye itself looks normal, but it is not
being used normally because the brain is favoring the other eye. This
condition is also sometimes called lazy eye.

How Common Is Amblyopia?

Amblyopia is the most common cause of visual impairment in
childhood. The condition affects approximately 2 to 3 out of every 100
children. Unless it is successfully treated in early childhood, amblyopia usually persists into adulthood, and is the most common cause
of monocular (one eye) visual impairment among children and young
and middle-aged adults.

What Causes Amblyopia?

Amblyopia may be caused by any condition that affects normal
visual development or use of the eyes. Amblyopia can be caused
by strabismus, an imbalance in the positioning of the two eyes.
Strabismus can cause the eyes to cross in (esotropia) or turn
out (exotropia). Sometimes amblyopia is caused when one eye is
more nearsighted, farsighted, or astigmatic than the other eye.
Occasionally, amblyopia is caused by other eye conditions such
as cataract.

How Is Amblyopia Treated in Children?

Treating amblyopia involves making the child use the eye with the reduced vision (weaker eye).

Currently, there are two ways used to do this:

1. **Atropine:** A drop of a drug called atropine is placed in the stronger eye once a day to temporarily blur the vision so that the child will prefer to use the eye with amblyopia. Treatment with atropine also stimulates vision in the weaker eye and helps the part of the brain that manages vision develop more completely.

2. **Patching:** An opaque, adhesive patch is worn over the stronger eye for weeks to months. This therapy forces the child to use the eye with amblyopia. Patching stimulates vision in the weaker eye and helps the part of the brain that manages vision develop more completely.

Previously, eye care professionals often thought that treating amblyopia in older children would be of little benefit. However, surprising results from a nationwide clinical trial show that many children age seven through 17 with amblyopia may benefit from treatments that are more commonly used on younger children. This study shows that age alone should not be used as a factor to decide whether or not to treat a child for amblyopia.

Can Amblyopia Be Treated in Adults?

Studies are very limited at this time and scientists don't know what the success rate might be for treating amblyopia in adults. During the first six to nine years of life, the visual system develops very rapidly. Complicated connections between the eye and the brain are created during that period of growth and development. Scientists are exploring whether treatment for amblyopia in adults can improve vision.

Section 11.2

Brown Syndrome

Brown syndrome—also known as Superior Oblique Tendon Sheath syndrome—is a rare condition affecting one of the muscles that control eye movement. The superior oblique muscle, which is connected to the outside of the eyeball by the superior oblique tendon, is unable to move properly. As a result, people with Brown syndrome have difficulty looking upward and inward toward the nose. Most cases of Brown syndrome are congenital (present from birth), although the condition is sometimes acquired later in life due to an eye injury or a different health issue. In 90 percent of cases it only affects one eye, usually the right. Brown syndrome is named after Dr. Harold W. Brown, the ophthalmologist who first described it in 1950.

What Causes Brown Syndrome?

Brown syndrome is a mechanical issue caused by abnormalities in the superior oblique muscle or tendon. The superior oblique muscle is the longest of the six muscles that control the movement of the eye. Rather than connecting directly to the eyeball from the eye socket like the other muscles, it passes through a ring of cartilage first. This creates a sharp angle in the muscle between its two attachment points. Some doctors believe that Brown syndrome develops because the superior oblique muscle is too short or too thick to move freely or contract properly.

The exact cause of congenital Brown syndrome is unknown. It occurs slightly more often in males than in females. Although a few cases appear to be hereditary, most cases appear spontaneously in people with no family history of the condition. However, a person with Brown syndrome has a 50 percent chance of passing the disorder on to their children.

Acquired Brown syndrome can occur at any age. The most common causes include trauma to the eye socket and diseases that create inflammation of tissues in the eye socket. People have developed Brown syndrome after being hit in the inside corner of the eye by a blunt object. People have also developed the condition following surgery on the eye, eyelid, sinus, or oral cavity. Inflammatory diseases such as rheumatoid arthritis and systemic lupus erythematosus have also been associated with the development of Brown syndrome.

What Are the Symptoms of Brown Syndrome?

The primary symptom of Brown syndrome is misalignment (strabismus) of the eyes when the person looks up and away from the affected side. The affected eye appears lower because its movement is restricted by the superior oblique tendon. In mild cases, the condition is not noticeable when the person looks straight ahead. In severe cases, however, the affected eye turns downward when the person looks straight ahead.

Other symptoms may include a droopy eyelid or crossed eyes. Some people with Brown syndrome develop a habit of tilting their heads backward to compensate for the limited movement of the affected eye. In most cases, people with Brown syndrome do not experience problems with vision. Some children with the condition may develop poor binocular vision or limited vision in the affected eye (amblyopia), while some may experience double vision.

How Is Brown Syndrome Diagnosed?

To diagnose Brown syndrome, an eye doctor will observe the patient's eye movements for evidence of misalignment or decreased ability to look upward. The doctor may also examine the patient's head position, since some people with Brown syndrome develop an abnormal head tilt to compensate for the limitation in their upward eye movement. In some cases the condition is diagnosed when the patient's affected eye becomes "stuck" in position after looking up or down for an extended period of time. The patient may feel a painful click when the tendon releases and the eye returns to its normal position.

How Is Brown Syndrome Treated?

The treatment options for Brown syndrome depend on the severity of the condition and whether it is congenital or acquired. In mild cases of congenital Brown syndrome, no treatment is usually required. Children with the disorder are monitored to ensure that their vision develops normally, and sometimes they must wear an eyepatch over the unaffected eye to encourage the brain to use both eyes equally. In some cases the condition improves over time, and it usually becomes less noticeable as children grow taller and no longer have to look upward as often.

Surgical treatment may be indicated in severe cases of Brown syndrome, when the patient exhibits one or more of the following symptoms:

- eye misalignment when looking straight ahead;

- pronounced abnormal head tilt;

- severe double vision; or

- compromised binocular vision affecting depth perception.

Surgical treatment involves removing a portion of the superior oblique tendon to allow the eye muscle to move more freely. Although the surgery usually produces good results, the condition may return, so multiple surgeries are sometimes necessary.

Nonsurgical treatment is usually recommended for acquired Brown syndrome. For cases that develop due to an inflammatory disease like lupus or rheumatoid arthritis, treatment usually focuses on the underlying disorder. For cases that develop due to trauma, corticosteroids and non-steroidal anti-inflammatory drugs (NSAIDs) are often prescribed to reduce inflammation of the superior oblique tendon and improve symptoms.

References

1. "Brown Syndrome," Moorfields Eye Hospital, 2011.

2. "Brown Syndrome," National Organization for Rare Diseases (NORD), 2003.

3. Tsakiris, Kleonikos A. "Brown Syndrome," American Academy of Ophthalmology (AAO), December 2, 2014.

4. "What Is Brown Syndrome?" American Association for Pediatric Ophthalmology and Strabismus (AAPOS), March 2015.

Section 11.3

Nystagmus

Text in this section is excerpted from "Nystagmus,"
© 2017 American Association for Pediatric Ophthalmology
and Strabismus (AAPOS). Reprinted with permission.

What Is Nystagmus?

Nystagmus is an involuntary, shaking, "to and fro" movement of the eyes. These jiggling or jerking movements are usually in horizontal or vertical directions.

What Are the Different Types of Nystagmus?

Nystagmus is typically classified as congenital or acquired, with multiple subcategories.

Congenital nystagmus onset is typically between 6 weeks and several months of age. If it starts after 6 months of age, this is considered acquired and may require imaging studies. Infantile nystagmus tends to be divided into two groups, depending on the underlying problem. One group arises from an abnormal afferent (or sensory) system, and the other from an abnormal efferent (motor) system. The efferent type is more common, but sometimes patients have early nystagmus due to afferent, or vision system, problems. In patients with early nystagmus secondary to afferent problems, conditions that limit their vision are thought to be responsible for the development of their nystagmus. The brain needs feedback from the eyes, through vision, to learn to keep them steady. Conditions that can be associated with this type of nystagmus include congenital cataracts, optic nerve hypoplasia, Leber's congenital amaurosis, achromatopsia, oculocutaneous albinism, aniridia, choroidal coloboma, severe refractive error, among others. Sensory nystagmus tends to occur by 2–3 months of life. More commonly, patients have nystagmus in the efferent group. congenital motor nystagmus tends to be horizontal, bilateral, and is sometimes inherited. For these patients, the jiggling may affect vision some, but usually not too much.

Acquired nystagmus occurs later, at least after the age of 6 months of age and can occur anytime thereafter. It can have many etiologies. Acquired nystagmus can be associated with serious medical conditions and will usually require further evaluation with imaging studies of the brain in order to determine a potential cause.

What Ocular/Medical Conditions Are Associated with Nystagmus?

- Cataract
- Strabismus
- Amblyopia
- Optic nerve hypoplasia
- Leber's congenital amaurosis
- Aniridia
- Achromatopsia
- Severe refractive error
- Retina coloboma
- Other optic nerve and retina disorders
- Albinism
- Medication use
- Vitamin deficiency
- Fetal alcohol syndrome
- Trauma
- Inner ear (vestibular) problems
- Stroke (most common cause in older people with acquired nystagmus)
- Brain tumor (rare cause of acquired nystagmus)

All children and adults with nystagmus should be evaluated by an ophthalmologist (and primary care physician) to determine if any association exists with other conditions.

Is Nystagmus Inheritable?

Nystagmus can be inheritable, sometimes with a strong family history. Dominant, recessive and X-linked patterns have been reported.

The severity of nystagmus often varies among members of an involved family.

How Does Nystagmus Affect a Child's Visual Development? What Will the Vision Be as an Adult?

The visual development of a child with nystagmus is quite variable. Some children with nystagmus have a mild reduction in visual acuity (20/50 or better), while others have severe visual disability (20/200 or worse). It is difficult to predict what the visual acuity will be as an adult; however, most individuals with nystagmus have some reduction of visual function.

What Does a Person with Nystagmus Actually See?

Children with nystagmus typically see the world similarly to other children, albeit with some blurriness. The world does not appear to "shake." Individuals with adult onset or acquired nystagmus often report the appearance of movement of the seen world (oscillopsia).

Why Do People with Nystagmus Tilt or Turn Their Head?

Nystagmus severity can vary upon direction of gaze; the eyes oscillate more when looking in certain directions. The gaze position of least eye movement is the "null point" and tends to be where vision is best. Tilting or turning the head into this direction where the movements are least can thus optimize vision.

Can Nystagmus Occur in One Eye?

Yes, but rarely. Spasmus nutans (triad of nystagmus, head bobbing or nodding, and a head turn or tilt) is often noted to have unilateral nystagmus. However, under close observation, the nystagmus is bilateral but highly asymmetric with a high-frequency "shimmering" movement.

Can Surgery Make Nystagmus Go Away?

Eye muscle surgery (strabismus surgery) may be indicated for some individuals with nystagmus. The goal of surgery in most instances is to help alleviate a significantly abnormal head position or to decrease the amplitude of nystagmus. Surgery can sometimes cause vision improvement but does not fully eliminate nystagmus.

What Non-Surgical Treatments Exist for Nystagmus?

Significant refractive error is corrected with glasses or contact lenses. Contact lenses, in some circumstances, can be more visually beneficial than spectacles. Variable success has been noted with medications used to dampen the severity of nystagmus. Unfortunately, the use of these medications is frequently limited by side effects. Botulinum toxin is helpful for some individuals with severe, intractable oscillopsia.

Section 11.4

Strabismus (Crossed Eyes)

Text in this section is excerpted from "Strabismus
(Crossed Eyes)," © 2017 American Optometric Association.
Reprinted with permission.

Crossed eyes, or strabismus, is a condition in which both eyes do not look at the same place at the same time. It usually occurs in people who have poor eye muscle control or are very farsighted.

Six muscles attach to each eye to control how it moves. The muscles receive signals from the brain that direct their movements. Normally, the eyes work together so they both point at the same place. When problems develop with eye movement control, an eye may turn in, out, up or down. The eye turning may occur all the time or may appear only when the person is tired, ill, or has done a lot of reading or close work. In some cases, the same eye may turn each time. In other cases, the eyes may alternate turning.

Proper eye alignment is important to avoid seeing double, for good depth perception, and to prevent the development of poor vision in the turned eye. When the eyes are misaligned, the brain receives two different images. At first, this may create double vision and confusion. But over time the brain will learn to ignore the image from the turned eye. Untreated eye turning can lead to permanently reduced vision in one eye. This condition is called amblyopia or lazy eye.

Some babies' eyes may appear to be misaligned, but they are actually both aiming at the same object. This is a condition called pseudostrabismus or false strabismus. The appearance of crossed eyes may be due to extra skin that covers the inner corner of the eyes or a wide bridge of the nose. Usually, the appearance of crossed eyes will go away as the baby's face begins to grow.

Strabismus usually develops in infants and young children, most often by age 3. But older children and adults can also develop the condition.

People often believe that a child with strabismus will outgrow the condition. However, this is not true. In fact, strabismus may get worse without treatment. An optometrist should examine any child older than 4 months whose eyes do not appear to be straight all the time.

Strabismus is classified by the direction the eye turns:

- Inward turning is called esotropia

- Outward turning is called exotropia

- Upward turning is called hypertropia

- Downward turning is called hypotropia

Other classifications of strabismus include:

- The frequency with which it occurs—either constant or intermittent

- Whether it always involves the same eye—unilateral

- If the turning eye is sometimes the right eye and other times the left eye—alternating

Treatment for strabismus may include eyeglasses, prisms, vision therapy, or eye muscle surgery. If detected and treated early, strabismus can often be corrected with excellent results.

What Causes Strabismus?

Strabismus can be caused by problems with the eye muscles, the nerves that transmit information to the muscles, or the control center in the brain that directs eye movements. It can also develop due to other general health conditions or eye injuries.

Risk factors for developing strabismus include:

- **Family history.** People with parents or siblings who have strabismus are more likely to develop it.

- **Refractive error.** People who have a significant amount of uncorrected farsightedness (hyperopia) may develop strabismus because of the additional eye focusing they must do to keep objects clear.

- **Medical conditions.** People with conditions such as Down syndrome and cerebral palsy or who have suffered a stroke or head injury are at a higher risk for developing strabismus.

Many types of strabismus can develop in children or adults, but the two most common forms are:

- **Accommodative esotropia** often occurs because of uncorrected farsightedness (hyperopia). The eye's focusing system is linked to the system that controls where the eyes point. So people who are farsighted are focusing extra hard to keep images clear. This may cause the eyes to turn inward. Symptoms of accommodative esotropia may include seeing double, closing or covering one eye when doing close work, and tilting or turning the head.

- **Intermittent exotropia** may develop when a person cannot coordinate both eyes together. The eyes may point beyond the object being viewed. People with intermittent exotropia may experience headaches, difficulty reading and eye strain. They also may close one eye when viewing at distance or in bright sunlight.

How Is Strabismus Diagnosed?

An optometrist can diagnose strabismus through a comprehensive eye exam. Testing for strabismus, with special emphasis on how the eyes focus and move, may include:

- **Patient history.** An optometrist will ask the patient or parent about any current symptoms. In addition, the optometrist will note any general health problems, medications or environmental factors that may be contributing to the symptoms.

- **Visual Acuity.** An optometrist will measure visual acuity to assess how much vision is being affected. For the test, you will be asked to read letters on reading charts that are near and at a distance. Visual acuity is written as a fraction, such as 20/40. The top number is the standard distance at which testing is done (20 feet). The bottom number is the smallest letter size you were able to read at the 20-foot distance. A person with 20/40 visual acuity would have to get within 20 feet of a letter that should be seen clearly at 40 feet. "Normal" distance visual acuity is 20/20. Your eye doctor has other methods of measuring vision in young children or patients who cannot speak or comprehend the visual acuity test.

- **Refraction.** An optometrist can conduct a refraction to determine the appropriate lens power you need to compensate for any refractive error (nearsightedness, farsightedness or astigmatism). Using an instrument called a phoropter, the optometrist places a series of lenses in front of your eyes and measures how they focus light using a handheld lighted instrument called a retinoscope. Or the doctor may use an automated or handheld instrument that evaluates the refractive power of the eye without the patient needing to answer any questions.

- **Alignment and focusing testing.** Your optometrist needs to assess how well your eyes focus, move and work together. In order to obtain a clear, single image of what you are viewing, your eyes must effectively change focus, move and work in unison. This testing will look for problems that keep your eyes from focusing effectively or make it difficult to use both eyes together.

- **Examination of eye health.** Using various testing procedures, your optometrist will observe the internal and external structures of your eyes to rule out any eye disease that may be contributing to strabismus. This testing will determine how the eyes respond under normal seeing conditions. For patients who can't respond verbally or when some of the eyes focusing power may be hidden, your optometrist may use eye drops. The eye drops temporarily keep the eyes from changing focus during testing.

Using the information obtained from these tests, along with results of other tests, your optometrist can determine if you have strabismus. Once testing is complete, your optometrist can discuss treatment options.

How Is Strabismus Treated?

People with strabismus have several treatment options to improve eye alignment and coordination. They include:

- **Eyeglasses or contact lenses.** This may be the only treatment needed for some patients.

- **Prism lenses.** These special lenses have a prescription for prism power in them. The prisms alter the light entering the eye and reduce how much turning the eye must do to view objects. Sometimes the prisms can eliminate the eye turning.

- **Vision therapy.** Your optometrist might prescribe a structured program of visual activities to improve eye coordination and eye focusing. Vision therapy trains the eyes and brain to work together more effectively. These eye exercises can help problems with eye movement, eye focusing and eye teaming and reinforce the eye-brain connection. Treatment can occur in your optometrist's office as well as at home.

- **Eye muscle surgery.** Surgery can change the length or position of the muscles around the eye so they appear straight. Often, people who have eye muscle surgery will also need vision therapy to improve eye coordination and to keep the eyes from becoming misaligned again.

Chapter 12

Eyeglasses

Chapter Contents

Section 12.1

How to Read Your Eyeglass Prescription

"How to Read Your Eyeglass Prescription,"
© 2017 Omnigraphics. Reviewed March 2017.

More than half of American adults—or around 150 million people—wear prescription eyeglasses to correct their vision. Yet few people understand the meaning behind the complicated series of letters, numbers, and symbols that appear on their eyeglass prescriptions. This shorthand code provides eyeglass manufacturers with specific information about a patient's vision, including the degree of nearsightedness, farsightedness, and astigmatism. This information enables the manufacturer to create custom eyeglasses to provide the patient with the best possible clarity of vision. Learning how to read an eyeglass prescription can provide patients with important knowledge about their eye health.

Terminology Used in Eyeglass Prescriptions

During an eye examination, the practitioner uses a process known as refraction to determine the exact amount of correction needed to give the patient clear vision. Refraction involves showing the patient a series of lenses using an instrument called a phoropter. As the patient repeatedly chooses the lens option that provides greater clarity of vision, the lens power is fine-tuned until the practitioner determines the final prescription for corrective lenses. The prescription is like a formula or equation for the eyeglass manufacturer to follow in creating the lenses. A written eyeglass prescription typically includes the following terminology:

OD and OS

OD is an abbreviation for the Latin term "oculus dexter," which means "right eye." OS is an abbreviation for the Latin term "oculus sinister," which means "left eye." When both of the patient's eyes require the same amount of correction, the abbreviation OU—short for "oculus uterque," meaning "both eyes"—may appear instead. Although these Latin terms have traditionally been used, some eye care practitioners have moved to the more modern abbreviations RE for "right eye" and LE for "left eye." The information for the right eye is always listed before the information for the left eye, because eye doctors work from left to right as they are facing a patient.

Sphere (SPH)

The sphere or SPH on an eyeglass prescription indicates the lens power the patient requires to achieve clear vision. The lens power is expressed in diopters (D), a unit of measure used to describe the refractive or light-bending ability of a lens. Prescriptions are usually measured in quarter-diopter increments and expressed in decimal form, such as 3.25 D. If the sphere begins with a minus sign (–), it means the patient is myopic (nearsighted) and needs corrective lenses to see distant objects clearly. If the sphere begins with a plus sign (+) or has no sign, it means the patient is hyperopic (farsighted) and needs corrective lenses to see near objects clearly. A higher sphere number indicates that the patient needs a higher power lens, and thus more correction.

Cylinder (CYL)

If CYL appears on an eyeglass prescription, it means that the patient has astigmatism. This common condition occurs when the eye, cornea, or lens has an irregular shape or curvature, rather than being perfectly round or spherical. Astigmatism can affect the way the eye focuses light, causing objects to appear blurry. The cylinder number indicates the amount of lens power required to correct the astigmatism. If the number is preceded by a minus sign, it refers to nearsighted astigmatism, or if it is preceded by a plus sign or no sign, it refers to farsighted astigmatism. If there is no cylinder number, then the patient does not have astigmatism or has very mild astigmatism that does not require correction.

Axis (X)

The axis (X) provides additional information to correct the vision of people with astigmatism. Due to the irregular shape of the eye, the cylinder lens power is not applied evenly to the entire eyeglass lens. Instead, the lens power is added those meridians of the eye where it is needed to correct the imperfect curvature. The axis number describes the location on the eye where the astigmatism correction is needed. The axis number is expressed in whole numbers between 0 and 180 degrees. It is determined by placing an imaginary protractor through the middle of the eye, with the flat side running horizontally through the pupil and the curved side following the arch of the eyebrow. The 90-degree line runs vertically through the eye. The axis value on an eyeglass prescription indicates the meridian that contains no cylinder power to correct astigmatism, while the lens meridian that is 90 degrees away contains the cylinder power.

Add

Add refers to magnifying power that is added to bifocal, trifocal, or progressive lenses to correct presbyopia, or blurry near vision. Many people develop presbyopia and need reading glasses as they reach middle age. The magnifying power is always positive. It usually ranges from +0.75 to +3.00 D and is the same for both eyes.

Prism (p.d.) and Base (B)

Prism and base appear on a small percentage of eyeglass prescriptions. These terms provide information needed to compensate for problems with eye alignment. The prismatic power is measured in prism diopters (p.d.) and may appear as a decimal or a fraction. The base (B) indicates the direction of the thickest part of the prism: BU (base up), BD (base down), BI (base in, toward the nose), or BO (base out, toward the ears).

Sample Eyeglass Prescription

As an example, a patient might receive the following eyeglass prescription:

| OD | -2.75 SPH | +1.50 add | 0.5 p.d. BD |
| OS | -2.00 -0.50 x 180 | +1.50 add | 0.5 p.d. BI |

In the left eye (OS), the practitioner has prescribed -2.00 D sphere to correct nearsightedness, plus -0.50 D cylinder to correct astigmatism. The axis for the cylinder power is 180, meaning the horizontal meridian of the eye has no added power for astigmatism, while the vertical (90-degree) meridian has -0.50 D applied.In the right eye (OD), the eye care practitioner has prescribed -2.75 D sphere to correct nearsightedness. SPH indicates that the right eye is only being prescribed spherical power. Since there is no astigmatism in the right eye, no cylinder power or axis is noted.

In both eyes, the practitioner has added +1.50 D magnification to correct presbyopia. Finally, the practitioner has included a prismatic correction of 0.5 p.d. in each eye, with the prism orientation base down (BD) in the right eye and base in (BI) in the left eye.

Eyeglass versus Contact Lens Prescriptions

It is important to note that separate prescriptions are needed for eyeglasses and contact lenses. Although both prescriptions may be provided at the same eye examination, they are not interchangeable. Eyeglass prescriptions only work for ordering eyeglasses, and contact lens prescriptions only work for ordering contact lenses.

The main reason the two types of prescriptions are different is that contact lenses are worn directly on the surface of the eyes, while glasses are positioned in frames at a distance from the eyes. The distance between the eye and the lens affects the power needed to provide clear vision. In addition, contact lens prescriptions include additional information about the lens diameter, curvature, and manufacturer or brand that can only be determined through a special contact lens fitting.

The Prescription Release Rule

Under a 1980 rule issued by the Federal Trade Commission (FTC), eye care practitioners are required to provide patients with a copy of their eyeglass prescription. The rule is intended to protect consumers' right to shop around for the best deal when purchasing eyeglasses, rather than being compelled to purchase glasses from the practitioner who performed the eye examination.

Under the Prescription Release Rule, eye care practitioners must provide a copy of the prescription whether the patient requests it or not. In addition, they cannot charge an extra fee or require the patient to meet any other conditions for the release of the prescription. Finally, practitioners cannot tell patients that the prescription may not be accurate if they purchase glasses from a different vendor. Practitioners who violate the rule face a $10,000 penalty from the FTC.

References

1. "Anatomy of an Eyeglass Prescription," FramesDirect, 2017.

2. Heiting, Gary. "How to Read Your Eyeglass Prescription," All About Vision, May 2016.

Section 12.2

Types of Eyeglasses

"Types of Eyeglasses," © 2017 Omnigraphics.
Reviewed March 2017.

The most basic eyeglasses—a pair of lenses mounted in a frame to hold them in position in front of the eyes—were invented more than 700 years ago. In recent years, however, technological advances have created new types of lenses and coatings that have made eyeglasses more comfortable, durable, and versatile than ever before. With stylish frame designs by the leading names in fashion, eyeglasses have moved beyond practical necessity to become decorative accessories.

The main purpose of prescription eyeglasses is to correct vision problems by adjusting the way the eye focuses light. The shape of the lens is what allows eyeglasses to correct vision problems. To correct nearsightedness (myopia), which makes it difficult for people to see distant objects clearly, the lens must be concave (curve inward). To correct farsightedness (hyperopia), which makes it difficult for people to see near objects clearly, the lens must be convex (curve outward). To correct astigmatism, which is caused by irregularities in eye shape, the lens must be cylindrical. In all of these cases, a wide variety of lens types, materials, and coatings are available to create perfect eyeglasses for any purpose or lifestyle.

Single Vision and Multifocal Lenses

Traditional, single-vision lenses contain the same prescription throughout the entire lens. They are designed to correct one type of vision problem, whether nearsightedness, farsightedness, astigmatism, or presbyopia (blurry near vision due to age-related changes

112

in the eyes). Single-vision reading glasses, with various powers of magnification, are available without a prescription for people with presbyopia. But many people have more than one vision problem, so the lenses in their eyeglasses must accommodate two or more prescriptions. In this case, they may choose multifocal lenses. There are three main types available: bifocals, trifocals, and progressive lenses.

Bifocals are lenses that are divided into two sections. The upper section contains a prescription to correct distance vision (10 feet or further), while the lower section contains a prescription to correct near vision (18 inches or closer). Many people get bifocals when they reach middle age and need reading glasses for presbyopia as well as glasses for distance. At one time bifocal lenses had an obvious line between the two sections, but in modern lenses the transition between the sections is often seamless.

Trifocals are lenses that are divided into three sections. The top and bottom sections work like the lenses in bifocals, while the middle section contains a prescription to correct intermediate distances. Trifocal lenses are designed to help people see computer screens and other objects within arm's reach as well as near and far objects.

Progressives are multifocal lenses that are divided into three sections, like trifocals, to correct distance, intermediate, and near vision. They are designed so that the different prescriptions blend together seamlessly to provide an uninterrupted transition from one section to the next.

Types of Lenses

Eyeglass lenses were once made of glass, which meant they were thick, heavy, and fragile. High-tech plastics have replaced glass in most modern lens applications, however, so they are thinner, lighter, and more durable than ever before. Some of the main options in terms of lens types include the following:

- **Polycarbonate lenses** are highly impact resistant, so they tend to work well for young children, people who wear glasses to play sports, and people who work in industrial or construction jobs where their glasses are likely to get damaged.

- **Trivex lenses** are made of a thin, lightweight plastic. Although they offer similar impact resistance to polycarbonate lenses, they also offer superior vision correction for some people.

- **High-index plastic lenses** are designed for people with strong prescriptions. They replace the thick, clunky "Coke-bottle" lenses with thinner, lightweight plastic.

- **Aspheric lenses** provide a larger useable surface because they are not spherical like traditional lenses. Instead, the degree of curvature varies across the surface of the lens. They can also be thinner and flatter than standard lenses.

- **Photochromic lenses** change color when exposed to sunlight. They work like clear prescription lenses indoors, and they change to tinted prescription lenses outdoors. Since the darkness of the lens adjusts to changing light conditions, it eliminates the need for sunglasses, reduces eye fatigue, and improves visual contrast.

- **Polarized lenses** are designed to reduce glare and improve contrast for outdoor sports and driving.

Lens Coatings

In addition to the new types of lenses, there are also a variety of coatings available to improve the appearance and performance of eyeglass lenses as well as protect the wearer's eyes. Some of the lens coating options include the following:

- **Scratch resistance** is applied to lenses to improve their durability.

- **Ultraviolet (UV) protection** is applied to reduce the eyes' exposure to damaging UV rays.

- **Anti-reflective (AR)** is applied to eliminate reflection, glare, or halos from the lens surface. It not only improves night vision and reduces eyestrain from electronic device screens, but it also gives eyeglasses a more flattering, transparent appearance.

- **Blue-light blocking** is available on intermediate-distance reading glasses designed for people who spend a lot of time working at a computer. These specialized computer glasses feature a tinted lens that protects the eyes from the blue light that radiates from electronic devices.

- **Tinted lenses** include a hint of color to increase visual contrast or to conceal signs of aging around the eyes.

- **Mirror coatings** are available in a range of colors to enhance the appearance of eyeglasses and hide the eyes from view.

Although modern eyeglasses are fairly durable, they can still be scratched, broken, or damaged if they are not handled with care. Experts recommend storing eyeglasses in a clean, dry case to protect them from damage. To get rid of spots, they suggest wiping gently with water and a lint-free cloth.

References

1. "Eyeglasses," Cleveland Clinic, 2017.

2. "Eyeglasses: Tips to Help You Pick the Right Lenses," WebMD, 2015.

Section 12.3

Fitting Glasses for Children

This section contains text excerpted from the following sources: Text beginning with the heading "What Type of Lenses Should Be Used?" is excerpted from "Glasses Fitting for Children," © 2017 American Association for Pediatric Ophthalmology and Strabismus (AAPOS). Reprinted with permission; Text under the heading "Using Sunglasses to Protect Your Eyes" is excerpted from "Reason #1 for Sunglasses: Protect Your Eyes," U.S. Department of Veterans Affairs (VA), April 17, 2015.

What Type of Lenses Should Be Used?

Polycarbonate (shatter proof) lenses are the ONLY type of lenses that should be prescribed to children unless your physician tells you differently. Polycarbonate lenses have built in U.V. protection to block harmful rays from the sun, they are light in weight and work well with strong prescriptions, and come with an anti-scratch coating.

Which Optical Shop Is Best?

Optical shops that frequently work with children are preferable. If frames and lenses are not fit properly, the endeavor of having a child wear glasses may be severely compromised. These optical shops also often have a superior selection of children's frames. Your local independent optician will work with your doctor to ensure proper power and continued good fit for your child.

Ask your optical shop about any frame or lens warranty that is available. If there is a warranty available, be sure to ask what it covers. Most warranties do not cover lost glasses.

What Frame Should Be Chosen?

Size is very important. Glasses must fit well so that they are comfortable and provide clear vision. If uncomfortable, a child may be reluctant to wear spectacles. Children should not be given adult frames to grow into. Some children wear straps to help keep glasses in place. Every child has a unique face and frames should be chosen to fit appropriately. One size does not fit all. Remember that your child will spend most waking hours wearing his or her glasses. Quality glasses will not only hold up better, but will be more comfortable for your child. The frame should be adjusted as needed for comfort and alignment on your child's face.

- Frames should preferably not touch the cheeks or eye lashes and the eyes should be centered in the lenses. The frame and nose pads can be adjusted for optimal fit.

- The horizontal line on bifocal lenses should go through the middle or immediately below the pupil (significantly higher than the typical bifocal position in adult glasses).

- Glasses for infants and toddlers often come with cable temples. This type of temple wraps around the ear. It is important that the cable not be too tight or the temple length too short. Children can grow out of cable frames very quickly, so ask about silicone temple tips for glasses as they work the same way as cables but are adjustable.

Do Children Love Glasses as Soon as They Get Them?

Nearsighted (myopic) children often enjoy their glasses immediately. However, far-sighted (hyperopic) and astigmatic children may take several weeks to adjust to wearing spectacles. If the child does not cooperate, the doctor may prescribe eye drops in an attempt to help the child adjust to the glasses.

How Do I Care for Glasses?

When not being worn, glasses should be placed in a case and should never be placed face down on a surface for fear of scratching the lenses. The motto for children is "Glasses stay on your face or they go in your case." Lenses may be cleaned with a soft cotton cloth or a special "lens cloth." If the frames are bent or do not fit well, take them to your optical shop for an adjustment. Do not try to adjust the frame yourself as breakage may occur.

Section 12.4

Using Sunglasses to Protect Your Eyes

This section contains text excerpted from the following sources: Text in this section begins with excerpts from "Keeping Your Eyes Healthy: Wear Sunglasses," National Eye Institute (NEI), February 10, 2015; Text beginning with the heading "Protect Your Eyes" is excerpted from "Reason #1 for Sunglasses: Protect Your Eyes," U.S. Department of Veterans Affairs (VA), April 17, 2015.

Most people know the sun's rays are bad for our skin. But did you know they're just as bad for our eyes?

Sunglasses are a great fashion accessory, but their most important job is to protect your eyes from the sun's ultraviolet (UV) rays. Some of the sun's effects on the eyes include:

- **Cataracts**, a clouding of the eye's lens that can blur vision. An estimated 20 percent of cases are caused by extended UV exposure.

- **Macular degeneration**, resulting from damage to the retina that destroys central vision. Macular degeneration is the leading cause of blindness in the United States.

- **Pterygium**, a tissue growth over the white part of the surface of the eye that can alter the curve of the eyeball, causing astigmatism.

When purchasing sunglasses, look for ones that block out 99 to 100 percent of both UVA and UVB radiation, so you can keep your vision sharp and eyes healthy. A wide-brimmed hat offers great protection, too!

Protect Your Eyes

UV radiation from the sun's rays can potentially cause skin cancer and affect your overall health. It can also be damaging to your eyes and potentially harm your vision.

According to Dr. Kelly Thomann, Chief of the Optometry Program at Hudson Valley Health Care System, "Long-term UV radiation exposure puts you at a greater risk of developing ocular conditions such as cataracts and macular degeneration. In fact, people with any ocular disease should be especially cautious about protecting themselves from the sun."

Dr. Thomann notes that while most elderly people will eventually develop cataracts, most people are not aware that increased UV radiation can result in cataracts developing earlier.

Good quality sunglasses are recommended when outdoors, even if it's for a few minutes at a time. The sunglass frame should be wide and adequately cover the eyes and fragile tissue around the eyes including the eyelids. Dr. Thomann reminds her patients that the fragile tissue around the eyelids can develop melanoma from UV radiation. Another reason to wear quality sunglasses whenever you are out in the sun.

A hat with a brim is also beneficial to block out those sun rays coming in over the top of your sunglasses.

Look for UV Protections on the Label

As Dr. Becky Forman points out, "When purchasing sunglasses, it is important to make sure there is both UVA and UVB protection, as both types contribute to dermatological and ocular disease." Dr. Forman is an Optometry Resident at Hudson Valley.

She adds that "It is important to understand that lens darkness does not correlate with the amount of UV protection, which is the key factor in adequate sun protection. Polarized sunglasses may be beneficial in patients who experience glare."

Most eye doctors recommend wraparound sunglasses for better protection. And while prescription sunglasses are better, standard off-the-rack sunglasses are okay if they provide full protection.

Dr. Forman says people should look for sunglasses that absorb at least 90 percent of UV radiation. "Look for the two categories of protection on the label—UVA and UVB."

Routine visits to your eye doctor will help determine your specific UV protection needs and new advances in sunglass wear.

Chapter 13

Contact Lenses

Chapter Contents

Section 13.1

Types of Contact Lenses

This section includes text excerpted from "Contact Lens Types,"
Centers for Disease Control and Prevention (CDC), July 23, 2015.

There are many different contact lens types available, all of which require a prescription from an eye care provider. Talk to your eye care provider if you're thinking about getting contact lenses or changing your contact lens type. To get a prescription for contact lenses, an eye care provider will:

- perform a complete examination of your eyes

- try contact lenses on your eyes

- determine how the contact lenses fit on your eyes

- test your vision through the contact lenses

- give you instructions on proper contact lens wear and care

Your eye care provider will help you get the best possible vision and comfort from contact lenses. Wearing contact lenses without a proper fitting and lens care instructions from an eye care provider can lead to eye injury, infection, or other complications. Contact lens types may differ based on what they are made from (lens material), how long they are designed for wearing each day (wear schedule), and how often they should be replaced (replacement schedule). The most common contact lens types include the following:

- **Lens Material:** Soft or Hard (Rigid Gas Permeable)

- **Wear Schedule:** Daily Wear or Extended Wear

- **Replacement Schedule (for soft contact lenses):** Daily Disposable or Planned Replacement

Less commonly, people wear other types of contact lenses for special reasons.

Lens Material

Soft

Soft contact lenses are made of soft, flexible plastics that allow oxygen to pass through to the cornea—the clear dome that covers the colored part of the eye. This lens material may be easier to adjust to and provide better initial comfort than hard, or rigid gas permeable, contact lenses. Soft contact lenses are the most common lens material worn.

Hard, or Rigid Gas Permeable (RGP)

Hard, or rigid gas permeable (RGP), contact lenses are more durable than soft contact lenses and are resistant to buildup of eye-produced deposits on the lens surface. Hard contact lenses generally provide clearer, crisper vision. They also tend to be less expensive over the life of the lens since they last longer than soft contact lenses. Hard contact lenses are easier to handle and less likely to tear. However, they may take a longer period of time to adjust to as compared to soft contact lenses. They also require a more complex cleaning and disinfection process than soft contact lenses.

Wear Schedule

Daily Wear

Daily wear contact lenses are intended for use during the day. They are not designed for overnight wear. Remove daily wear contact lenses each night, rub and rinse with contact lens solution, and place in a clean contact lens storage case filled with fresh contact lens solution to disinfect them. Sleeping in daily wear contact lenses can increase the chances of getting a serious eye infection.

Extended Wear

Extended wear contact lenses are available for overnight wear ranging from one to six nights or up to 30 days. Extended wear contact lenses are usually made of soft plastics that allow more oxygen to pass through to the cornea. There are also a few brands of hard contact lenses designed and approved for overnight wear. Length of continuous wear depends on the contact lens type and your eye care provider's evaluation of your tolerance for overnight wear. It's important for the eyes to have a rest without lenses for at least one night following each scheduled removal. Talk with your eye care provider before considering this option, as overnight contact lens wear has been linked to serious eye infections.

Replacement Schedule

The majority of soft contact lens wearers must replace their contact lenses according to a schedule prescribed by an eye care provider.

Daily Disposable

Disposable contact lenses—as defined by the U.S. Food and Drug Administration (FDA)—are used once and then thrown away. With a true daily disposable schedule, a brand new pair of lenses is used each day. Wearing daily disposable contact lenses for more than one day may cause eye discomfort or other complications. Discard daily disposable contact lenses at the end of each day, and put in a new pair the next day.

Planned Replacement

Some soft contact lenses are labeled as "disposable," but they may be removed nightly and re-worn for multiple days. Replacement schedules for these contact lenses can vary from seven to 30 days. Talk to your eye care provider about the proper schedule for replacing your specific type of contact lens. Follow these tips to clean, disinfect, and store your contact lenses each time you remove them. Replace your contact lenses as often as your eye care provider tells you. Wearing contact lenses longer than the recommended replacement schedule can lead to eye discomfort or other complications.

Special Contact Lens Types

The types of contact lenses listed above correct vision in the same way that glasses do, only they are in contact with the eye. There are additional contact lens types that people may use to enhance eye color, correct special vision problems or even treat eye diseases.

Hybrid

Hybrid contact lenses have a rigid gas-permeable center attached to an outer "skirt" made of soft contact lens material. The soft, outer part of the lens increases comfort and helps the lens to stay centered on the eye, while the rigid gas permeable center provides clear vision. This design is intended for people who have irregular corneas. Because this is a newer type of contact lens, there are fewer options available and fewer eye care providers who fit these contact lenses as compared to soft or hard contact lenses.

Orthokeratology (Ortho-K)

Orthokeratology, or Ortho-K, uses specially designed hard contact lenses to change the shape of the cornea. This contact lens temporarily corrects vision and is mainly used in patients who are nearsighted. Ortho-K lenses are most often prescribed to be worn while sleeping. They are usually removed in the morning and not worn during the day. Most people can go all day without their glasses or contact lenses. For others, vision correction will wear off later in the day. Ortho-K lenses must be worn every night—or on some other prescribed schedule—in order to maintain the treatment effect. Your eye care provider will determine the best maintenance schedule for you.

Scleral

A scleral lens is a larger type of hard, or rigid gas permeable (RGP), contact lens. Scleral lenses rest on the sclera—the white part of the eye—and not the cornea. Fluid collects in the small amount of space between the lens and cornea. This fluid protects the cornea and can also help heal damaged corneas. Scleral lenses are often prescribed to patients with damaged corneas or patients with severe dry eye conditions. People who wear scleral lenses should carefully follow their eye care providers' instructions for proper wear and care.

Decorative

Some people choose to wear contact lenses to enhance or change the color of the eye. Decorative contact lenses are available with and without vision correction, but all contact lenses require a prescription from an eye care provider. FDA regulations and medical device law deem all contact lenses to be medical devices whether they correct vision or not. Visit an eye care provider for a prescription and follow-up examination to make sure the contact lenses fit properly.

Section 13.2

Contact Lens Risks

This section contains text excerpted from the following sources: Text
in this section begins with excerpts from "Contact Lens Risks," U.S.
Food and Drug Administration (FDA), August 24, 2015; Text under
the heading "Germs and Infections" is excerpted from "Healthy
Contact Lens Wear and Care: Germs and Infections," Centers for
Disease Control and Prevention (CDC), April 17, 2014; and text
under the heading "Other Complications" is excerpted from "Healthy
Contact Lens Wear and Care: Other Complications," Centers for
Disease Control and Prevention (CDC), March 14, 2014.

Wearing contact lenses puts you at risk of several serious conditions including eye infections and corneal ulcers. These conditions
can develop very quickly and can be very serious. In rare cases, these
conditions can cause blindness.

You can not determine the seriousness of a problem that develops
when you are wearing contact lenses. You have to get help from an
eye care professional to determine your problem.

If you experience any symptoms of eye irritation or infection,

- remove your lenses immediately and do not put them back in
  your eyes.

- contact your eye care professional right way.

- don't throw away your lenses. Store them in your case and take
  them to your eye care professional. He or she may want to use
  them to determine the cause of your symptoms.

- report serious eye problems associated with your lenses to the
  FDA's MedWatch reporting program.

Symptoms of Eye Irritation or Infection

- Discomfort

- Excess tearing or other discharge

- Unusual sensitivity to light

- Itching, burning, or gritty feelings
- Unusual redness
- Blurred vision
- Swelling
- Pain

Serious Hazards of Contact Lenses

Symptoms of eye irritation can indicate a more serious condition. Some of the possible serious hazards of wearing contact lenses are corneal ulcers, eye infections, and even blindness.

Corneal ulcers are open sores in the outer layer of the cornea. They are usually caused by infections. To reduce your chances of infection, you should:

- **Rub and rinse** your contact lenses as directed by your eye care professional.
- Clean and disinfect your lenses properly according to the labeling instructions.
- **Do not "top-off" the solutions in your case.** Always discard all of the leftover contact lens solution after each use. Never reuse any lens solution.
- **Do not expose your contact lenses to any water: tap, bottled, distilled, lake or ocean water.** Never use non-sterile water (distilled water, tap water or any homemade saline solution). Tap and distilled water have been associated with *Acanthamoeba* keratitis, a corneal infection that is resistant to treatment and cure.
- Remove your contact lenses before swimming. There is a risk of eye infection from bacteria in swimming pool water, hot tubs, lakes and the ocean.
- Replace your contact lens storage case every 3 months or as directed by your eye care professional.

Other Risks of Contact Lenses

- Pink eye (conjunctivitis)
- Corneal abrasions
- Eye irritation

Germs and Infections

Being able to see well is a vital aspect of performing daily activities for most people. Worldwide, many people rely on contact lenses (as well as glasses and eye surgery) to improve their sight. Contact lenses can provide many benefits, but they are not risk-free—especially if contact lens wearers don't practice healthy habits and take care of their contact lenses and supplies. If patients seek care quickly, most complications can be easily treated by an eye doctor. However, more serious infections can cause pain and even permanent vision loss, depending on the cause and how long the patient waits to seek treatment.

Keratitis

Contact lens wear is linked to higher risk of keratitis, or inflammation of the cornea (the clear dome that covers the colored part of the eye). Many contact lens wearers do not care for their contact lenses and supplies as instructed, which increases their risk of eye problems like keratitis.

Keratitis in contact lens wearers can be caused by many factors. One type of keratitis, called microbial keratitis, can occur when germs invade the cornea. These germs—such as viruses, bacteria, fungi, or parasites (amoebae)—are more likely to invade the eyes when contact lenses are worn for too long or are not cared for correctly. Microbial keratitis is a serious type of eye infection in contact lens wearers, which can lead to blindness or the need for corneal transplant in the most severe cases.

Types of Microbial Keratitis

- Bacterial Keratitis
- Fungal Keratitis
- Parasitic/Amebic Keratitis
- Viral Kveratitis

Prevention

Microbial keratitis can usually be prevented through healthy habits and proper care of contact lenses and supplies. Keep your eyes healthy while wearing contact lenses, and always be sure to carry a pair of glasses with you—just in case you have to take out your contact lenses.

Other Complications

Rare infections of the cornea (the clear dome covering the colored part of the eye), called microbial keratitis, are among the most serious complications related to contact lens wear. Other complications that are commonly linked to contact lenses usually cause milder symptoms, or no symptoms at all. They may resolve through temporarily not wearing contact lenses, or with eye drops prescribed by an eye doctor. Some of these complications include:

- **Allergies** affecting the eyes

- **Giant Papillary Conjunctivitis:** bumps that appear underneath the eyelid

- **Corneal abrasion:** a scratch or scrape on the cornea

- **Contact Lens-induced Acute Red Eye (CLARE):** red, irritated eyes

- **Corneal infiltrates:** irritation of the cornea indicating inflammation and possible infection

- **Dry eyes**

- **Neovascularization:** new blood vessels growing onto the cornea, sometimes causing eye redness

Section 13.3

Proper Care of Contact Lenses

This section includes text excerpted from "Healthy Contact Lens Wear and Care: Show Me the Science," Centers for Disease Control and Prevention (CDC), September 14, 2016.

Wearing and caring for contact lenses properly is critical to keeping the eyes healthy and preventing eye infections; however, the majority of contact lens wearers do not practice proper contact lens hygiene. In the United States there have been outbreaks of *Acanthamoeba* keratitis *and Fusarium* keratitis—both of which are very serious and sometimes blinding types of eye infections. These outbreaks have brought attention to contact lens wearer hygiene and the need for consistent information about how to wear and care for contact lenses to help prevent such infections.

Centers for Disease Control and Prevention (CDC)—with feedback from experts in optometry, ophthalmology, opticianry, and infectious diseases—encourages contact lens wearers to follow these recommendations, which are based on data from a number of studies.

Your Habits

Wash your hands with soap and water. Dry them well with a clean cloth before touching your contact lenses every time.

Why? Not washing hands with soap and water prior to touching your contact lenses is a risk factor for complications related to contact lens wear, as germs from the hands are transferred to the contact lenses and the lens case. Because microbes that cause eye infections are found in the water, you should dry your hands first before touching your contact lenses. Washing hands with soap and water, and drying them with a clean, lint-free cloth, is essential each time that contact lenses are inserted and removed.

Don't sleep in your contact lenses unless prescribed by your eye doctor.

Why? Sleeping in any type of contact lens increases by 6 to 8 times the risk of getting a serious type of corneal infection called microbial keratitis. Out of every 10,000 people who sleep overnight in their contact lenses in an average year, 18–20 infections of microbial keratitis will occur. Several companies make contact lenses that are approved by the U.S. Food and Drug Administration (FDA) to wear during the day and to sleep in (often called "extended wear," "continuous wear," or "overnight wear"); however, contact lens wearers who choose this type of lens should be informed that sleeping in any type of contact lenses increases the risk of serious eye infections.

Keep water away from your contact lenses. Avoid showering in contact lenses, and remove them before using a hot tub or swimming.

Why? Contact lenses are a known risk factor for *Acanthamoeba* keratitis, a severe type of eye infection caused by a free-living ameba that is commonly found in water. Infection from *Acanthamoeba* is relatively rare, with 1–21 infections per million contact lens wearers, depending on the geographical location. It can be difficult to treat and extremely painful—in the worst cases causing blindness. Activities such as showering, using a hot tub, and swimming while wearing contact lenses may increase the risk of this infection, as well as other types of infections. Due to regional differences in environmental factors and water quality worldwide contact lens wearers should always avoid exposure of contact lenses to water—both at home and when traveling.

Your Supplies

Your Contact Lenses

Rub and rinse your contact lenses with contact lens disinfecting solution—never water or saliva—to clean them each time you remove them.

Why? Improper cleaning of contact lenses raises the risk of complications among contact lens wearers. Rubbing contact lenses with a clean finger and rinsing them with disinfecting solution is the most effective way to remove deposits and microbes from soft contact lenses. Rinsing contact lenses with multipurpose solution and soaking them overnight without rubbing them first is not as effective at removing microbes. Regardless of the type of contact lens worn, rubbing and rinsing the lenses daily is an important step in maintaining contact lens and eye health.

Never store your contact lenses in water.

Why? For the same reason that showering, using a hot tub, and swimming should be avoided while wearing contact lenses, contacts should not be stored in water at any time. Exposing contact lenses to water may increase the risk of different types of eye infections. One serious type of contact lens-related eye infection, *Acanthamoeba* keratitis, is caused by a microscopic ameba commonly found in water. Even though infection from *Acanthamoeba* is rare, it can be difficult to treat and extremely painful—in the worst cases causing blindness.

Replace your contact lenses as often as recommended by your eye doctor.

Why? While the effects of not replacing contact lenses as regularly as recommended by an eye care provider have not been fully examined, studies have shown that contact lens wearers who do not follow recommended replacement schedules have more complications and self-reported discomfort than contact lens wearers who follow the replacement recommendations. Some contact lens wearers have also reported poorer vision as a result of wearing contact lenses longer than indicated by their eye care providers.

Your Contact Lens Case

Rub and rinse your contact lens case with contact lens solution—never water—and then empty and dry with a clean tissue. Store upside down with the caps off after each use.

Why? Contaminated contact lens cases have been linked to rare but serious eye infections in contact lens wearers in recent years. An invisible layer in the case called a biofilm can become a breeding ground for microscopic germs that can cause infections. Biofilms in contact lens cases can be best removed by rubbing and rinsing the case with disinfecting solution, and wiping dry with a tissue, and then allowing to air-dry face down with the caps off. Fewer than half of contact lens wearers report always cleaning their contact lens cases, even though the number of moderate to severe contact lens-related infections could be cut in half through improved lens case cleaning procedures.

Replace your contact lens case at least once every three months.

Why? Infrequent replacement of contact lens cases, along with poor cleaning of cases, has been linked to serious eye infections in contact lens wearers. A significant number of contact lens wearers report not changing their lens case on a regular basis. Even when cleaned properly by rubbing and rinsing the case with disinfecting solution, contact lens cases can still be contaminated with microscopic germs that can cause infections when they come into contact with the eye. The ideal frequency for lens case replacement has not been scientifically established, but there is agreement among experts in the vision care field that cases should be replaced every three months, or when a new bottle of solution is purchased that comes with a case—whichever comes sooner.

Your Contact Lens Solution

Don't "top off" solution. Use only fresh contact lens disinfecting solution in your case—never mix fresh solution with old or used solution.

Why? Topping off solution—or mixing fresh solution with used solution in the case for storing contact lenses—has been an important risk factor in serious outbreaks of contact lens-associated infections. Used solution in the case can become contaminated by germs that are on contact lenses or in the contact lens case. An invisible layer called a biofilm can grow in the case. The presence of biofilms can make contact lens disinfecting solution less effective at killing germs that can cause serious eye infections, and adding new solution to used solution can lower germ-killing power. It is important to use only fresh solution—never water—in the contact lens case when storing contact lenses overnight to help prevent infections.

Use only the contact lens solution recommended by your eye doctor.

Why? It is important to use the type or brand of contact lens solution recommended by your eye care provider. An eye doctor or optician recommends a contact lens solution based on each patient's eyes and medical history. In addition, certain types of contact lenses and solutions may interact and cause eye irritation when used together. An eye doctor can help determine the best solution for each type of contact lens. Eye doctors should be consulted before changing the type or brand of contact lens solution, and contact lens wearers should always be sure to read the package insert carefully before using any type of solution.

Your Eye Doctor

Visit your eye doctor yearly or as often as he or she recommends.

Why? The eye care community generally agrees that yearly eye exams are recommended for contact lens wearers in order to keep their eyes as healthy as possible while wearing contact lenses—particularly given that wearing contact lenses increases the risk for eye infections and complications. Additionally, contact lens wearers often need to have a yearly exam to confirm their prescription so that they may order new supplies of contact lenses. In some instances, eye doctors may recommend that patients return more frequently for eye exams.

Section 13.4

Contact Lens Care Systems and Solutions

This section includes text excerpted from "Contact
Lens Care Systems and Solutions," Centers for Disease
Control and Prevention (CDC), March 21, 2016.

Lens care systems and solutions are products you use to clean, disinfect, and store your contact lenses. Proper contact lens care is important for keeping your eyes healthy and free from infection. Only your eye care provider can determine which contact lens care system is best for you. Talk to your eye care provider before using a new contact lens care system.

What Is the Difference between Cleaning and Disinfection?

Cleaning is the removal of deposits, debris and some germs from the surface of the contact lens.

Disinfection is the killing of germs present on the contact lens, some of which can cause serious eye infections.

Multipurpose Solution

Multipurpose solution is an all-in-one care system used to clean, rinse, disinfect, and store soft contact lenses. This solution is the most commonly used care system among soft contact lens wearers. Follow these steps for proper use of multipurpose solution:

- Rub and rinse your contact lenses and store them in fresh solution every time you take them out.

- Never mix fresh solution with old or used solution in the case—a practice called "topping off"—since it reduces the effectiveness of disinfection.

- Rub and rinse your contact lens storage case with fresh solution—never water—every day.

134

- Empty all excess solution out of the case, and dry it with a fresh, clean tissue.

- Store the clean case upside down on a fresh, clean tissue with the caps off after each use 8 in order to prevent germs from building up in the case.

Hydrogen Peroxide-Based Systems

Hydrogen peroxide-based systems clean, disinfect, and store contact lenses. An eye care provider may prescribe this care system if you have an allergy to ingredients in multipurpose solution that causes redness or irritation of the eye. Systems that use this type of solution require the use of a special case that comes with the solution when you buy it. The special case reacts with the hydrogen peroxide, converting it to harmless saline solution over time. Never use another type of case with hydrogen peroxide-based solution, as the solution will not convert to saline and will cause burning, stinging, and redness upon inserting the contact lenses.

- Carefully follow all instructions on the label for proper use of hydrogen peroxide-based systems

- Put the contact lenses in the special case with fresh solution. Never mix fresh solution with old or used solution.

- Wait at least 4 to 6 hours—depending on the label's instructions—before inserting your contact lenses.

- Never rinse your contact lenses with hydrogen peroxide-based solutions and directly insert into your eyes, as this can cause burning, stinging, and redness.

Saline

Saline solution does not disinfect contact lenses. Only use saline for rinsing contact lenses after cleaning and disinfecting with another care system. For example, some hydrogen peroxide-based systems suggest rinsing contact lenses with saline prior to insertion. Talk to your eye care provider about whether or not you need to use saline with your care system.

Daily Cleaners

Daily cleaner is intended for cleaning—not disinfecting—your contact lenses. The cleaner loosens and removes deposits and debris from the contact lens. Place a few drops in the palm of your hand and carefully rub the contact lens for as long as directed on both sides. You must use additional products, such as multipurpose solution, for rinsing the daily cleaner off, disinfecting, and storing the contact lenses.

Enzymatic Protein Removers

Enzymatic protein removers clean off material that your eyes deposit on the contact lenses over time. Depending on the type of contact lenses you wear and the amount of deposits that build up on the lens surface, your eye care provider may recommend you use a product for removing the buildup. Enzymatic protein removers are available in liquid and tablet forms and are used on a daily or weekly basis depending on the product. Ask your eye care provider before using this product.

Rigid Gas Permeable (RGP) Care Systems

Care systems for rigid gas permeable, or hard, contact lenses are different from care systems used with soft contact lenses. Hard contact lenses typically require several different solutions for wetting, cleaning, and disinfecting. If you wear hard contact lenses, talk to your eye care provider about which care system is best for you. Never use hard contact lens care products on soft contact lenses.

Talk to your eye care provider for more information about contact lens care systems. Your eye care provider can help you determine which care system will work best with your eyes and your contact lens type.

Section 13.5

Things to Know about Decorative Contact Lenses

This section includes text excerpted from ""Colored" and Decorative Contact Lenses: A Prescription Is a Must," U.S. Food and Drug Administration (FDA), February 2016.

"Colored" and Decorative Contact Lenses: A Prescription Is a Must

Decorative contact lenses (sometimes called "fashion," "costume," or "colored" contact lenses) don't correct vision—they just change how your eyes look. But you need a prescription to avoid eye injury. Before buying decorative lenses, here's what you should know.

They are not cosmetics or over-the-counter merchandise. They are medical devices regulated by the U.S. Food and Drug Administration (FDA). Places that advertise them as cosmetics or sell them over-the-counter, without a prescription, are breaking the law.

They are not "one size fits all." An eye doctor (ophthalmologist or optometrist) must measure each eye to properly fit the lenses and evaluate how your eye responds to contact lens wear. A poor fit can cause serious eye damage, including:

- scratches on the cornea (the clear dome of tissue over the iris— the part of the eye that gives you your eye color)

- corneal infection (an ulcer or sore on the cornea)

- conjunctivitis (pink eye)

- decreased vision

- blindness

Places that sell decorative lenses without a prescription may give you few or no instructions on how to clean and care for your lenses. Failure to use the proper solution to keep contact lenses clean and moist can lead to infections, says Bernard P. Lepri, O.D., M.S., M.Ed., an FDA optometrist in the agency's Contact Lens and Retinal Devices Branch. "Bacterial infections can be extremely rapid, result in corneal ulcers, and cause blindness—sometimes within as little as 24 hours if not diagnosed and treated promptly."

"The problem isn't with the decorative contacts themselves," adds Lepri. "It's the way people use them improperly—without a valid prescription, without the involvement of a qualified eye care professional, or without appropriate follow-up care."

Where NOT to Buy Contact Lenses

FDA is aware that many places illegally sell decorative contact lenses to consumers without valid prescriptions for as little as $20. You should never buy lenses from:

- street vendors
- salons or beauty supply stores
- boutiques
- flea markets
- novelty stores
- Halloween stores
- record or video stores
- convenience stores
- beach shops
- Internet sites that do not require a prescription

These are not authorized distributors of contact lenses, which are prescription devices by federal law. You can talk with your eye care provider if you have questions. And if you find a website you think is illegally selling contact lenses over the Web, you should report it to FDA (www.fda.gov/Safety/ReportaProblem/ucm059315.htm).

How to Safely Wear Decorative Contact Lenses

Get an eye exam from a licensed eye doctor (ophthalmologist or optometrist), even if you feel your vision is perfect.

Get a valid prescription that includes the brand name, lens measurements, and an expiration date.

Don't buy anime or circle lenses—and don't expect your eye doctor to prescribe them. These bigger-than-normal lenses that give the wearer a wide-eyed, doll-like look have not been cleared by the FDA.

Buy the lenses from a seller that requires you to provide a prescription, whether you purchase them in person or shop online.

Follow all directions for cleaning, disinfecting, and wearing the lenses, and visit your eye doctor for follow-up eye exams. It's especially important to read and follow all instructions because you can injure your eyes if you do not use these medical device products according to the labeling.

See your eye doctor right away if you have signs of possible eye infection:

- redness

- eye pain that doesn't go away after a short time

- decrease in vision

Section 13.6

Contact Lenses for Children

This section includes text excerpted from "What to Know If Your Child Wants Contact Lenses," U.S. Food and Drug Administration (FDA), February 26, 2016.

What to Know If Your Child Wants Contact Lenses

These days, eyeglasses can look pretty cool. Still, the day may come when your son or daughter asks you for contact lenses.

There are pros to consider—and cons.

The U.S. Food and Drug Administration (FDA) regulates contact lenses and certain contact lens care products as medical devices. Contact lenses have benefits, says Bernard P. Lepri, O.D., M.S., M.Ed., an FDA optometrist in the agency's Contact Lens and Retinal Devices Branch.

"They can be better for sports activities, because they don't break as frames and the lenses of glasses can. And they provide better peripheral vision for sports, or driving, if your teen is of driving age," Lepri explains. Moreover, in some cases, contact lenses improve the quality of vision in comparison to eyeglasses, especially when a child is very nearsighted, says Lepri.

"On the other hand, you have to remember that contact lenses are medical devices, not cosmetics," Lepri says. "Like any medical device, contact lenses should be used only if they can be used safely and responsibly. And only under the supervision of your eye care professional." Serious injury to the eye can result, particularly if the contact lenses are not removed at the first hint of a problem.

Contact Lens Risks and Safety Tips

Kids and contact lenses are not always the best fit.

"Eye care professionals typically don't recommend contacts for kids until they are 12 or 13, because the risks are often greater than the benefits for younger children," Lepri says. "But age isn't the only issue. It's also a question of maturity."

Lepri suggests that parents who are considering contacts for their kids take a look at how well they handle other responsibilities, especially personal hygiene. "It takes vigilance on the part of the parents," he says. "You need to constantly be looking over your child's shoulder to make sure they are properly caring for their lenses."

As many an eye care professional can attest, kids find all sorts of ways to be less than hygienic. Common, dangerous behaviors include wearing another child's lens; using saliva to moisten a lens; and wearing decorative lenses purchased from flea markets, beauty supply stores, the Internet and other sources. These behaviors can result in injury.

The problems from contact lenses include infections and eye abrasions—meaning that your eye can be bruised from contact lenses. The reasons? Hygiene and responsibility. Or rather, Lepri says, the lack thereof. He adds that it's essential for all people who wear contact lenses to follow their eye care professional's advice "to the letter." That means observing all hygienic precautions.

Even lenses without corrective power, such as decorative or so-called "colored" or "costume" contact lenses, are still medical devices and have all the risks other contact lenses do, says Lepri. "Never buy decorative/costume contact lenses without a prescription from your eye doctor," he adds.

If considering contact lenses, your child should be able to follow the following safety tips.

- Always wash your hands before cleaning or inserting lenses, and carefully dry your hands with a clean, lint-free cloth.

- Rub, rinse, clean and disinfect your contact lenses as directed and only with the products and solutions recommended by your eye care professional.

- Never expose your contact lenses to any kind of water or saliva.

- Do not wear your lenses for longer than the prescribed wearing schedule. This means that you should not sleep in lenses that were not prescribed to be worn this way.

- Never wear someone else's lenses.

- Always have a prescription for any lenses you wear.

- When playing sports, wear safety goggles or glasses over your lenses.

- In general, always have a pair of back-up glasses handy.

- Never put a contact lens into an eye that is red.

- Don't ignore eye itching, burning, irritation or redness that could signal potentially dangerous infection. Remove the lenses and contact your eye care professional. Apply cosmetics after inserting lenses, and remove your lenses before removing makeup.

Not taking the necessary safety precautions can result in ulcers (sores) of the cornea—which is the front of the eye that shields it from germs, dust, and other harmful material—and even blindness.

"Even an experienced lens wearer can scratch a cornea while putting in or taking out a lens," Lepri notes.

What Else Should You Know?

Eye care professionals generally do not recommend extended wear lenses for kids and teens because they can increase the incidence of corneal ulcers, which can lead to permanent loss of vision.

Although they are a bit more expensive, daily disposable lenses can reduce some of the risks since the wearer is using a new pair of lenses every day.

In addition, children with seasonal allergies are usually not good candidates for wearing contact lenses. The lenses may only increase the itching and burning caused by their allergies.

You can talk with your child about the risks and responsibilities of wearing contact lenses and whether she or he is able to handle these responsibilities. Then talk with your eye care provider to determine if your child is a good candidate for wearing contact lenses.

Chapter 14

Laser-Assisted In Situ Keratomileusis (LASIK) Surgery

Chapter Contents

Section 14.1

LASIK: The Basics

This section contains text excerpted from the following sources:
Text in this section begins with excerpts from "LASIK," U.S. Food
and Drug Administration (FDA), June 9, 2014; Text under the
heading "The Eye and Vision Errors" is excerpted from "What Is
LASIK?" U.S. Food and Drug Administration (FDA), September 6,
2016; and text under the heading "When Is LASIK Not for Me?" is
excerpted from "When Is LASIK Not for Me?" U.S. Food and Drug
Administration (FDA), June 9, 2014.

LASIK is a surgical procedure intended to reduce a person's dependency on glasses or contact lenses. LASIK stands for Laser-Assisted *In Situ* Keratomileusis and is a procedure that permanently changes the shape of the cornea, the clear covering of the front of the eye, using an excimer laser. A mechanical microkeratome (a blade device) or a laser keratome (a laser device) is used to cut a flap in the cornea. A hinge is left at one end of this flap. The flap is folded back revealing the stroma, the middle section of the cornea. Pulses from a computer-controlled laser vaporize a portion of the stroma and the flap is replaced. There are other techniques and many new terms related to LASIK that you may hear about.

The Eye and Vision Errors

The cornea is a part of the eye that helps focus light to create an image on the retina. It works in much the same way that the lens of a camera focuses light to create an image on film. The bending and focusing of light is also known as refraction. Usually the shape of the cornea and the eye are not perfect and the image on the retina is out-of-focus (blurred) or distorted. These imperfections in the focusing power of the eye are called refractive errors.

There are three primary types of refractive errors: myopia, hyperopia and astigmatism.

- Persons with **myopia**, or nearsightedness, have more difficulty seeing distant objects as clearly as near objects.

- Persons with **hyperopia**, or farsightedness, have more difficulty seeing near objects as clearly as distant objects.

- **Astigmatism** is a distortion of the image on the retina caused by irregularities in the cornea or lens of the eye.

Combinations of myopia and astigmatism or hyperopia and astigmatism are common. Glasses or contact lenses are designed to compensate for the eye's imperfections. Surgical procedures aimed at improving the focusing power of the eye are called refractive surgery. In LASIK surgery, precise and controlled removal of corneal tissue by a special laser reshapes the cornea changing its focusing power.

Other Types of Refractive Surgery

Radial Keratotomy or RK and Photorefractive Keratectomy or PRK are other refractive surgeries used to reshape the cornea. In RK, a very sharp knife is used to cut slits in the cornea changing its shape. PRK was the first surgical procedure developed to reshape the cornea, by sculpting, using a laser. Later, LASIK was developed. The same type of laser is used for LASIK and PRK. Often the exact same laser is used for the two types of surgery. The major difference between the two surgeries is the way that the stroma, the middle layer of the cornea, is exposed before it is vaporized with the laser. In PRK, the top layer of the cornea, called the epithelium, is scraped away to expose the stromal layer underneath. In LASIK, a flap is cut in the stromal layer and the flap is folded back.

Another type of refractive surgery is thermokeratoplasty in which heat is used to reshape the cornea. The source of the heat can be a laser, but it is a different kind of laser than is used for LASIK and PRK. Other refractive devices include corneal ring segments that are inserted into the stroma and special contact lenses that temporarily reshape the cornea (orthokeratology).

When Is LASIK Not for Me?

You are probably NOT a good candidate for refractive surgery if:

- **You are not a risk taker.** Certain complications are unavoidable in a percentage of patients, and there are no long-term data available for current procedures.

- **It will jeopardize your career.** Some jobs prohibit certain refractive procedures. Be sure to check with your employer/ professional society/military service before undergoing any procedure.

- **Cost is an issue.** Most medical insurance will not pay for refractive surgery. Although the cost is coming down, it is still significant.

- **You required a change in your contact lens or glasses prescription in the past year.** This is called refractive instability. Patients who are in their early 20s or younger, whose hormones are fluctuating due to disease such as diabetes, who are pregnant or breastfeeding, or who are taking medications that may cause fluctuations in vision are more likely to have refractive instability and should discuss the possible additional risks with their doctor.

- **You have a disease or are on medications that may affect wound healing.** Certain conditions, such as autoimmune diseases (e.g., lupus, rheumatoid arthritis), immunodeficiency states (e.g., HIV) and diabetes, and some medications (e.g., retinoic acid and steroids) may prevent proper healing after a refractive procedure.

- **You actively participate in contact sports.** You participate in boxing, wrestling, martial arts or other activities in which blows to the face and eyes are a normal occurrence.

- **You are not an adult.** Currently, no lasers are approved for LASIK on persons under the age of 18.

Precautions

The safety and effectiveness of refractive procedures has not been determined in patients with some diseases. Discuss with your doctor if you have a history of any of the following:

- herpes simplex or herpes zoster (shingles) involving the eye area

- glaucoma, glaucoma suspect, or ocular hypertension

- eye diseases, such as uveitis/iritis (inflammations of the eye)

- eye injuries or previous eye surgeries

- keratoconus

Other Risk Factors

Your doctor should screen you for the following conditions or indicators of risk:

- **Blepharitis.** Inflammation of the eyelids with crusting of the eyelashes, that may increase the risk of infection or inflammation of the cornea after LASIK.

- **Large pupils.** Make sure this evaluation is done in a dark room. Although anyone may have large pupils, younger patients and patients on certain medications may be particularly prone to having large pupils under dim lighting conditions. This can cause symptoms such as glare, halos, starbursts, and ghost images (double vision) after surgery. In some patients these symptoms may be debilitating. For example, a patient may no longer be able to drive a car at night or in certain weather conditions, such as fog.

- **Thin corneas.** The cornea is the thin clear covering of the eye that is over the iris, the colored part of the eye. Most refractive procedures change the eye's focusing power by reshaping the cornea (for example, by removing tissue). Performing a refractive procedure on a cornea that is too thin may result in blinding complications.

- **Previous refractive surgery (e.g., RK, PRK, LASIK).** Additional refractive surgery may not be recommended. The decision to have additional refractive surgery must be made in consultation with your doctor after careful consideration of your unique situation.

- **Dry Eyes.** LASIK surgery tends to aggravate this condition.

Section 14.2

Risks in LASIK

This section includes text excerpted from "LASIK,"
U.S. Food and Drug Administration (FDA), June 9, 2014.

Most patients are very pleased with the results of their refractive surgery. However, like any other medical procedure, there are risks involved. That's why it is important for you to understand the limitations and possible complications of refractive surgery.

Before undergoing a refractive procedure, you should carefully weigh the risks and benefits based on your own personal value system, and try to avoid being influenced by friends that have had the procedure or doctors encouraging you to do so.

- **Some patients lose vision.** Some patients lose lines of vision on the vision chart that cannot be corrected with glasses, contact lenses, or surgery as a result of treatment.

- **Some patients develop debilitating visual symptoms.** Some patients develop glare, halos, and/or double vision that can seriously affect nighttime vision. Even with good vision on the vision chart, some patients do not see as well in situations of low contrast, such as at night or in fog, after treatment as compared to before treatment.

- **You may be undertreated or overtreated.** Only a certain percent of patients achieve 20/20 vision without glasses or contacts. You may require additional treatment, but additional treatment may not be possible. You may still need glasses or contact lenses after surgery. This may be true even if you only required a very weak prescription before surgery. If you used reading glasses before surgery, you may still need reading glasses after surgery.

- **Some patients may develop severe dry eye syndrome.** As a result of surgery, your eye may not be able to produce enough tears to keep the eye moist and comfortable. Dry eye not only causes discomfort, but can reduce visual quality due to intermittent blurring and other visual symptoms. This condition may be permanent. Intensive drop therapy and use of plugs or other procedures may be required.

- **Results are generally not as good in patients with very large refractive errors of any type.** You should discuss your expectations with your doctor and realize that you may still require glasses or contacts after the surgery.

- **For some farsighted patients, results may diminish with age.** If you are farsighted, the level of improved vision you experience after surgery may decrease with age. This can occur if your manifest refraction (a vision exam with lenses before dilating drops) is very different from your cycloplegic refraction (a vision exam with lenses after dilating drops).

- **Long-term data are not available.** LASIK is a relatively new technology. The first laser was approved for LASIK eye surgery in 1998. Therefore, the long-term safety and effectiveness of LASIK surgery is not known.

Additional Risks If You Are Considering the Following

Monovision

Monovision is one clinical technique used to deal with the correction of presbyopia, the gradual loss of the ability of the eye to change focus for close-up tasks that progresses with age. The intent of monovision is for the presbyopic patient to use one eye for distance viewing and one eye for near viewing. This practice was first applied to fit contact lens wearers and more recently to LASIK and other refractive surgeries. With contact lenses, a presbyopic patient has one eye fit with a contact lens to correct distance vision, and the other eye fit with a contact lens to correct near vision. In the same way, with LASIK, a presbyopic patient has one eye operated on to correct the distance vision, and the other operated on to correct the near vision. In other words, the goal of the surgery is for one eye to have vision **worse than** 20/20, the commonly referred to goal for LASIK surgical correction of distance vision. Since one eye is corrected for distance viewing and the other eye is corrected for near viewing, the two eyes no longer work together. This results in poorer quality vision and a decrease in depth perception. These effects of monovision are most noticeable in low lighting conditions and when performing tasks requiring very sharp vision. Therefore, you may need to wear glasses or contact lenses to fully correct both eyes for distance or near when performing visually demanding tasks, such as driving at night, operating dangerous equipment, or performing occupational tasks requiring very sharp close vision (e.g., reading small print for long periods of time).

Many patients cannot get used to having one eye blurred at all times. Therefore, if you are considering monovision with LASIK, make sure you go through a trial period with contact lenses to see if you can tolerate monovision, before having the surgery performed on your eyes. Find out if you pass your state's driver's license requirements with monovision.

In addition, you should consider how much your presbyopia is expected to increase in the future. Ask your doctor when you should expect the results of your monovision surgery to no longer be enough for you to see nearby objects clearly without the aid of glasses or contacts, or when a second surgery might be required to further correct your near vision.

Bilateral Simultaneous Treatment

You may choose to have LASIK surgery on both eyes at the same time or to have surgery on one eye at a time. Although the convenience of having surgery on both eyes on the same day is attractive, this practice is riskier than having two separate surgeries.

If you decide to have one eye done at a time, you and your doctor will decide how long to wait before having surgery on the other eye. If both eyes are treated at the same time or before one eye has a chance to fully heal, you and your doctor do not have the advantage of being able to see how the first eye responds to surgery before the second eye is treated.

Another disadvantage to having surgery on both eyes at the same time is that the vision in both eyes may be blurred after surgery until the initial healing process is over, rather than being able to rely on clear vision in at least one eye at all times.

Complications during and after Surgery

Even the best screened patients under the care of most skilled surgeons can experience serious complications.

- **During surgery.** Malfunction of a device or other error, such as cutting a flap of cornea through and through instead of making a hinge during LASIK surgery, may lead to discontinuation of the procedure or irreversible damage to the eye.

- **After surgery.** Some complications, such as migration of the flap, inflammation or infection, may require another procedure and/or intensive treatment with drops. Even with aggressive therapy, such complications may lead to temporary loss of vision or even irreversible blindness.

Finding the Right Doctor

If you are considering refractive surgery, make sure you:

- **Compare.** The levels of risk and benefit vary slightly not only from procedure to procedure, but from device to device depending on the manufacturer, and from surgeon to surgeon depending on their level of experience with a particular procedure.

- **Don't base your decision simply on cost** and don't settle for the first eye center, doctor, or procedure you investigate. Remember that the decisions you make about your eyes and refractive surgery will affect you for the rest of your life.

- Be wary of eye centers that advertise, "20/20 vision or your money back" or "package deals." There are **never any guarantees** in medicine.

- **Read.** It is important for you to read the patient handbook provided to your doctor by the manufacturer of the device used to perform the refractive procedure. Your doctor should provide you with this handbook and be willing to discuss his/her outcomes (successes as well as complications) compared to the results of studies outlined in the handbook.

Even the best screened patients under the care of most skilled surgeons can experience serious complications.

- **During surgery.** Malfunction of a device or other error, such as cutting a flap of cornea through and through instead of making a hinge during LASIK surgery, may lead to discontinuation of the procedure or irreversible damage to the eye.

- **After surgery.** Some complications, such as migration of the flap, inflammation or infection, may require another procedure and/or intensive treatment with drops. Even with aggressive therapy, such complications may lead to temporary loss of vision or even irreversible blindness.

Under the care of an experienced doctor, carefully screened candidates with reasonable expectations and a clear understanding of the risks and alternatives are likely to be happy with the results of their refractive procedure.

Advertising

Be cautious about "slick" advertising and/or deals that sound "too good to be true." Remember, they usually are. There is a lot of competition resulting in a great deal of advertising and bidding for your business. Do your homework.

Section 14.3

LASIK Surgery Checklist

This section includes text excerpted from "LASIK Surgery Checklist," U.S. Food and Drug Administration (FDA), June 9, 2014.

Know What Makes You a Poor Candidate

- **Career impact**—does your job prohibit refractive surgery?

- **Cost**—can you really afford this procedure?

- **Medical conditions**—e.g., do you have an autoimmune disease or other major illness? Do you have a chronic illness that might slow or alter healing?

- **Eye conditions**—do you have or have you ever had any problems with your eyes other than needing glasses or contacts?

- **Medications**—do you take steroids or other drugs that might prevent healing?

- **Stable refraction**—has your prescription changed in the last year?

- **High or Low refractive error**—do you use glasses/contacts only some of the time? Do you need an unusually strong prescription?

- **Pupil size**—are your pupils extra large in dim conditions?

- **Corneal thickness**—do you have thin corneas?

- **Tear production**—do you have dry eyes?

Know All the Risks and Procedure Limitations

- **Overtreatment or undertreatment**—are you willing and able to have more than one surgery to get the desired result?

- **May still need reading glasses**—do you have presbyopia?

- **Results may not be lasting**—do you think this is the last correction you will ever need? Do you realize that long-term results are not known?

- **May permanently lose vision**—do you know some patients may lose some vision or experience blindness?

- **Dry eyes**—do you know that if you have dry eyes they could become worse, or if you don't have dry eyes before you could develop chronic dry eyes as a result of surgery?

- **Development of visual symptoms**—do you know about glare, halos, starbursts, etc., and that night driving might be difficult?

- **Contrast sensitivity**—do you know your vision could be significantly reduced in dim light conditions?

- **Bilateral treatment**—do you know the additional risks of having both eyes treated at the same time?

- **Patient information**—have you read the patient information booklet about the laser being used for your procedure?

Know Preoperative, Operative, and Postoperative Expectations

- **No contact lenses prior to evaluation and surgery**—can you go for an extended period of time without wearing contact lenses?

- **Have a thorough exam**—have you arranged not to drive or work after the exam?

- **Read and understand the informed consent**—has your doctor given you an informed consent form to take home and answered all your questions?

- **No makeup before surgery**—can you go 24–36 hours without makeup prior to surgery?

- **Arrange for transportation**—can someone drive you home after surgery?

- **Plan to take a few days to recover**—can you take time off to take it easy for a couple of days if necessary?

- **Expect not to see clearly for a few days**—do you know you will not see clearly immediately?

- **Know sights, smells, sounds of surgery**—has your doctor made you feel comfortable with the actual steps of the procedure?

- **Be prepared to take drops/medications**—are you willing and able to put drops in your eyes at regular intervals?

- **Be prepared to wear an eye shield**—do you know you need to protect the eye for a period of time after surgery to avoid injury?

- **Expect some pain/discomfort**—do you know how much pain to expect?

- **Know when to seek help**—do you understand what problems could occur and when to seek medical intervention?

- **Know when to expect your vision to stop changing**—are you aware that final results could take months?

- **Make sure your refraction is stable before any further surgery**—if you don't get the desired result, do you know not to have an enhancement until the prescription stops changing?

Section 14.4

What to Expect before, during, and after LASIK Surgery

This section includes text excerpted from "LASIK," U.S. Food and Drug Administration (FDA), October 20, 2015.

What to expect before, during, and after surgery will vary from doctor to doctor and patient to patient. This section is a compilation of patient information developed by manufacturers and healthcare professionals, but cannot replace the dialogue you should have with your doctor.

Before Surgery

If you decide to go ahead with LASIK surgery, you will need an initial or baseline evaluation by your eye doctor to determine if you are a good candidate. This is what you need to know to prepare for the exam and what you should expect:

If you wear contact lenses, it is a good idea to stop wearing them before your baseline evaluation and switch to wearing your glasses full-time. Contact lenses change the shape of your cornea for up to several weeks after you have stopped using them depending on the type of contact lenses you wear. Not leaving your contact lenses out long enough for your cornea to assume its natural shape before surgery can have negative consequences. These consequences include inaccurate measurements and a poor surgical plan, resulting in poor vision after surgery. These measurements, which determine how much corneal tissue to remove, may need to be repeated at least a week after your initial evaluation and before surgery to make sure they have not changed, especially if you wear RGP or hard lenses. If you wear:

- soft contact lenses, you should stop wearing them for 2 weeks before your initial evaluation.

- toric soft lenses or rigid gas permeable (RGP) lenses, you should stop wearing them for at least 3 weeks before your initial evaluation.

- hard lenses, you should stop wearing them for at least 4 weeks before your initial evaluation.

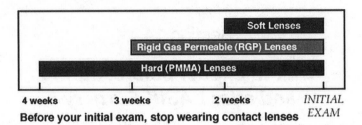

Before your initial exam, stop wearing contact lenses

Figure 14.1. *Before Your Initial Exam, Stop Wearing Contact Lenses*

You should tell your doctor:

- about your past and present medical and eye conditions
- about all the medications you are taking, including over-the-counter medications and any medications you may be allergic to

Your doctor should perform a thorough eye exam and discuss:

- whether you are a good candidate
- what the risks, benefits, and alternatives of the surgery are
- what you should expect before, during, and after surgery
- what your responsibilities will be before, during, and after surgery

You should have the opportunity to ask your doctor questions during this discussion. Give yourself plenty of time to think about the risk/benefit discussion, to review any informational literature provided by your doctor, and to have any additional questions answered by your doctor before deciding to go through with surgery and before signing the informed consent form.

You should not feel pressured by your doctor, family, friends, or anyone else to make a decision about having surgery. Carefully consider the pros and cons.

The day before surgery, you should stop using:

- creams
- lotions
- makeup
- perfumes

These products as well as debris along the eyelashes may increase the risk of infection during and after surgery. Your doctor may ask you to scrub your eyelashes for a period of time before surgery to get rid of residues and debris along the lashes.

Also before surgery, arrange for transportation to and from your surgery and your first follow-up visit. On the day of surgery, your doctor may give you some medicine to make you relax. Because this medicine impairs your ability to drive and because your vision may be blurry, even if you don't drive make sure someone can bring you home after surgery.

During Surgery

The surgery should take less than 30 minutes. You will lie on your back in a reclining chair in an exam room containing the laser system. The laser system includes a large machine with a microscope attached to it and a computer screen.

A numbing drop will be placed in your eye, the area around your eye will be cleaned, and an instrument called a lid speculum will be used to hold your eyelids open.

Your doctor may use a **mechanical microkeratome** (a blade device) to cut a flap in the cornea.

If a mechanical microkeratome is used, a ring will be placed on your eye and very high pressures will be applied to create suction to the cornea. Your vision will dim while the suction ring is on and you may feel the pressure and experience some discomfort during this part of the procedure. The microkeratome, a cutting instrument, is attached to the suction ring. Your doctor will use the blade of the microkeratome to cut a flap in your cornea. Microkeratome blades are meant to be used only once and then thrown out. The microkeratome and the suction ring are then removed.

Your doctor may use a **laser keratome** (a laser device), instead of a mechanical microkeratome, to cut a flap on the cornea.

If a laser keratome is used, the cornea is flattened with a clear plastic plate. Your vision will dim and you may feel the pressure and experience some discomfort during this part of the procedure. Laser energy is focused inside the cornea tissue, creating thousands of small bubbles of gas and water that expand and connect to separate the tissue underneath the cornea surface, creating a flap. The plate is then removed.

You will be able to see, but you will experience fluctuating degrees of blurred vision during the rest of the procedure. The doctor will then lift the flap and fold it back on its hinge, and dry the exposed tissue.

The laser will be positioned over your eye and you will be asked to stare at a light. This is not the laser used to remove tissue from the cornea. This light is to help you keep your eye fixed on one spot once the laser comes on. **NOTE: If you cannot stare at a fixed object for at least 60 seconds, you may not be a good candidate for this surgery.**

When your eye is in the correct position, your doctor will start the laser. At this point in the surgery, you may become aware of new sounds and smells. The pulse of the laser makes a ticking sound. As the laser removes corneal tissue, some people have reported a smell similar to burning hair. A computer controls the amount of laser energy delivered to your eye. Before the start of surgery, your doctor will have programmed the computer to vaporize a particular amount of tissue based on the measurements taken at your initial evaluation. After the pulses of laser energy vaporize the corneal tissue, the flap is put back into position.

A shield should be placed over your eye at the end of the procedure as protection, since no stitches are used to hold the flap in place. It is important for you to wear this shield to prevent you from rubbing your eye and putting pressure on your eye while you sleep, and to protect your eye from accidentally being hit or poked until the flap has healed.

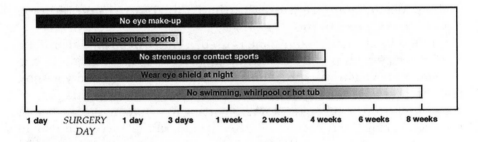

Figure 14.2. *Good Practices to Follow before and after Surgery*

After Surgery

Immediately after the procedure, your eye may burn, itch, or feel like there is something in it. You may experience some discomfort, or in some cases, mild pain and your doctor may suggest you take a mild pain reliever. Both your eyes may tear or water. Your vision will probably be hazy or blurry. You will instinctively want to rub your eye, but don't! Rubbing your eye could dislodge the flap, requiring further treatment. In addition, you may experience sensitivity to light, glare, starbursts or halos around lights, or the whites of your eye may look red or bloodshot. These symptoms should improve considerably within the first few days after surgery. You should plan on taking a few days off from work until these symptoms subside. **You should contact your doctor immediately** and not wait for your scheduled visit, if you experience severe pain, or if your vision or other symptoms get worse instead of better.

You should see your doctor within the **first 24 to 48 hours** after surgery and at regular intervals after that for at least the first six months. At the first postoperative visit, your doctor will remove the eye shield, test your vision, and examine your eye. Your doctor may give you one or more types of eye drops to take at home to help prevent infection and/or inflammation. You may also be advised to use artificial tears to help lubricate the eye. Do not resume wearing a contact lens in the operated eye, even if your vision is blurry.

You should wait **one to three days** following surgery before beginning any non-contact sports, depending on the amount of activity required, how you feel, and your doctor's instructions.

To help prevent infection, you may need to wait for up to **two weeks after surgery or until your doctor advises you otherwise** before using lotions, creams, or makeup around the eye. Your doctor may advise you to continue scrubbing your eyelashes for a period of time after surgery. You should also avoid swimming and using hot tubs or whirlpools for 1–2 months.

Strenuous contact sports such as boxing, football, karate, etc., should not be attempted for **at least four weeks** after surgery. It is important to protect your eyes from anything that might get in them and from being hit or bumped.

During the **first few months** after surgery, your vision may fluctuate.

- It may take up to three to six months for your vision to stabilize after surgery.

- Glare, halos, difficulty driving at night, and other visual symptoms may also persist during this stabilization period. If further correction or enhancement is necessary, you should wait until your eye measurements are consistent for two consecutive visits at least 3 months apart before re-operation.

- It is important to realize that although distance vision may improve after re-operation, it is unlikely that other visual symptoms such as glare or halos will improve.

- It is also important to note that no laser company has presented enough evidence for the U.S. Food and Drug Administration

(FDA) to make conclusions about the safety or effectiveness of enhancement surgery.

Contact your eye doctor immediately, if you develop any new, unusual or worsening symptoms at any point after surgery. Such symptoms could signal a problem that, if not treated early enough, may lead to a loss of vision.

Section 14.5

LASIK FAQs

This section includes text excerpted from "LASIK—FAQs (Frequently Asked Questions)," U.S. Food and Drug Administration (FDA), June 9, 2014.

Q: Can you refer me to a good LASIK surgeon in my area?
A: While U.S. Food and Drug Administration (FDA) regulates medical devices and drugs, FDA does not regulate the practice of medicine and does not have a registry of doctors. FDA does not know of any government agency that can provide a referral for any medical procedure. You may want to go to your library and see if there is a local community services magazine that may provide comparison information of services for doctors in your area.

Q: How do I report a bad experience or who do I notify about a 'bad' doctor?
A: If you had a bad experience or sustained an injury, you should file a voluntary MedWatch report (800-FDA-1088) to the FDA. Also, you could contact your state medical licensing board and file a complaint with them. In addition, you could contact your state health department or consumer complaint organization (e.g., Better Business Bureau).

Q: How much does LASIK cost?
A: The FDA regulates the safety and effectiveness of medical devices for their intended use. The FDA does not regulate the marketing of or any fees associated with the use of that product. Again, you may want to go to your library and see if there is a local community services

magazine that may provide comparison information of services for doctors in your area.

Q: How can I find out if a particular laser has been approved to treat my refractive error (nearsightedness, farsightedness and/or astigmatism)?

A: You can find approved devices, their approval date, and a synopsis of the approved indications on the FDA-Approved Lasers page (www.fda.gov/MedicalDevices/ProductsandMedicalProcedures/SurgeryandLifeSupport/LASIK/ucm192109.htm).

Q: If the laser I am interested in has not yet been approved for a particular indication, how can I find out when it will be approved?

A: Confidentiality restrictions prohibit FDA from commenting on the status of a device under regulatory review, but you can try asking the laser company for this information.

Q: Which laser is the best for treating my refractive error?

A: FDA does not provide comparisons between refractive lasers. FDA approves the safety and effectiveness of a device independent of any other product. However, you are encouraged to review the approval documents to assess the capabilities of specific laser systems and make your own comparisons. Discuss any concerns you may have with your doctor.

Q: How does wavefront LASIK compare to conventional LASIK?

A: Wavefront adds an automatic measurement of more subtle distortions (called higher order aberrations) than just nearsightedness, farsightedness, and astigmatism corrected by conventional LASIK. However, these "higher order aberrations" account for only a small amount (probably no more than 10%) of the total refractive error of the average person's eye. Conventional LASIK increases higher order aberrations. Although wavefront-guided treatments attempt to eliminate higher order aberrations, results from the clinical studies have shown that the average aberrations still increase, but less than they do after conventional LASIK. In a few studies comparing wavefront-guided LASIK to conventional LASIK, a slightly larger percentage of subjects treated with wavefront LASIK achieved 20/20 vision without glasses or contact lenses compared to subjects treated with conventional LASIK. Patient selection and the experience and competence of the surgeon are still the most important considerations.

Q: What is "All-Laser LASIK" and how does it compare to traditional LASIK surgery?

A: The difference between traditional LASIK and "All-Laser LASIK" (also known as "Bladeless LASIK") is the method by which the LASIK flap is created. In "All-Laser LASIK," a laser device called a laser keratome, is used to cut a corneal flap for LASIK surgery. This is a newer method to create a corneal flap than the traditional method of using a microkeratome, a mechanical device with a blade. There is no absolute agreement among eye surgeons on the better choice for flap creation. Some of the factors a surgeon considers when choosing a preferred method of flap creation during LASIK are as follows:

- quality of vision

- rate of complications

- pain during and after surgery

- precision of flap size and thickness

- time to recovery of vision

- expense

Discuss with your doctor any questions and concerns you have about how they chose their preferred method of flap creation.

Chapter 15

Photorefractive Keratectomy (PRK) Eye Surgery

Photorefractive keratectomy (PRK) is a type of vision correction eye surgery in which a laser is used to reshape the cornea. The cornea is a clear layer in the front of the eye that helps to focus light images on the retina at the back of the eye. Errors in the way the cornea bends or refracts light through the eye create vision problems. PRK can be used to permanently correct refractive errors that cause nearsightedness (myopia), farsightedness (hyperopia), and astigmatism (irregularities in the shape of the eye).

In comparison to laser-assisted in situ keratomileusis (LASIK)—the most popular type of laser eye surgery—PRK is less invasive because the excimer laser is used on the surface of the cornea rather than deep within the cornea. Both types of surgery are highly effective in correcting mild to moderate vision problems, although PRK generally requires a longer recovery time. PRK is often used for people who are ineligible for LASIK or whose corneas were previously treated with LASIK.

What to Expect

Before PRK Surgery

Before having PRK surgery, a patient must undergo a comprehensive eye examination to evaluate whether they are a suitable

---

"Photorefractive Keratectomy (PRK) Eye Surgery," © 2017 Omnigraphics. Reviewed March 2017.

candidate for the procedure. The eye surgeon will ask questions about the patient's overall health, whether they have any medical conditions such as diabetes or arthritis, and what medications they are taking. The eye surgeon will also measure the thickness of the cornea, determine the amount of refractive error to be corrected in each eye, and use imaging technology to create a corneal map showing the precise curvature of the surface of each eye. Since contact lenses can affect the shape of the cornea, patients who wear rigid, gas permeable contact lenses may need to stop wearing them about three weeks before the initial eye examination, while those who wear soft contact lenses should avoid wearing them for three days before the initial visit.

Preparing for PRK Surgery

The PRK procedure is performed under local anesthesia, so patients are allowed to eat a light meal beforehand and take any prescribed medications. Patients should avoid wearing eye makeup and any hats or hair accessories that could interfere with the position of their head under the laser. The eyes are prepared for surgery by applying a topical anesthetic in the form of eye drops to numb the surface. A device called a lid speculum will be used to prevent the eyelids from closing during the procedure. The patient may also receive an oral sedative to promote relaxation.

During PRK Surgery

The PRK procedure itself only takes 10 to 15 minutes to treat both eyes. As the patient stares straight ahead, the surgeon begins by using an alcohol solution or a surgical instrument to carefully remove a layer of surface cells known as epithelium from the cornea. Next, the surgeon uses a computer-controlled excimer laser to direct pulses of ultraviolet light on the cornea. The laser energy removes microscopic amounts of tissue in a precise pattern to reshape the cornea to the specifications of the patient's prescription. In most cases the procedure is completely painless, although some patients experience a feeling of pressure. Most patients elect to have both eyes treated on the same day, one immediately after the other, while some decide to have the second eye treated a few weeks after the first.

After PRK Surgery

Once the surgery is completed, the surgeon will place a bandage contact lens over the treated cornea to protect it while the epithelial cells grow back. The surgeon will also prescribe topical antibiotics, anti-inflammatory medications, and eye lubrication drops to reduce swelling and minimize discomfort. The patient can go home the same day with an escort to drive them, although they must return for several follow-up appointments over the next few weeks so the surgeon can monitor the healing process. The bandage contact lens is typically removed after 4 to 6 days.

Recovery from PRK Surgery

Recovery from PRK can take a few weeks. Most patients experience some discomfort, irritation, and sensitivity to light for the first few days. Many patients find that their vision is blurry at first but gradually improves enough to drive a car within 1 to 3 weeks. It can take up to 6 months, however, for the patient's eyesight to be completely clear and stable. Around 90 percent of patients who undergo PRK have 20/20 vision without glasses or contact lenses one year after the surgery.

Long-Term Results and Possible Complications

PRK laser eye surgery has been performed millions of times around the world since the 1980s, and it is considered safe and effective. Nearly all patients who undergo PRK experience significant improvements in the clarity of their vision. Although serious side effects and complications are rare, patients should be aware of the potential for the following:

- glare, starbursts, or halos around lights at night;

- abnormal corneal healing resulting in the formation of opaque cells that cause hazy vision;

- regression or partial loss of treatment effect in patients who have PRK to correct large amounts of farsightedness or astigmatism.

In addition, most patients who have PRK surgery still require reading glasses with magnification to correct presbyopia (age-related loss of near vision) once they reach middle age. Some patients opt for a process called monovision, in which one eye is corrected for distance vision and the other is corrected for near vision, whether through contact lenses or laser surgery.

Advantages and Disadvantages

PRK is often compared to LASIK, the most popular form of laser eye surgery used to correct nearsightedness, farsightedness, and astigmatism. The two procedures use the same modern laser technologies and offer the same long-term results. The main difference between PRK and LASIK involves how much of the cornea is disturbed. In PRK procedures, only the epithelial layer or "skin" of the cornea is removed. This thin outer surface of the cornea grows back within a few days after the surgery, although patients may experience some discomfort and blurry vision during this time.

In LASIK procedures, the surgeon makes an incision with a microkeratome or a femtosecond laser to create a thin flap on the cornea. This flap is lifted so the underlying corneal tissue can be reshaped with an excimer laser. Although the flap is replaced at the end of the procedure, it can remain vulnerable to tearing or injury. The main reason LASIK is more popular is that patients experience little to no discomfort and achieve clear vision almost immediately.

PRK is often recommended for patients whose corneas are too thin for LASIK, or who have irregularities in the surface of their corneas that might complicate LASIK. In addition, PRK is often performed on patients who have already undergone LASIK but require additional correction to achieve clear vision.

References

1. Kozarsky, Alan. "Photorefractive Keratectomy Eye Surgery," WebMD, November 25, 2015.

2. "Photorefractive Keratectomy (PRK) Eye Surgery," Cleveland Clinic, 2015.

3. Wachler, Brian Boxer. "PRK Laser Eye Surgery," All About Vision, September 2016.

Chapter 16

Laser Epithelial Keratomileusis (LASEK) Surgery

Laser epithelial keratomileusis (LASEK) is a type of vision correction eye surgery in which a laser is used to reshape the cornea. LASEK can be used to permanently correct vision problems like nearsightedness (myopia), farsightedness (hyperopia), and astigmatism (irregularities in the shape of the eye). LASEK is a variation of two other laser eye surgery procedures, photorefractive keratectomy (PRK) and laser-assisted in situ keratomileusis (LASIK). The main difference between the procedures involves the way in which the eye is prepared for the laser treatment:

- In PRK procedures, the eye surgeon removes and discards a very thin layer of epithelial cells from the surface of the cornea. This "skin" layer of the cornea regenerates within a few days after the surgery, but the healing process creates discomfort and occasionally results in hazy vision.

- In LASIK procedures, the eye surgeon creates a thicker, circular flap of corneal tissue, performs the laser treatment underneath it, and then replaces it. Although this process allows for minimal discomfort and a shorter recovery time than PRK, it can result in dry eyes, and the flap may be vulnerable to traumatic injury.

- LASEK procedures resemble PRK procedures because the eye surgeon removes a very thin surface layer of cells from the cornea. Rather than discarding the epithelium, however, the surgeon replaces the flap following the laser treatment, as in LASIK procedures. LASEK is intended to reduce the discomfort and risk of corneal haze associated with PRK, as well as to avoid potential problems related to the thicker flap created in LASIK.

LASEK, PRK, and LASIK all offer similar success rates and long-term vision outcomes. LASIK is the most popular type of laser eye surgery because it allows for minimal discomfort and provides clear vision almost immediately. Still, LASEK may be a good option for patients who are not good candidates for LASIK because they have thin corneas, or for patients who have already undergone LASIK but require additional correction to achieve clear vision. LASEK may be preferable to PRK for patients who have refractive errors greater than 6.00 diopters because it reduces the risk of corneal haze. A qualified eye surgeon can provide individualized advice about the best type of laser eye surgery for a patient's circumstances.

What to Expect

Before LASEK Surgery

Before having LASEK surgery, a patient must undergo a comprehensive eye examination to evaluate whether they are a suitable candidate for the procedure. The eye surgeon will ask questions about the patient's overall health, whether they have any medical conditions such as diabetes or arthritis, and what medications they are taking. The eye surgeon will also measure the thickness of the cornea, determine the amount of refractive error to be corrected in each eye, and use imaging technology to create a corneal map showing the precise curvature of the surface of each eye. Since contact lenses can affect the shape of the cornea, patients who wear rigid, gas permeable contact lenses may need to stop wearing them about three weeks before the initial eye examination, while those who wear soft contact lenses should avoid wearing them for three days before the initial visit.

Preparing for LASEK Surgery

The LASEK procedure is performed under local anesthesia, so patients are allowed to eat a light meal beforehand and take any prescribed medications. Patients should avoid wearing eye makeup and any hats or hair accessories that could interfere with the position of their head under the laser. The eyes are prepared for surgery by applying a topical anesthetic in the form of eye drops to numb the surface. A device called a lid speculum will be used to prevent the eyelids from closing during the procedure. The patient may also receive an oral sedative to promote relaxation.

During LASEK Surgery

During the LASEK procedure, the eye surgeon uses a fine blade called a trephine to make a circular incision in the epithelium. Next, the surgeon places a diluted alcohol solution over the eye to loosen the edges of the epithelium flap so it can be moved gently to the side. The corneal tissue underneath the flap is then reshaped with an excimer laser to the patient's exact prescription. Following the laser treatment, the top layer of cells is returned to its original position on the eye, and a special contact lens bandage is put in place to protect the wound. In some cases, the thin flap of "skin" is too fragile and cannot be replaced on the eye. When the epithelial layer must be removed, the surgery technically becomes a PRK procedure rather than a LASEK procedure.

After LASEK Surgery

The main advantage of preserving the top layer of cells is that the patient experiences less discomfort following LASEK surgery than PRK surgery. However, the recovery process is similar for the two procedures, and slower than for a LASIK procedure. The patient wears the protective contact lens bandage for 4 to 6 days while the epithelium heals. The surgeon will also prescribe topical antibiotics, anti-inflammatory medications, and eye lubrication drops to reduce swelling and minimize discomfort. The patient can go home the same day with an escort to drive them, although they must return for several follow-up appointments over the next few weeks so the surgeon can monitor the healing process.

Recovery from LASEK Surgery

Patients who undergo LASEK surgery usually regain clear vision within a week, although it may take several weeks for the eyesight to stabilize. Around 90 percent of patients who undergo LASEK have 20/20 vision without glasses or contact lenses one year after the surgery.

Long-Term Results and Possible Complications

LASEK laser eye surgery is considered safe and effective. Nearly all patients who undergo LASEK experience significant improvements in the clarity of their vision. Although serious side effects and complications are rare, patients should be aware of the potential for the following:

- blurry vision, glare, or halos around lights at night;
- eye infection;
- dry eyes;
- regression or partial loss of treatment effect.

In addition, most patients who have LASEK surgery still require reading glasses with magnification to correct presbyopia (age-related loss of near vision) once they reach middle age. Some patients opt for a process called monovision, in which one eye is corrected for distance vision and the other is corrected for near vision, whether through contact lenses or laser surgery.

Advantages and Disadvantages

Although LASEK is considered a safe and effective alternative to LASIK or PRK, it is mainly used in patients who are not good candidates for the other procedures. LASEK is preferable to LASIK for people with thin corneas, dry eyes, or jobs and hobbies that put them at high risk of injury to the corneal flap. Many people opt for LASIK, however, because it offers minimal discomfort and a quick visual recovery.

LASEK is comparable to PRK in terms of visual recovery. Whereas eye surgeons once believed that replacing the epithelial level would lead to quicker healing, in practice it takes the cornea less time to regrow a new layer of "skin." As a result, PRK is more popular than LASEK except for people with very strong prescriptions who face a higher risk of corneal hazing from PRK.

References

1. Hagele, Glenn. "LASEK—Laser Assisted Sub-Epithelial Keratomileusis," USA Eyes, 2013.

2. "LASEK Eye Surgery," WebMD, 2016.

3. Wachler, Brian Boxer. "LASEK Eye Surgery: How It Works," All About Vision, April 2016.

Chapter 17

Phakic Intraocular Lenses

Chapter Contents

Section 17.1

Phakic Lenses Basics

This section includes text excerpted from "Phakic Intraocular
Lenses: What Are Phakic Lenses?" U.S. Food and Drug
Administration (FDA), October 20, 2015.

Phakic intraocular lenses, or phakic lenses, are lenses made of plastic or silicone that are implanted into the eye permanently to reduce a person's need for glasses or contact lenses. Phakic refers to the fact that the lens is implanted into the eye without removing the eye's natural lens. During phakic lens implantation surgery, a small incision is made in the front of the eye. The phakic lens is inserted through the incision and placed just in front of or just behind the iris.

What Do They Treat?

Phakic lenses are used to correct refractive errors, errors in the eye's focusing power. All phakic lenses approved by the U.S. Food and Drug Administration (FDA) are for the correction of nearsightedness (myopia).

The cornea and natural lens of the eye focus light to create an image on the retina, much like the way the lens of a camera focuses light to create an image on film. The bending and focusing of light is also known as refraction. Imperfections in the focusing power of the eye, called refractive errors, cause images on the retina to be out of focus or blurred.

People who are nearsighted have more difficulty seeing distant objects than near objects. For these people, the images of distant objects come to focus in front of the retina instead of on the retina.

Ideally, phakic lenses cause light entering the eye to be focused on the retina providing clear distance vision without the aid of glasses or contact lenses.

Surgery is not required to correct nearsightedness. You can wear glasses or contact lenses instead to correct your vision. Depending on how nearsighted you are, and other conditions of your eye, other refractive surgery (surgery to correct refractive errors) options may be available to you, including PRK (Photorefractive Keratectomy) and LASIK (Laser Assisted In-Situ Keratomileusis).

Can They Be Removed?

Phakic lenses are intended to be permanent. While the lenses can be surgically removed, return to your previous level of vision or condition of your eye cannot be guaranteed.

What Is the Difference between Phakic Intraocular Lenses and Intraocular Lenses Following Cataract Surgery?

Phakic intraocular lenses are implanted in the eye without removing the natural lens. This is in contrast to intraocular lenses that are implanted into eyes after the eye's cloudy natural lens (cataract) has been removed during cataract surgery.

Section 17.2

Are Phakic Lenses for You?

This section includes text excerpted from "Phakic Intraocular Lenses: Are Phakic Lenses for You?" U.S. Food and Drug Administration (FDA), June 12, 2014.

You are probably NOT a good candidate for phakic lenses if:

- **You are not an adult.** There are no phakic lenses approved by the U.S. Food and Drug Administration (FDA) for persons under the age of 21.

- **You are not a risk taker.** Certain complications are unavoidable in a percentage of patients, and there are no long-term data available for phakic lenses.

- **You required a change in your contact lens or glasses prescription in the last 6 to 12 months in order to obtain the best possible vision for you.** This is called refractive instability. Patients who are:

  - in their early 20s or younger,

- whose hormones are fluctuating due to disease such as diabetes,

- who are pregnant or breastfeeding, or

- who are taking medications that may cause fluctuations in vision,

are more likely to have refractive instability and should discuss the possible additional risks with their doctor.

- **You may jeopardize your career.** Some jobs prohibit certain refractive procedures. Be sure to check with your employer/ professional society/military service before undergoing any procedure.

- **Cost is an issue.** Most medical insurance will not pay for refractive surgery.

- **You have a disease or are on medications that may affect wound healing.** Certain conditions, such as autoimmune diseases (e.g., lupus, rheumatoid arthritis), immunodeficiency states (e.g., human immunodeficiency virus (HIV)) and diabetes, and some medications (e.g., retinoic acid and steroids) may prevent proper healing after intraocular surgery.

- **You have a low endothelial cell count or abnormal endothelial cells.** If the cells that pump the fluid out of your cornea, the endothelial cells, are low in number relative to your age, or if your endothelial cells are abnormal, you have a higher risk of developing a cloudy cornea and requiring a corneal transplant.

- **You actively participate in sports with a high risk of eye trauma.** Your eye may be more susceptible to damage should you receive a blow to the face or eye, such as a blow to the head during boxing or hit in the eye by a ball during baseball. Your eye may be more susceptible to rupture or retinal detachment, and the phakic lens may dislocate.

- **You only have one eye with potentially good vision.** If you only have one eye with good vision with glasses or contact lenses, due to disease, irreparable damage, or amblyopia (eye with poor vision since childhood that cannot be corrected with glasses or contact lenses), you and your doctor should consider the risk of possible damage and/or loss of vision to your better eye as a result phakic lens implantation.

- **You have large pupils.** If your pupil dilates in low lighting conditions to a size that is larger than the size of the lens, you have a higher risk of experiencing visual disturbances after surgery that may affect your ability to function comfortably or normally under such conditions (e.g., while driving at night).

- **You have a shallow anterior chamber.** If the space between the cornea and the iris, the anterior chamber, is narrow, you have a higher risk of developing complications, such as greater endothelial cell loss, due to implantation of the phakic lens.

- **You have an abnormal iris.** If your pupil is irregularly shaped you have a higher risk of developing visual disturbances.

- **You have had uveitis.** If you have had inflammation in your eye, you may have a recurrence or worsening of your disease and/or may develop additional complications, such as glaucoma, as a result of surgery.

- **You have had problems with the posterior part of your eye.** If you have had any problems in the back part of your eye or are at risk for such problems, for example, proliferative diabetic retinopathy (growth of abnormal vessels in the back of the eye due to diabetes) or retinal detachment, you may not be a good candidate for phakic lens implantation. The phakic lens may not allow your eye doctor to get a clear view of the back part of your eye, preventing or delaying detection of a new or worsening problem, and/or the phakic lens may prevent or make treatment of a problem in the back of your eye more difficult.

The safety and effectiveness of phakic lenses have NOT been studied in patients with certain conditions. If any of the following apply to you, make sure you discuss them with your doctor:

- **You have glaucoma** (damage to the nerve of the eye resulting in loss of peripheral and then central vision due to too high pressure inside the eye), **ocular hypertension** (high eye pressure), or **glaucoma suspect** (some indications, but not clear, that patient has glaucoma). You may have a higher risk of developing or worsening of glaucoma as a result of phakic lens implantation.

- You have **pseudoexfoliation syndrome** (abnormal deposits of material in the eye visible on the structures in the front part of the eye, such as on the front of the natural lens and the back of the cornea). This syndrome is associated with glaucoma and weakness of the structures holding the natural lens in place (the zonules). You may have a higher risk of surgical complications and/or complications after surgery if you have this syndrome.

- **You have had an eye injury or previous eye surgery.**

- **Your need for visual correction is outside the range for which the phakic lens has been approved.** Ask your eye doctor if the phakic lens that he or she recommends for you has been approved to treat your refractive error and/or check FDA-approved Phakic Lenses for the approved refractive range.

- **You are over the age of 45 years old.** Some phakic lenses have not been studied in patients over the age of 45.

Section 17.3

The Risks of Phakic Lenses

This section includes text excerpted from "Phakic Intraocular Lenses: What Are the Risks?" U.S. Food and Drug Administration (FDA), June 12, 2014.

Implanting a phakic lens involves a surgical procedure. As in any other medical procedure, there are risks involved. That's why it is important for you to understand the limitations and risks of phakic intraocular lens implant surgery.

Before undergoing surgery for implantation of a phakic intraocular lens, you should carefully weigh the risks and benefits and try to avoid being influenced by other people encouraging you to do it.

Risks

- **You may lose vision.** Some patients lose vision as a result of phakic lens implant surgery that cannot be corrected with glasses, contact lenses, or another surgery. The amount of vision loss may be severe.

- **You may develop debilitating visual symptoms.** Some patients develop glare, halos, double vision, and/or decreased vision in situations of low level lighting that can cause difficulty with performing tasks, such as driving, particularly at night or under foggy conditions.

- **You may need additional eye surgery to reposition, replace or remove the phakic lens implant.** These surgeries may be necessary for your safety or to improve your visual function. If the lens power is not right, then a phakic lens exchange may be needed. You may also have to have the lens repositioned, removed, or replaced, if the lens does not stay in the right place, is not the right size, and/or causes debilitating visual symptoms. Every additional surgical procedure has its own risks.

- **You may be undertreated or overtreated.** Many treated patients do not achieve 20/20 vision after surgery. The power of the implanted phakic lens may be too strong or too weak. This is because of the difficulties with determining exactly what power lens you need. This means that you will probably still need glasses or contact lenses to perform at least some tasks. For example, you may need glasses for reading, even if you did not need them before surgery. This also means that you may need a second surgery to replace the lens with another, if the power of the originally implanted lens was too far from what you needed.

- **You may develop increased intraocular pressure.** You may experience increased pressure inside the eye after surgery, which may require surgery or medication to control. You may need long-term treatment with glaucoma medications. If the pressure is too high for too long, you may lose vision.

- **Your cornea may become cloudy.** The endothelial cells of your cornea are a thin layer of cells responsible for pumping fluid out of the cornea to keep it clear. If the endothelial cells become too few in number, the endothelial cell pump will fail and the cornea will become cloudy, resulting in loss of vision. You start with a certain number of cells at birth, and this number continuously decreases as you age, since these cells are not replenished. Normally, you die from old age before the number of endothelial cells becomes so low that your cornea becomes cloudy. Some lens designs have shown that their implantation causes endothelial cells to be lost at a faster rate than normal. If the number of endothelial cells drops too low and your cornea becomes cloudy, you will lose vision and you may require a corneal transplant in order to see more clearly.

- **You may develop a cataract.** You may get a cataract, clouding of the natural lens. The amount of time for a cataract to develop can vary greatly. If your cataract develops and progresses enough to significantly decrease your vision, you may require cataract surgery your doctor will have to remove both your natural and your phakic lenses.

- **You may develop a retinal detachment.** The retina is the tissue that lines the inside of the back of your eyeball. It contains the light-sensing cells that collect and send images to your brain, much like the film in a camera. The risk of the retina becoming detached from the back of your eye increases after intraocular surgery. It is not known at this time by how much your risk of retinal detachment will increase as a result of phakic intraocular lens implantation surgery.

- **You may experience infection, bleeding, or severe inflammation (pain, redness, and decreased vision).** These are rare complications that can sometimes lead to permanent loss of vision or loss of the eye.

- **Long-term data are not available.** Phakic lenses are a new technology and have only recently been approved by the U.S. Food and Drug Administration (FDA). Therefore, there may be other risks to having phakic lenses implanted that we don't yet know about.

Section 17.4

Phakic Lens Implantation Surgery— What to Expect

This section includes text excerpted from "Phakic Intraocular Lenses: Before, during, and after Surgery," U.S. Food and Drug Administration (FDA), October 20, 2015.

This section gives you a general idea of what you might expect if you decide to have phakic intraocular lens implantation surgery. What to expect before, during and after surgery will vary according to:

- the type of phakic lens implanted

- the practices of the medical facility where the surgery will be performed and of the doctor who will be providing your care

- your unique health circumstances and body's response

The information provided here may not apply to your particular situation and should not replace an in-depth discussion with your doctor.

What Should I Expect before Surgery?

Initial Visit

Before deciding to have phakic intraocular lens implantation surgery, you will need an initial examination to make sure your eye is healthy and suitable for surgery. Your doctor will take a complete history about your medical and eye health and perform a thorough examination of both eyes, which will include measurements of your pupils, anterior chamber depth (the distance between your cornea and iris), and endothelial cell counts (the number of cells on the back of your cornea).

If you wear contact lenses, your doctor may ask you to stop wearing them before your initial examination (from the day of to a few weeks before), so that your refraction (measure of how much your eye bends light) and central keratometry readings (measure of how much the cornea curves) are more accurate.

At this time, **you should tell your doctor** if you:

- take any medications, including over-the-counter medications, vitamins and other supplements

- have any allergies

- have had any eye conditions

- have undergone any previous eye surgery

- have had any medical conditions.

Deciding to Have Surgery

To help you decide whether phakic lenses are right for you, talk to your doctor about your expectations and whether there are elements of your medical history, eye history, or eye examination that might increase your risk or prevent you from having the outcome you expect. Before you sign an informed consent document (a form giving permission to your doctor to operate on your eye), you should discuss with your doctor:

- whether you are a good candidate,

- what are the risks, benefits and alternatives of the surgery,

- what you should expect before, during and after surgery, and

- what your responsibilities will be before, during and after surgery.

You should have the opportunity to ask your doctor questions during this discussion. Ask your doctor for the Patient Labeling of the lens that he or she recommends for you. Give yourself plenty of time to think about the risk/benefit discussion, to review any informational literature provided by your doctor, and to have any additional questions answered by your doctor before deciding to go through with surgery and before signing the informed consent document. You should not feel pressured by anyone to make a decision about having surgery. Carefully consider the pros and cons.

Preparing for Surgery

Within Weeks of Surgery

About one to two weeks before surgery, your eye doctor may schedule you for a **laser iridotomy** to prepare your eye for implantation of the phakic lens. Before the procedure, your eye doctor may put drops in your eye to make the pupil small and to numb the eye. While you are seated, you doctor will rest a large lens on your eye. He or she will then make a small hole (or holes) in the extreme outer edge of the iris (the colored part of your eye) with a laser. This hole (holes) are to prevent fluid buildup and pressure in the back chamber of your eye after phakic lens implantation surgery. This procedure is usually performed in an office or clinic setting, not in an operating room, and usually only takes a few minutes.

After the iridotomy procedure, the doctor may have you wait around awhile before checking your eye pressure and letting you go home. The procedure should not prevent you from driving home, but you should check with your eye doctor when you schedule your appointment. You will be given a prescription for steroid drops to put in your eye at home for several days to reduce inflammation from the iridotomy procedure. It is important that you follow all instructions your doctor gives you after the iridotomy procedure.

Possible complications of laser iridotomy include:

- iritis (inflammation in the front part of the eye)

- increase in eye pressure (usually within 1 to 4 hours after the procedure)

- cataract (clouding of the natural lens) from the laser

- hyphema (bleeding into the anterior chamber of the eye, behind the cornea and in front of the iris, that can cause high pressure inside the eye)

- injury to the cornea from the laser that can result in clouding of the cornea

- incomplete opening of the hole all the way through the iris

- closure of the new opening

- rarely, retinal burns

Your doctor may ask you to **stop wearing contact lenses** before your surgery (anywhere from the day of the surgery to a few weeks before).

Before your surgery, your eye doctor may ask you to **temporarily stop taking certain medications that increase the risk of bleeding during surgery**. How long before surgery you may need to stop these medications depends upon which medications you are using and the conditions they are treating. You and your eye doctor may need to discuss stopping certain medications with the doctor who prescribed them, since you may need some of these medications to prevent life-threatening events. For example, you may need medications that stop blood clotting to keep from having a stroke.

Within Days of Surgery

Your doctor may give you prescriptions for antibiotic drops to prevent infection and/or anti-inflammatory drops to prevent inflammation to put in your eye for a few days **before surgery**.

Arrange for transportation to and from surgery and to your follow-up doctor's appointment the day after surgery, since you will be unable to drive. Your doctor will let you know when it is safe for you to drive again.

Your eye doctor will probably tell you **not to eat or drink anything** after midnight the night **before your surgery**.

What Should I Expect during Surgery?

The Day of Surgery

Just before surgery, drops will be put in your eye. You will have to lie down for the surgery and remain still. If you cannot lie down flat on your back, you may not be a good candidate for this surgery. Usually, patients are not put to sleep for this type of surgery, but you may be given a sedative or other medication to make you relax and an IV may be started. Your doctor may inject medication around the eye to numb the eye. The doctor also may give you an injection around the eye to also prevent you from being able to move your eye or see out of your eye. You will have to ask your doctor to find out exactly which of these types of anesthesia will be used in your case. Your eye and the surrounding area will be cleaned and an instrument called a lid speculum will be used to hold your eyelids open.

The doctor will make an incision in your cornea, sclera (the white part of your eye), or limbus (where the cornea meets the sclera). He or she will place a lubricant into your eye to help protect the back of the cornea (the endothelial cells) during the insertion of the phakic lens. The doctor will insert the phakic lens through the incision in the eye into the anterior chamber, behind the cornea and in front of the iris. Depending upon the type of phakic lens, the doctor will either attach the lens to the front of the iris in the anterior chamber of the eye or move it through the pupil into position behind the iris and in front of the lens in the posterior chamber of the eye. The doctor will remove the lubricant and may close the incision with tiny stitches, depending upon the type of incision. Your doctor will place some eye drops or ointment in your eye and cover your eye with a patch and/or a shield. The surgery will probably take around 30 minutes.

After the surgery is over, you may be brought to a recovery room for a couple of hours before you will be allowed to go home. You will be given prescriptions for antibiotic and anti-inflammatory drops to use at home as directed. You will be given an Implant Identification Card, which you should keep as a permanent record of the lens that was implanted in your eye. Make sure you show this card to anyone who takes care of your eyes in the future. You will be asked to go home and take it easy for the rest of the day.

What Should I Expect after Surgery?

Immediately after Surgery

After the surgical procedure, you may be sensitive to light and have a feeling that something is in your eye. You may experience minor discomfort after the procedure. Your doctor may prescribe pain medication to make you more comfortable during the first few days after the surgery. **You should contact your eye doctor immediately if you have severe pain.**

You should see your eye doctor the day after surgery. Your doctor will remove the patch and/or shield and will check your vision and the condition of your eye. Your doctor will instruct you on how to use the eye drops that you were prescribed for **after the surgery**. You will need to take these drops for up to a few weeks after surgery to decrease inflammation and help prevent infection. Your doctor may instruct you to continue wearing the shield all day and all night or just at night. You should wear the shield until your doctor tells you that you no longer have to do so. The shield is meant to prevent you from rubbing your eye or putting pressure on your eye while you sleep and to protect your eye from accidentally being hit or poked while it is healing.

As You Recover

Your vision will probably be somewhat hazy or blurry for the first several days after surgery. Your vision should start to improve after the first several days, but may continue to fluctuate for the next several weeks. It usually takes about 2 to 4 weeks for the vision to stabilize. Do NOT rub your eyes, especially for the first 3 to 5 days. You may also experience sensitivity to light, glare, starbursts or halos around lights, or the whites of your eye may look red or bloodshot. These symptoms should decrease as your eye recovers over the next several weeks.

You should contact your doctor immediately if you develop severe pain or if your vision or other symptoms get worse instead of better. Follow all postoperative instructions given to you by your surgeon and surgical center.

Remember to:

- Wash your hands before putting drops in your eye.

- Use the prescribed medications to help minimize the risk of infection and inflammation. Serious infection or inflammation can result in loss of vision.

- Try not to get water in your eyes until your doctor says it is okay to do so.

- Try not to bend from the waist to pick up objects on the floor, as this can cause undue pressure to your eyes. Do not lift any heavy objects.

- Do not engage in any strenuous activity until your doctor says it is okay to do so. It will take about 8 weeks for your eye to heal.

Long-Term

Your doctor will instruct you to return for additional follow-up visits to monitor your progress. Initially, these visits will be closer together (a few days to a few weeks apart) and then they will be spread out (several weeks to several months apart). It is important to go to all these appointments, even if you think you are doing well, so that the doctor can check for complications that you may not be aware of.

Because you will have a permanent implant in your eye with long-term risks, and especially since all these risks are not known at this time, **you will need to be followed by an eye doctor on a regular basis for the rest of your life. Endothelial cell counts will have to be performed on a regular basis. You and/or your doctor should maintain records of these measurements, so as to be able to estimate the rate of cell loss.** It is especially important for you to have your endothelial cells counted before you and your eye doctor consider any other intraocular procedures, such as cataract surgery, that will decrease the endothelial cell count even further.

Annual eye exams are usually recommended. However, if you have any problems with your vision or your eyes, such as flashing lights, floating spots, or blank spots in your vision (symptoms of a retinal detachment), you should see an eye doctor right away and inform him or her that you have a phakic lens implant. When participating in sports or other activities during which you might injure your eye, like home improvement work, always wear protective eyewear, such as safety goggles.

Part Three

Understanding and Treating Disorders of the Cornea, Conjunctiva, Sclera, Iris, and Pupil

Chapter 18

The Cornea and Corneal Disease: An Overview

What Is the Cornea?

The cornea is the eye's outermost layer. It is the clear, dome-shaped surface that covers the front of the eye. It plays an important role in focusing your vision.

What Are the Parts of the Cornea?

Although the cornea may look clear and seem to lack substance, it is a highly organized tissue. Unlike most tissues in the body, the cornea contains no blood vessels to nourish or protect it against infection. Instead, the cornea receives its nourishment from tears and the aqueous humor (a fluid in the front part of the eye that lies behind the cornea).

The tissues of the cornea are arranged in three basic layers, with two thinner layers, or membranes, between them. Each of these five layers has an important function. These layers are:

This chapter includes text excerpted from "Facts about the Cornea and Corneal Disease," National Eye Institute (NEI), May 2016.

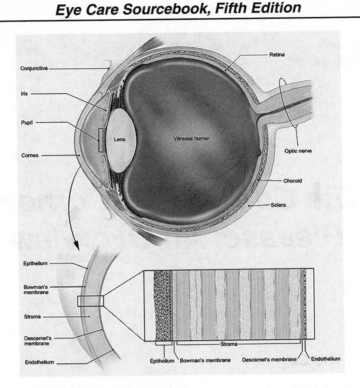

Figure 18.1. *Structures of the Eye*

Epithelium

The epithelium is the cornea's outermost layer. Its primary functions are to:

- block the passage into the eye of foreign material, such as dust, water, and bacteria; and

- provide a smooth surface to absorb oxygen and nutrients from tears, which are then distributed to the other layers of the cornea.

The epithelium is filled with thousands of tiny nerve endings, which is why your eye may hurt when it is rubbed or scratched. The part of the epithelium that epithelial cells anchor and organize themselves to is called the basement membrane.

Bowman Membrane

The next layer behind the basement membrane of the epithelium is a transparent film of tissue called Bowman layer, composed of protein fibers called collagen. If injured, Bowman layer can form a scar as it heals. If these scars are large and centrally located, they may cause vision loss.

Stroma

Behind Bowman layer is the stroma, which is the thickest layer of the cornea. It is composed primarily of water and collagen. Collagen gives the cornea its strength, elasticity, and form. The unique shape, arrangement, and spacing of collagen proteins are essential in producing the cornea's light-conducting transparency.

Descemet Membrane

Behind the stroma is Descemet membrane, a thin but strong film of tissue that serves as a protective barrier against infection and injuries. Descemet membrane is composed of collagen fibers that are different from those of the stroma, and are made by cells in the endothelial layer of the cornea. Descemet membrane repairs itself easily after injury.

Endothelium

The endothelium is the thin, innermost layer of the cornea. Endothelial cells are important in keeping the cornea clear. Normally, fluid leaks slowly from inside the eye into the stroma. The endothelium's primary task is to pump this excess fluid out of the stroma. Without this pumping action, the stroma would swell with water and become thick and opaque.

In a healthy eye, a perfect balance is maintained between the fluid moving into the cornea and the fluid pumping out of the cornea. Unlike the cells in Descemet membrane, endothelial cells that have been destroyed by disease or trauma are not repaired or replaced by the body.

Why Are Tears Important to the Cornea?

Every time we blink, tears are distributed across the cornea to keep the eye moist, help wounds heal, and protect against infection. Tears form in three layers:

- An outer, oily (lipid) layer that keeps tears from evaporating too quickly and helps tears remain on the eye;

- A middle (aqueous) layer that nourishes the cornea and the conjunctiva—the mucous membrane that covers the front of the eye and the inside of the eyelids;

- A bottom (mucin) layer that helps spread the aqueous layer across the eye to ensure that the eye remains wet.

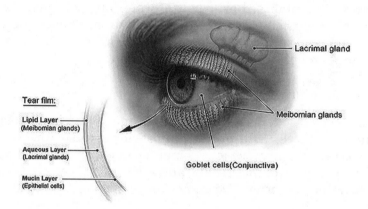

Tear film:

Lipid Layer
(Meibomian glands)

Aqueous Layer
(Lacrimal glands)

Mucin Layer
(Epithelial cells)

Lacrimal gland

Meibomian glands

Goblet cells(Conjunctiva)

Figure 18.2. *Structures Involved in Tear Production*

What Does the Cornea Do?

The cornea acts as a barrier against dirt, germs, and other particles that can harm the eye. The cornea shares this protective task with the eyelids and eye sockets, tears, and the sclera (white part of the eye). The cornea also plays a key role in vision by helping focus the light that comes into the eye. The cornea is responsible for 65–75 percent of the eye's total focusing power.

The cornea and lens of the eye are built to focus light on the retina, which is the light-sensitive tissue at the back of the eye. When light strikes the cornea, it bends—or refracts—the incoming light onto the lens. The lens refocuses that light onto the retina, which starts the translation of light into vision. The retina converts light into electrical impulses that travel through the optic nerve to the brain, which interprets them as images.

The refractive process the eye uses is similar to the way a camera takes a picture. The cornea and lens in the eye act as the camera lens. The retina is like the film (in older cameras), or the image sensor (in digital cameras). If the image is not focused properly, the retina makes a blurry image.

The cornea also serves as a filter that screens out damaging ultra-violet (UV) light from the sun. Without this protection, the lens and the retina would be exposed to injury from UV rays.

What Are Some Common Conditions That Affect the Cornea?

Injuries

After minor injuries or scratches, the cornea usually heals on its own. Deeper injuries can cause corneal scarring, resulting in a haze on the cornea that impairs vision. If you have a deep injury, or a corneal disease or disorder, you could experience:

- pain in the eye
- sensitivity to light
- reduced vision or blurry vision
- redness or inflammation in the eye
- headache, nausea, fatigue

If you experience any of these symptoms, seek help from an eye care professional.

Allergies

The most common allergies that affect the eye are those related to pollen, particularly when the weather is warm and dry. Symptoms in the eye include redness, itching, tearing, burning, stinging, and watery discharge, although usually not severe enough to require medical attention. Antihistamine decongestant eye drops effectively reduce these symptoms. Rain and cooler weather, which decreases the amount of pollen in the air, can also provide relief.

Keratitis

Keratitis is an inflammation of the cornea. Noninfectious keratitis can be caused by a minor injury, or from wearing contact lenses too long. Infection is the most common cause of keratitis. Infectious keratitis can be caused by bacteria, viruses, fungi or parasites. Often, these infections are also related to contact lens wear, especially improper cleaning of contact lenses or overuse of old contact lenses that should be discarded. Minor corneal infections are usually treated with antibacterial eye drops. If the problem is severe, it may require more intensive antibiotic or antifungal treatment to eliminate the infection, as well as steroid eye drops to reduce inflammation.

Dry Eye

Dry eye is a condition in which the eye produces fewer or lower quality tears and is unable to keep its surface lubricated.

The main symptom of dry eye is usually a scratchy feeling or as if something is in your eye. Other symptoms include stinging or burning in the eye, episodes of excess tearing that follow periods of dryness, discharge from the eye, and pain and redness in the eye.

Sometimes people with dry eye also feel as if their eyelids are very heavy or their vision is blurred.

What Are Corneal Dystrophies?

A corneal dystrophy is a condition in which one or more parts of the cornea lose their normal clarity due to a buildup of material that clouds the cornea. These diseases:

- are usually inherited

- affect both eyes

- progress gradually

- don't affect other parts of the body, and aren't related to diseases affecting other parts of the eye or body

- happen in otherwise healthy people.

Corneal dystrophies affect vision in different ways. Some cause severe visual impairment, while a few cause no vision problems and are only discovered during a routine eye exam. Other dystrophies may cause repeated episodes of pain without leading to permanent vision loss. Some of the most common corneal dystrophies include keratoconus, Fuchs dystrophy, lattice dystrophy, and map-dot-fingerprint dystrophy.

Keratoconus

Keratoconus is a progressive thinning of the cornea. It is the most common corneal dystrophy in the United States, affecting one in every 2,000 Americans. It is most prevalent in teenagers and adults in their 20s.

Keratoconus causes the middle of the cornea to thin, bulge outward, and form a rounded cone shape. This abnormal curvature of the cornea can cause double or blurred vision, nearsightedness, astigmatism, and increased sensitivity to light.

The causes of keratoconus aren't known, but research indicates it is most likely caused by a combination of genetic susceptibility along with environmental and hormonal influences. About 7 percent of those with the condition have a history of keratoconus in their family. Keratoconus is diagnosed with a slit-lamp exam. Your eye care professional will also measure the curvature of your cornea.

Keratoconus usually affects both eyes. At first, the condition is corrected with glasses or soft contact lenses. As the disease progresses, you may need specially fitted contact lenses to correct the distortion of the cornea and provide better vision.

In most cases, the cornea stabilizes after a few years without causing severe vision problems. A small number of people with keratoconus may develop severe corneal scarring or become unable to tolerate a contact lens. For these people, a corneal transplant may become necessary.

Fuchs Dystrophy

Fuchs dystrophy is a slowly progressing disease that usually affects both eyes and is slightly more common in women than in men. It can cause your vision to gradually worsen over many years, but most people with Fuchs dystrophy won't notice vision problems until they reach their 50s or 60s.

Fuchs dystrophy is caused by the gradual deterioration of cells in the corneal endothelium; the causes aren't well understood. Normally, these endothelial cells maintain a healthy balance of fluids within the cornea. Healthy endothelial cells prevent the cornea from swelling and keep the cornea clear. In Fuchs dystrophy, the endothelial cells slowly die off and cause fluid buildup and swelling within the cornea. The cornea thickens and vision becomes blurred.

As the disease progresses, Fuchs dystrophy symptoms usually affect both eyes and include:

- glare, which affects vision in low light

- blurred vision that occurs in the morning after waking and gradually improves during the day

- distorted vision, sensitivity to light, difficulty seeing at night, and seeing halos around light at night

- painful, tiny blisters on the surface of the cornea
- a cloudy or hazy looking cornea

The first step in treating Fuchs dystrophy is to reduce the swelling with drops, ointments, or soft contact lenses. If you have severe disease, your eye care professional may suggest a corneal transplant.

Lattice Dystrophy

Lattice dystrophy gets its name from a characteristic lattice-like pattern of deposits in the stroma layer of the cornea. The deposits are made of amyloid, an abnormal protein fiber. Over time, the deposits increase and the lattice lines grow opaque, take over more of the stroma, and gradually converge to impair vision.

Although lattice dystrophy can occur at any time in life, it most commonly begins in childhood between the ages of 2 and 7. In some people, amyloid deposits can accumulate under the epithelium of the cornea. This can erode the epithelium, and cause a condition known as recurrent epithelial erosion. This erosion alters the cornea's normal curvature and causes temporary vision problems. It can also expose the nerves that line the cornea and cause severe pain.

To ease this pain, an eye care professional may prescribe eye drops and ointments to reduce the friction of the eyelid against the cornea. In some cases, an eye patch may be used to immobilize the eyelid. The erosions usually heal within days, although you may have some pain for the next six to eight weeks.

By age 40, some people with lattice dystrophy have scarring under the epithelium that can impact vision to such an extent that the most effective treatment will be a corneal transplant. Although the early results of corneal transplantation are typically good, lattice dystrophy may reappear later and require long-term treatment.

Map-Dot-Fingerprint Dystrophy

Map-Dot-Fingerprint dystrophy, also known as epithelial basement membrane dystrophy, occurs when the basement membrane develops abnormally and forms folds in the tissue. The folds create gray shapes that look like continents on a map. There also may be clusters of opaque dots underneath or close to the maplike patches. Less frequently, the folds form concentric lines in the central cornea that resemble small fingerprints.

Symptoms include blurred vision, pain in the morning that lessens during the day, sensitivity to light, excessive tearing, and a feeling that there's something in the eye.

Map-dot-fingerprint dystrophy usually occurs in both eyes and affects adults between the ages of 40 and 70, although it can develop earlier in life. Typically, map-dot-fingerprint dystrophy will flare up now and then over the course of several years and then go away, without vision loss. Some people can have map-dot-fingerprint dystrophy but not experience any symptoms.

Others with the disease will develop recurring epithelial erosions, in which the epithelium's outermost layer rises slightly, exposing a small gap between the outermost layer and the rest of the cornea. These erosions alter the cornea's normal curvature and cause blurred vision. They may also expose the nerve endings that line the tissue, resulting in moderate to severe pain over several days.

The discomfort of epithelial erosions can be managed with topical lubricating eye drops and ointments. If drops or ointments don't relieve the pain and discomfort, there are outpatient surgeries including:

- anterior corneal puncture, which help the cells adhere better to the tissue

- corneal scraping to remove eroded areas of the cornea and allow healthy tissue to regrow

- laser surgery to remove surface irregularities on the cornea

What Other Diseases Can Affect the Cornea?

Herpes Zoster (Shingles)

Shingles is a reactivation of the varicel-lazoster virus, the same virus that causes chickenpox. If you have had chickenpox, the virus can live on within your nerve cells for years after the sores have gone away. In some people, the varicel-lazoster virus reactivates later in life, travels through the nerve fibers, and emerges in the cornea. If this happens, your eye care professional may prescribe oral anti-viral treatment to reduce the risk of inflammation and scarring in the cornea. Shingles can also cause decreased sensitivity in the cornea.

Corneal problems may arise months after the shingles are gone from the rest of the body. If you experience shingles in your eye, or nose, or on your face, it's important to have your eyes examined several months after the shingles have cleared.

Ocular Herpes

Herpes of the eye, or ocular herpes, is a recurrent viral infection that is caused by the herpes simplex virus (HSV-1). This is the same virus that causes cold sores. Ocular herpes can also be caused by the sexually transmitted herpes simplex virus (HSV-2) that causes genital herpes.

Ocular herpes can produce sores on the eyelid or surface of the cornea and over time the inflammation may spread deeper into the cornea and eye, and develop into a more severe infection called stromal keratitis. There is no cure for ocular herpes, but it can be controlled with antiviral drugs.

Iridocorneal Endothelial Syndrome

Iridocorneal endothelial syndrome (ICE) is more common in women and usually develops between ages 30–50. ICE has three main features:

- visible changes in the iris, the colored part of the eye

- swelling of the cornea

- glaucoma

ICE is usually present in only one eye. It is caused by the movement of endothelial cells from the cornea to the iris. This loss of cells from the cornea leads to corneal swelling and distortion of the iris and pupil. This cell movement also blocks the fluid outflow channels of the eye, which causes glaucoma.

There is no treatment to stop the progression of ICE, but the glaucoma is treatable. If the cornea becomes so swollen that vision is significantly impaired, a corneal transplant may be necessary.

Pterygium

A pterygium is a pinkish, triangular tissue growth on the cornea. Some pterygia (plural for pterygium) grow slowly throughout a lifetime, while others stop growing. A pterygium rarely grows so large that it covers the pupil of the eye.

Pterygia are more common in sunny climates and in adults 20–40 years of age. It's unclear what causes pterygia. However, since people who develop pterygia usually have spent significant time outdoors, researchers believe chronic exposure to UV light from the sun may be a factor.

To protect yourself from developing pterygia, wear sunglasses, or a wide-brimmed hat in places where the sunlight is strong. If you have one or more pterygia, lubricating eye drops may be recommended to reduce redness and soothe irritation.

Because a pterygium is visible, some people might want to have it removed for cosmetic reasons. However, unless it affects vision, surgery to remove a pterygium is not recommended. Even if it is surgically removed, a pterygium may grow back, particularly if removed before age 40.

Stevens-Johnson Syndrome

Stevens-Johnson Syndrome (SJS), also called erythema multiforme major, is a disorder of the skin that also affects the eyes. SJS is characterized by painful blisters on the skin and the mucous membranes of the mouth, throat, genitals, and eyelids.

Often, SJS begins with flu-like symptoms, followed by a painful red or purplish rash of blisters that spread. SJS can cause severe conjunctivitis, iritis (an inflammation inside the eye), corneal blisters and erosions, and corneal holes. In some cases, SJS can lead to significant vision loss.

The most commonly cited cause of SJS is an allergic reaction to a drug or medication, particularly sulfa drugs. It is also associated with viral infections.

Treatment for the eye may include artificial tears or lubricating eye drops, antibiotics, or corticosteroids. About one-third of those who develop SJS will have one or more episodes of the disease. SJS occurs twice as often in men as in women, and most often affects children and young adults under 30, although it can develop at any age.

What Treatments Are There for Advanced Corneal Disease?

Laser Surgery

Phototherapeutic keratectomy (PTK) is a surgical technique that uses UV light and laser technology to reshape and restore the cornea. PTK has been used to treat recurrent erosions and corneal dystrophies, such as map-dot-fingerprint dystrophy and basal membrane dystrophy. PTK helps delay or postpone corneal grafting or replacement.

Corneal Transplant Surgery

Corneal transplant surgery removes the damaged portion of the cornea and replaces it with healthy donor tissue. Corneas are the most commonly transplanted tissue worldwide. More than 47,000 corneal transplants were performed in the United States in 2014.

In the past, the standard approach to corneal transplants was to surgically replace the entire cornea with donor tissue, a technique known as **penetrating keratoplasty**. This is called a full thickness transplant, and may still be the only option for people with advanced keratoconus and scarring, severe herpetic scarring, or traumatic injury that affects the whole cornea.

However, most people who need a cornea transplant undergo a newer procedure called **lamellar keratoplasty**. This is called a partial thickness transplant. In this procedure, the surgeon selectively removes and replaces the diseased layer(s) of the cornea and leaves the healthy tissue in place. Replacing only diseased layers with a donor graft leaves the cornea more structurally intact and leads to a lower rate of complications and better visual improvement.

Anterior lamellar keratoplasty removes damaged stromal tissue and replaces it with healthy stroma from a donor. This procedure is used for:

- keratoconus

- severe corneal scarring

- corneal dystrophies that affect the stroma

Endothelial lamellar keratoplasty removes diseased endothelial tissue and replaces it with healthy endothelium from a donor. This procedure is used for:

- Fuchs dystrophy

- post-cataract edema

- corneal failure after surgery for cataract, glaucoma or retinal detachment

Corneal transplants are generally done under local anesthetic as an outpatient procedure. With full thickness transplants, the damaged cornea is removed and replaced with a donor cornea. Tiny stitches secure the transplant. Partial thickness transplants use fewer stitches. Either type of surgery usually takes 30 minutes.

Artificial Cornea

A keratoprosthesis (KPro) is an artificial cornea. A KPro may be the only option available for people who have not had success with corneal tissue implants or who have a high risk of tissue rejection (such as those with Stevens-Johnson syndrome or severe chemical burns).

The Boston type-1 KPro is the most used keratoprosthesis. It is made of clear plastic and consists of three parts, with donor cornea tissue clamped between front and back plates. When fully assembled it has the shape of a collar button. The procedure to insert a KPro is performed by an ophthalmologist, usually on an outpatient basis.

Current Corneal Research

Improved **corneal wound healing** could have an impact on many disorders and injuries of the cornea. National Eye Institute (NEI) researchers are conducting studies to better understand how the cornea naturally heals after injury, which involves the release of proteins that act together to move the epithelial layer over the wound. This research could lead to new therapeutic strategies for transplantation and other treatments to repair corneal damage.

Other research seeks to improve the success of **corneal grafts**. For example, one study is looking at immune system factors that influence whether or not a graft will integrate and attach successfully. Identifying these factors could lead to new ways to promote graft survival without the use of strong immunosuppressive medications that can put people at risk for infections.

There is an increasing need for development and refinement of **artificial (prosthetic) corneas**. The demand for human corneal tissue is growing, but the supply is falling due to the popularity of LASIK surgeries, which weaken the corneal stroma and make it unsuitable for donation.

Researchers supported by NEI are looking to bypass this shortage by developing tissue-engineered corneas that combine clear silk protein films with live corneal cells.

A clinical study funded by NEI is testing the effectiveness and safety of a folding, injectable artificial cornea that can be implanted through an opening one-tenth the size of the usual incision. This smaller incision size is expected to decrease the amount of time required for surgery and recovery.

The development of **endothelial stem cell** lines is an area of research being explored by a number of NEI-supported investigators. The goal of this research is to create stem cells that can be used as a laboratory model to test potential therapies, or used as therapies on their own to promote regrowth of healthy corneal tissue. For example, one group of researchers is developing a source of human corneal endothelial stem cells, and a procedure to implant them into the eye and restore clear vision.

Research to **improve the diagnosis of corneal diseases and disorders** is another priority for NEI. For example, keratoconus is the most common degenerative disease affecting the cornea. In its earliest stages, keratoconus is difficult to detect and may go untreated.

- One group of NEI-supported researchers seeks to improve detection of keratoconus with a technique that uses high resolution ultrasound to measure the thickness of corneal layers, combined with other measurements of corneal elasticity, irregularities in the corneal surface, and epithelial thickness.

- Another study is testing how genetic risk factors for keratoconus influence the function and health of corneal cells grown in the lab. The results of these studies will help advance our understanding of genetic susceptibility to keratoconus, and may result in novel treatment options to slow its progression.

Fuchs dystrophy accounts for most of the corneal transplants performed each year in the United States. To identify new treatment approaches, NEI-supported researchers are searching for genetic mutations that are associated with Fuchs dystrophy. Such genes could be targets for future therapies.

Herpetic stromal keratitis caused by herpes simplex virus (HSV) infection is the most common cause of corneal blindness in the developed world. One group of researchers is developing a vaccine that, if successful, will lead to a significant reduction in the transmission of HSV to the cornea.

NEI is supporting a number of clinical trials in the United States to confirm that corneal **collagen cross-linking (CXL)** is safe and effective. CXL is a minimally-invasive surgical procedure that combines a photosensitive solution applied to the cornea with a low dose of UV light. The photosensitive solution reacts with the UV light to create new collagen bonds (cross-links) that strengthen the cornea. CXL has been approved in Europe and Canada for treating keratoconus.

Chapter 19

Cataract

Cataracts Basics

What Is a Cataract?

A cataract is a clouding of the lens in the eye that affects vision. Most cataracts are related to aging. Cataracts are very common in older people. By age 80, more than half of all Americans either have a cataract or have had cataract surgery.

A cataract can occur in either or both eyes. It cannot spread from one eye to the other.

What Is the Lens?

The lens is a clear part of the eye that helps to focus light, or an image, on the retina. The retina is the light-sensitive tissue at the back of the eye.

In a normal eye, light passes through the transparent lens to the retina. Once it reaches the retina, light is changed into nerve signals that are sent to the brain.

The lens must be clear for the retina to receive a sharp image. If the lens is cloudy from a cataract, the image you see will be blurred.

This chapter includes text excerpted from "Facts about Cataract," National Eye Institute (NEI), September 2015.

What Causes Cataracts?

The lens lies behind the iris and the pupil. It works much like a camera lens. It focuses light onto the retina at the back of the eye, where an image is recorded. The lens also adjusts the eye's focus, letting us see things clearly both up close and far away. The lens is made of mostly water and protein. The protein is arranged in a precise way that keeps the lens clear and lets light pass through it.

But as we age, some of the protein may clump together and start to cloud a small area of the lens. This is a cataract. Over time, the cataract may grow larger and cloud more of the lens, making it harder to see.

Researchers suspect that there are several causes of cataract, such as smoking and diabetes. Or, it may be that the protein in the lens just changes from the wear and tear it takes over the years.

How Do Cataracts Affect Vision?

Age-related cataracts can affect your vision in two ways:

1. Clumps of protein reduce the sharpness of the image reaching the retina.

The lens consists mostly of water and protein. When the protein clumps up, it clouds the lens and reduces the light that reaches the retina. The clouding may become severe enough to cause blurred vision. Most age-related cataracts develop from protein clumpings.

When a cataract is small, the cloudiness affects only a small part of the lens. You may not notice any changes in your vision. Cataracts tend to "grow" slowly, so vision gets worse gradually. Over time, the cloudy area in the lens may get larger, and the cataract may increase in size. Seeing may become more difficult. Your vision may get duller or blurrier.

2. The clear lens slowly changes to a yellowish/brownish color, adding a brownish tint to vision.

As the clear lens slowly colors with age, your vision gradually may acquire a brownish shade. At first, the amount of tinting may be small and may not cause a vision problem. Over time, increased tinting may make it more difficult to read and perform other routine activities. This gradual change in the amount of tinting does not affect the sharpness of the image transmitted to the retina.

If you have advanced lens discoloration, you may not be able to identify blues and purples. You may be wearing what you believe to be a pair of black socks, only to find out from friends that you are wearing purple socks.

When Are You Most Likely to Have a Cataract?

The term "age-related" is a little misleading. You don't have to be a senior citizen to get this type of cataract. In fact, people can have an age-related cataract in their 40s and 50s. But during middle age, most cataracts are small and do not affect vision. It is after age 60 that most cataracts cause problems with a person's vision.

Who Is at Risk for Cataract?

The risk of cataract increases as you get older. Other risk factors for cataract include:

- certain diseases (for example, diabetes)
- personal behavior (smoking, alcohol use
- the environment (prolonged exposure to ultraviolet sunlight)

What Are the Symptoms of a Cataract?

The most common symptoms of a cataract are:

- Cloudy or blurry vision.
- Colors seem faded.
- Glare. Headlights, lamps, or sunlight may appear too bright. A halo may appear around lights.
- Poor night vision.
- Double vision or multiple images in one eye. (This symptom may clear as the cataract gets larger.)
- Frequent prescription changes in your eyeglasses or contact lenses.

These symptoms also can be a sign of other eye problems. If you have any of these symptoms, check with your eye care professional.

Are There Different Types of Cataract?

Yes. Although most cataracts are related to aging, there are other types of cataract:

205

1. **Secondary cataract.** Cataracts can form after surgery for other eye problems, such as glaucoma. Cataracts also can develop in people who have other health problems, such as diabetes. Cataracts are sometimes linked to steroid use.

2. **Traumatic cataract.** Cataracts can develop after an eye injury, sometimes years later.

3. **Congenital cataract.** Some babies are born with cataracts or develop them in childhood, often in both eyes. These cataracts may be so small that they do not affect vision. If they do, the lenses may need to be removed.

4. **Radiation cataract.** Cataracts can develop after exposure to some types of radiation.

How Is a Cataract Detected?

Cataract is detected through a comprehensive eye exam that includes:

1. **Visual acuity test.** This eye chart test measures how well you see at various distances.

2. **Dilated eye exam.** Drops are placed in your eyes to widen, or dilate, the pupils. Your eye care professional uses a special magnifying lens to examine your retina and optic nerve for signs of damage and other eye problems. After the exam, your close-up vision may remain blurred for several hours.

3. **Tonometry.** An instrument measures the pressure inside the eye. Numbing drops may be applied to your eye for this test.

Your eye care professional also may do other tests to learn more about the structure and health of your eye.

Treatment of Cataracts

How Is a Cataract Treated?

The symptoms of early cataract may be improved with new eyeglasses, brighter lighting, anti-glare sunglasses, or magnifying lenses. If these measures do not help, surgery is the only effective treatment. Surgery involves removing the cloudy lens and replacing it with an artificial lens.

A cataract needs to be removed only when vision loss inter-feres with your everyday activities, such as driving, reading, or watching TV. You and your eye care professional can make this deci-sion together. Once you understand the benefits and risks of surgery, you can make an informed decision about whether cataract surgery is right for you. In most cases, delaying cataract surgery will not cause long-term damage to your eye or make the surgery more difficult. You do not have to rush into surgery.

Sometimes a cataract should be removed even if it does not cause problems with your vision. For example, a cataract should be removed if it prevents examination or treatment of another eye problem, such as age-related macular degeneration or diabetic retinopathy.

If you choose surgery, your eye care professional may refer you to a specialist to remove the cataract.

If you have cataracts in both eyes that require surgery, the surgery will be performed on each eye at separate times, usually four weeks apart.

Is Cataract Surgery Effective?

Cataract removal is one of the most common operations performed in the United States. It also is one of the safest and most effective types of surgery. In about 90 percent of cases, people who have cataract surgery have better vision afterward.

What Are the Risks of Cataract Surgery?

As with any surgery, cataract surgery poses risks, such as infection and bleeding. Before cataract surgery, your doctor may ask you to temporarily stop taking certain medications that increase the risk of bleeding during surgery. After surgery, you must keep your eye clean, wash your hands before touching your eye, and use the prescribed medications to help minimize the risk of infection. Serious infection can result in loss of vision.

Cataract surgery slightly increases your risk of retinal detachment. Other eye disorders, such as high myopia (nearsightedness), can fur-ther increase your risk of retinal detachment after cataract surgery. One sign of a retinal detachment is a sudden increase in flashes or floaters. Floaters are little "cobwebs" or specks that seem to float about in your field of vision. If you notice a sudden increase in floaters or flashes, see an eye care professional immediately. **A retinal detach-ment is a medical emergency.** If necessary, go to an emergency service or hospital. Your eye must be examined by an eye surgeon as soon as possible. **A retinal detachment causes no pain.** Early treatment for retinal detachment often can prevent permanent loss of vision. The sooner you get treatment, the more likely you will regain good vision. Even if you are treated promptly, some vision may be lost.

Talk to your eye care professional about these risks. Make sure cataract surgery is right for you.

What If I Have Other Eye Conditions and Need Cataract Surgery?

Many people who need cataract surgery also have other eye conditions, such as age-related macular degeneration or glaucoma. If you have other eye conditions in addition to cataract, talk with your doctor. Learn about the risks, benefits, alternatives, and expected results of cataract surgery.

Is Cataract Surgery Right For You?*

Once you understand the benefits and risks of surgery, you can make an informed decision about whether cataract surgery is right for you. In most cases, delaying cataract surgery will not cause long-term damage to your eye or make the surgery more difficult. You do not have to rush into surgery.

Sometimes a cataract should be removed even if it does not cause problems with your vision. For example, a cataract should be removed if it prevents examination or treatment of another eye problem, such as age-related macular degeneration or diabetic retinopathy.

If you choose surgery, your eye care professional may refer you to a specialist to remove the cataract. If you have cataracts in both eyes that require surgery, the surgery will be performed on each eye at separate times, usually four to eight weeks apart.

Cataract removal is one of the most common operations performed in the United States. It also is one of the safest and most effective types of surgery. In about 90 percent of cases, people who have cataract surgery have better vision afterward.

Types of Cataract Surgery*

There are two types of cataract surgery, phacoemulsification and extracapsular surgery. Your doctor can explain the differences and help determine which is better for you.

With phacoemulsification, or phaco, a small incision is made on the side of the cornea, the clear, dome-shaped surface that covers the front of the eye. Your doctor inserts a tiny probe into the eye. This device emits ultrasound waves that soften and break up the lens so that it can be removed by suction. Most cataract surgery today is done by phacoemulsification, also called small incision cataract surgery.

With extracapsular surgery, your doctor makes a longer incision on the side of the cornea and removes the cloudy core of the lens in one piece. The rest of the lens is removed by suction.

* *Text excerpted from "Cataract: Treatment And Prevention," National Institute on Aging (NIA), National Institutes of Health (NIH), January 14, 2017.*

What Happens before Surgery?

A week or two before surgery, your doctor will do some tests. These tests may include measuring the curve of the cornea and the size and shape of your eye. This information helps your doctor choose the right type of intraocular lens (IOL).

You may be asked not to eat or drink anything 12 hours before your surgery.

What Happens during Surgery?

At the hospital or eye clinic, drops will be put into your eye to dilate the pupil. The area around your eye will be washed and cleansed.

The operation usually lasts less than one hour and is almost painless. Many people choose to stay awake during surgery. Others may need to be put to sleep for a short time. If you are awake, you will have an anesthetic to numb the nerves in and around your eye.

After the operation, a patch may be placed over your eye. You will rest for a while. Your medical team will watch for any problems, such as bleeding. Most people who have cataract surgery can go home the same day. You will need someone to drive you home.

What Happens after Surgery?

Itching and mild discomfort are normal after cataract surgery. Some fluid discharge is also common. Your eye may be sensitive to light and touch. If you have discomfort, your doctor can suggest treatment. After one or two days, moderate discomfort should disappear.

For a few weeks after surgery, your doctor may ask you to use eye drops to help healing and decrease the risk of infection. Ask your doctor about how to use your eye drops, how often to use them, and what effects they can have. You will need to wear an eye shield or eyeglasses to help protect your eye. Avoid rubbing or pressing on your eye.

When you are home, try not to bend from the waist to pick up objects on the floor. Do not lift any heavy objects. You can walk, climb stairs, and do light household chores.

In most cases, healing will be complete within eight weeks. Your doctor will schedule exams to check on your progress.

Protecting Vision

Wearing sunglasses and a hat with a brim to block ultraviolet sunlight may help to delay cataract. If you smoke, stop. Researchers also believe good nutrition can help reduce the risk of age-related cataract. They recommend eating green leafy vegetables, fruit, and other foods with antioxidants.

If you are age 60 or older, you should have a comprehensive dilated eye exam at least once every two years. In addition to cataract, your eye care professional can check for signs of age-related macular degeneration, glaucoma, and other vision disorders. Early treatment for many eye diseases may save your sight.

Studies on Cataracts

The National Eye Institute (NEI) is conducting and supporting a number of studies focusing on factors associated with the development of age-related cataract. These studies include:

- The effect of sunlight exposure, which may be associated with an increased risk of cataract.

- Vitamin supplements, which have shown varying results in delaying the progression of cataract.

- Genetic studies, which show promise for better understanding cataract development.

Chapter 20

Corneal Transplant

A corneal transplant, formally known as a keratoplasty, is a surgical procedure used to replace damaged or diseased corneal tissue with healthy donor tissue. The cornea is a clear layer in the front of the eye that helps to focus light images on the retina at the back of the eye. When an unhealthy cornea becomes scarred, swollen, or misshapen so that it cannot admit light into the eye properly, the person's vision becomes blurry and distorted. Corneal eye disease is a common cause of blindness, affecting an estimated 10 million people around the world. Fortunately, corneal transplant surgery restores the functional vision of around 50,000 people in the United States each year.

Conditions that Require Transplants

Corneal transplants are performed to improve the function of a diseased or damaged cornea in order to restore a patient's vision and relieve pain. Some of the health conditions that may require a transplant include the following:

- trichiasis, a condition in which eyelashes grow inward and rub against the surface of the eye;

- infections like herpes or fungal keratitis that can cause scarring of the eye tissue;

- keratoconus, an eye disease that causes the cornea to become thin and lose its shape;

- blunt force injuries or chemical burns to the eye;

- Fuchs dystrophy, lattice dystrophy, and other hereditary eye conditions that affect the cornea;

- complications from laser eye surgery or cataract surgery resulting in corneal failure;

- rejection of the donor tissue following an earlier corneal transplant.

The best candidates for corneal transplant surgery have problems with their functional vision that interfere with their activities of daily living and cannot be corrected with less invasive measures.

Types of Transplant Procedures

There are three main types of corneal transplant procedures, which differ mainly in the amount of donor tissue that is transferred to the recipient. The type of procedure that an individual patient needs depends on which parts of the cornea are damaged and must be replaced.

Penetrating keratoplasty (PK), also known as a full-thickness corneal transplant, is the traditional type of surgery that has been performed since the 1960s. The eye surgeon uses a surgical cutting tool called a trephine to remove a button-shaped section that includes all layers of tissue in the diseased or damaged cornea. Next, the eye surgeon removes a matching section of healthy cornea from the donor eye and attaches it to the patient's eye using tiny sutures. The traditional, full-thickness PK procedure is typically used with patients who have severe damage or disease affecting the majority of their corneal tissue.

Endothelial keratoplasty (EK), sometimes known as a back-layer corneal transplant, involves replacing only the deepest, innermost layers of the cornea while leaving the outer, healthy tissue layers intact. The endothelium layer, which controls the fluid balance in the cornea, is among those that are replaced. EK is often used in patients with disorders that cause corneal swelling, such as Fuchs dystrophy. The procedure involves inserting a thin disc of donor tissue containing a healthy endothelial layer into the patient's cornea through a tiny incision. Compared to PK, EK offers faster recovery of vision, reduced risk of complications, and less susceptibility to eye injury.

Lamellar keratoplasty (LK) is a relatively new procedure in which the eye surgeon selectively replaces only the inner or outer layers of the cornea, rather than the full thickness. The specific LK technique varies depending on which layers are replaced. In general, LK procedures are less invasive than PK or EK procedures and offer faster recovery and fewer complications. They are mainly used when the disease or damage is limited to certain layers of the cornea.

What to Expect

Before a Corneal Transplant

The healthy corneal tissue used in transplant procedures comes from deceased human donors. Patients who are approved for a corneal transplant are placed on a list at a local eye bank to wait for a suitable donor eye to become available. This process can take anywhere from a few days to several weeks. Eye banks ensure that donor eyes meet strict medical standards before they are released for use in transplant surgery.

During a Corneal Transplant

Most corneal transplant procedures are performed on an outpatient basis, and they generally last about an hour. The patient can be placed under local or general anesthesia, depending on their age, health, and preference. The eye surgeon will use eye drops to numb the surface of the eye as well as an injection to relax the eye muscles and control eye movements. A device called a lid speculum is used to hold the eyelids open. Most patients do not experience any discomfort during the procedure.

Recovery from a Corneal Transplant

The time required for full recovery from a corneal transplant can be a year or more. Patients should expect their vision to be blurry at first and improve gradually as the cornea heals. They will have to wear a protective patch over the eye, use eye drops to prevent infection or rejection, and avoid contact sports or heavy lifting for several weeks. The sutures may remain in place for 3 to 18 months following the procedure.

Long-Term Results and Possible Complications

Corneal transplants are the most successful type of tissue transplant. Although the results vary depending on the underlying cause

213

of the cornea damage or disease, the majority of patients experience significant vision improvement that lasts for at least ten years. Every surgical procedure involves some risks, but most patients find that the benefits of restored functional vision outweigh the possible complications.

Depending on the type of transplant surgery and the number of layers of tissue transferred, some of the potential complications include infection, bleeding, scarring, damage to other parts of the eye, and problems related to the use of sutures. Many recipients have refractive errors with their new cornea because its curvature does not exactly match the natural curvature of their eye. As a result, they may need eyeglasses or contact lenses to correct nearsightedness (myopia) or astigmatism (irregular shape of the eye). Since it takes a few months for vision to stabilize following transplant surgery, however, it is best to wait until the cornea is fully healed before getting a new corrective lens prescription. Some patients later undergo laser eye surgery to improve their vision.

Rejection of the donor tissue is the most serious potential complication of corneal transplant surgery. Fortunately, rejection is relatively rare because the cornea has no blood vessels and is thus unlikely to be recognized as a foreign body and attacked by the immune system. Although rejection occurs in between 5 percent and 30 percent of transplant patients, 90 percent of corneal tissue rejections can be reversed when the symptoms are detected early. Doctors have devised the acronym RSVP to help patients recognize the main warning signs of corneal transplant rejections, which may appear days, months, or even years after the surgery:

- **R**edness
- **S**ensitivity to light
- **V**ision decline
- **P**ain

Corneal transplant surgery can be repeated if the tissue is rejected, although the rejection rates increase with each successive procedure. Patients who have undergone multiple failed corneal transplants using human donor tissue may be candidates for a transplant using artificial or biosynthetic cornea tissues, which are experimental materials under development.

References

1. "Cornea Transplant," NHS Choices, May 15, 2015.

2. Kozarsky, Alan. "Cornea Transplant Surgery: What You Need to Know," WebMD, September 20, 2016.

3. Wachler, Brian Boxer. "Corneal Transplants: What to Expect," All About Vision, May 2015.

Chapter 21

Disorders of the Conjunctiva, Sclera, and Pupil

Chapter Contents

Section 21.1

Conjunctivitis

This section includes text excerpted from "Conjunctivitis (Pink Eye)," Centers for Disease Control and Prevention (CDC), June 30, 2016.

Conjunctivitis is often called "pink eye" because it can cause the white of the eye to take on a pink or red color. Symptoms of pink eye can vary but typically include redness or swelling of the white of the eye.

Causes of Conjunctivitis

The most common causes of conjunctivitis (pink eye) are

- viruses
- bacteria
- allergens

It can also be caused by

- chemicals
- contact lens wear (especially wearing lenses overnight)
- foreign bodies in the eye (like a loose eyelash)
- indoor and outdoor air pollution caused, for example, by chemical vapors, fumes, smoke, or dust
- fungi

It can be difficult to determine the exact cause of conjunctivitis because some symptoms may be the same no matter the cause.

Viral Conjunctivitis

- Caused by infection of the eye with a virus.
- Can be caused by a number of different viruses, such as adenoviruses.

218

- Very contagious.
- Sometimes can result in large outbreaks depending on the virus.

Bacterial Conjunctivitis

- Caused by infection of the eye with certain bacteria.
- Can be caused by *Staphylococcus aureus*, *Streptococcus pneumoniae*, *Haemophilus species*, or, less commonly, *Chlamydia trachomatis*.
- Very contagious.
- A leading cause of children being absent from daycare or school.
- More common in kids than adults.

Allergic Conjunctivitis

- The result of the body's reaction to allergens, such as pollen from trees, plants, grasses, and weeds; dust mites; molds; dander from pets; medicines, or cosmetics.
- Not contagious.
- Occurs more frequently among people with other allergic conditions, such as hay fever, asthma, and eczema.
- Can occur seasonally, when allergens such as pollen counts are high.
- Can also occur year-round due to indoor allergens, such as dust mites and animal dander.
- May result, in some people, from exposure to certain drugs and cosmetics.

Conjunctivitis Caused by Irritants

- Caused by irritation from a foreign body in the eye or contact with chemicals, fumes, smoke, or dust.
- Not contagious.
- Can occur when contact lenses are worn too long or not cleaned properly.

Symptoms of Conjunctivitis

Some of the common signs and symptoms of conjunctivitis (pink eye) can include

- Pink or red color in the white of the eye(s)
- Swelling of the conjunctiva (the thin layer that lines the white part of the eye and the inside of the eyelid) and/or eyelids
- Increased tear production
- Feeling like a foreign body is in the eye(s) or an urge to rub the eye(s)
- Itching, irritation, and/or burning
- Discharge (pus or mucus)
- Crusting of eyelids or lashes, especially in the morning
- Contact lenses that do not stay in place on the eye and/or feel uncomfortable

Depending on the cause, other symptoms may occur.

Viral Conjunctivitis

- Can occur with symptoms of a cold, flu, or other respiratory infection
- Usually begins in one eye and may spread to the other eye within days
- Discharge from the eye is usually watery rather than thick

Bacterial Conjunctivitis

- Usually begins in one eye and sometimes spreads to the other eye
- More commonly associated with discharge of pus, especially a yellow-green color
- Sometimes occurs with an ear infection

Allergic Conjunctivitis

- Usually occurs in both eyes
- Can produce intense itching, tearing, and swelling in the eyes

- May occur with symptoms of allergy, such as an itchy nose, sneezing, a scratchy throat, or asthma

Conjunctivitis Caused by Irritants

- Can produce watery eyes and mucus discharge

Transmission of Conjunctivitis

How It Spreads

Several viruses and bacteria can cause conjunctivitis (pink eye). Both viral and bacterial conjunctivitis are highly contagious. Each of these types of germs can spread from person to person in different ways. They are usually spread from an infected person to others through

- close personal contact, such as touching or shaking hands
- the air by coughing and sneezing
- touching an object or surface with germs on it, then touching your eyes before washing your hands

When to Go Back to Work or School

If you have conjunctivitis, you may be allowed to remain at work or school with your doctor's approval. However, if you still have symptoms, and your activities at work or school are such that you can't avoid close contact with other people, you should not attend.

Diagnosis of Conjunctivitis

A doctor can often determine whether conjunctivitis (pink eye) is caused by a virus, bacterium, or allergen based on patient history, symptoms, and an examination of the eye. Conjunctivitis always involves eye redness or swelling, but it also has other symptoms that can vary depending on the cause. These symptoms can help a healthcare professional diagnose the cause of conjunctivitis. However, it can sometimes be difficult to make a firm diagnosis because some symptoms are the same no matter the cause.

It can also sometimes be difficult to diagnose without doing laboratory testing. Although not routinely done, your healthcare provider may collect a sample of eye discharge from the infected eye and send it to the laboratory to help them determine which form of infection you have and how best to treat it.

Viral Conjunctivitis

The cause is likely a virus if

- conjunctivitis accompanies a common cold or respiratory tract infection, and
- discharge from the eye is watery rather than thick

Bacterial Conjunctivitis

The cause may be bacterial if

- conjunctivitis occurs at the same time as an ear infection, and
- discharge from the eye is thick rather than watery

Allergic Conjunctivitis

The cause is likely allergic if

- conjunctivitis occurs seasonally when pollen counts are high
- the patient's eyes itch intensely
- it occurs in someone with other signs of allergic disease, such as hay fever, asthma, or eczema

Prevention of Conjunctivitis

Preventing the Spread of Conjunctivitis

Viral and bacterial conjunctivitis (pink eye) are very contagious. They can spread easily from person to person. You can greatly reduce the risk of getting conjunctivitis or spreading it to someone else by following some simple good-hygiene steps.

If You Have Conjunctivitis

If you have conjunctivitis, you can help limit its spread to other people by following these steps:

- Wash your hands often with soap and warm water. Wash them especially well before and after cleaning, or applying eye drops or ointment to, your infected eye. If soap and water are not available, use an alcohol-based hand sanitizer.

- Avoid touching or rubbing your eyes. This can worsen the condition or spread it to your other eye.

- With clean hands, wash any discharge from around your eye(s) several times a day using a clean, wet washcloth or fresh cotton ball. Throw away cotton balls after use, and wash used washcloths with hot water and detergent, then wash your hands again with soap and warm water.

- Do not use the same eye drop dispenser/bottle for your infected and noninfected eyes.

- Wash pillowcases, sheets, washcloths, and towels often in hot water and detergent; wash your hands after handling such items.

- Stop wearing contact lenses until your eye doctor says it's okay to start wearing them again.

- Clean eyeglasses, being careful not to contaminate items (like hand towels) that might be shared by other people.

- Clean, store, and replace your contact lenses as instructed by your eye doctor.

- Do not share personal items, such as pillows, washcloths, towels, eye drops, eye makeup, face makeup, makeup brushes, contact lenses and, contact lens containers, or eyeglasses.

- Do not use swimming pools.

If You Are around Someone with Conjunctivitis

If you are around someone with conjunctivitis, you can reduce your risk of infection by following these steps:

- Wash your hands often with soap and warm water. If soap and warm water are not available, use an alcohol-based hand sanitizer.

- Wash your hands after contact with an infected person or items he or she uses; for example, wash your hands after applying eye drops or ointment to an infected person's eye(s) or after putting their bed linens in the washing machine.

- Avoid touching your eyes with unwashed hands.

- Do not share items used by an infected person; for example, do not share pillows, washcloths, towels, eye drops, eye or face

makeup, makeup brushes, contact lenses, contact lens containers, or eyeglasses.

Avoid Getting Sick Again

In addition, if you have conjunctivitis, there are steps you can take
to avoid re-infection once the infection goes away:

- Throw away and replace any eye or face makeup you used while
  infected.

- Throw away contact lens solutions that you used while your eyes
  were infected.

- Throw away disposable contact lenses and cases that you used
  while your eyes were infected.

- Clean extended wear lenses as directed.

- Clean eyeglasses and cases that you used while infected.

There is no vaccine that prevents all types of conjunctivitis. However, there are vaccines to protect against some viral and bacterial
diseases that are associated with conjunctivitis:

- rubella

- measles

- chickenpox

- shingles

- pneumococcal

- *Haemophilus influenzae* type b (Hib)

Conjunctivitis caused by allergens or irritants is not contagious
unless a secondary viral or bacterial infection develops.

Treatment of Conjunctivitis

There are times when it is important to seek medical care for conjunctivitis (pink eye), as the treatment sometimes depends on the
cause. However, this is not always necessary. To help relieve some of
the inflammation and dryness caused by conjunctivitis, you can use
cold compresses and artificial tears, which you can purchase over the
counter without a prescription. You should also stop wearing contact
lenses until your eye doctor says it's okay to start wearing them again.

When to Seek Medical Care

You should see a healthcare provider if you have conjunctivitis along with any of the following:

- pain in the eye(s)
- sensitivity to light or blurred vision that does not improve when discharge is wiped from the eye(s)
- intense redness in the eye(s)
- symptoms that get worse or don't improve, including pink eye thought to be caused by bacteria which does not improve after 24 hours of antibiotic use
- a weakened immune system, for example from human immuno-deficiency virus (HIV) infection, cancer treatment, or other medical conditions or treatments

Newborns with symptoms of conjunctivitis should see a doctor right away.

Viral Conjunctivitis

Most cases of viral conjunctivitis are mild. The infection will usually clear up in 7 to 14 days without treatment and without any long-term consequences. But in some cases, viral conjunctivitis can take 2 to 3 weeks or more to clear up.

A doctor can prescribe antiviral medication to treat more serious forms of conjunctivitis for which there is a specific treatment, such as those caused by herpes simplex virus or varicella-zoster virus. Antibiotics will not improve viral conjunctivitis; these drugs are not effective against viruses.

Bacterial Conjunctivitis

Antibiotics, usually given topically as eye drops or ointment, can help shorten the length of bacterial conjunctivitis, reduce complications, and reduce the spread of infection to others. If your doctor prescribes antibiotic eye drops or ointment, the infection should clear within several days.

However, mild bacterial conjunctivitis may get better without antibiotic treatment and without any complications. It often improves in 2 to 5 days without treatment but can last up to 2 or 3 weeks. The use of antibiotics is associated with increased antibiotic resistance and increased costs, and should be a shared decision between the doctor and the patient.

Allergic Conjunctivitis

Conjunctivitis caused by an allergen (such as pollen or animal dander) usually improves when the allergen is removed from the person's environment. Allergy medications and certain eye drops (topical antihistamine and vasoconstrictors), including some prescription eye drops, can also provide relief from allergic conjunctivitis. In some cases, a combination of drugs may be needed to improve symptoms. Your doctor can help if you have conjunctivitis caused by an allergy.

Section 21.2

Dry Eye

This section contains text excerpted from the following sources:
Text under the heading "Facts about Dry Eye" is excerpted from
"Facts about Dry Eye," National Eye Institute (NEI), February 2013.
Reviewed March 2017; Text under the heading "Condition of Dry
Eyes and Mouth" is excerpted from "Dry Eyes and Mouth?"
NIH News in Health, National Institutes of Health (NIH),
March 2012. Reviewed March 2017.

Dry Eye Basics

What Is Dry Eye?

Dry eye occurs when the eye does not produce tears properly, or when the tears are not of the correct consistency and evaporate too quickly.

In addition, inflammation of the surface of the eye may occur along with dry eye. If left untreated, this condition can lead to pain, ulcers, or scars on the cornea, and some loss of vision. However, permanent loss of vision from dry eye is uncommon.

Dry eye can make it more difficult to perform some activities, such as using a computer or reading for an extended period of time, and it can decrease tolerance for dry environments, such as the air inside an airplane.

Other names for dry eye include dry eye syndrome, keratoconjunctivitis sicca (KCS), dysfunctional tear syndrome, lacrimal keratoconjunctivitis, evaporative tear deficiency, aqueous tear deficiency, and LASIK-induced neurotrophic epitheliopathy (LNE).

What Are the Types of Dry Eye?

1. Aqueous tear-deficient dry eye is a disorder in which the lacrimal glands fail to produce enough of the watery component of tears to maintain a healthy eye surface.

2. Evaporative dry eye may result from inflammation of the meibomian glands, also located in the eyelids. These glands make the lipid or oily part of tears that slows evaporation and keeps the tears stable.

Dry eye can be associated with:

*   inflammation of the surface of the eye, the lacrimal gland, or the conjunctiva;

*   any disease process that alters the components of the tears;

*   an increase in the surface of the eye, as in thyroid disease when the eye protrudes forward;

*   cosmetic surgery, if the eyelids are opened too widely.

Frequently Asked Questions about Dry Eye

What Is the Cornea?

The cornea is the clear, dome-shaped outer surface that covers the eye in front of the iris, the colored part of the eye. The cornea helps protect the rest of the eye from germs, dust, and other harmful matter. The cornea bends, or refracts, light entering the eye, and accounts for most of the eye's total focusing power. It also serves as a filter to screen out most of the damaging ultraviolet (UV) wavelengths in sunlight.

The cornea is a highly organized, clear structure made up of a group of cells and proteins precisely arranged in layers, but it has no blood vessels to nourish or protect it against infection. Instead, it receives its nourishment from the tears and the watery fluid (aqueous humor) that fills the chamber behind it.

What Are Tears, and How Do They Relate to Dry Eye?

Tears, made by the lacrimal gland, are necessary for overall eye health and clear vision. Tears bathe the surface of the eye, keeping it moist, and wash away dust and debris. They also help protect the eye from bacterial and other types of infections.

Tears are composed of three major components:

1. outer, oily, lipid layer produced by the meibomian glands;

2. middle, watery, lacrimal layer produced by the lacrimal glands; and

3. inner, mucous or mucin layer produced by goblet cells located within a thin transparent layer over the white part of the eye and covering the inner surface of the eyelids.

Tears are made of proteins (including growth factors), electrolytes, and vitamins that are critical to maintain the health of the eye surface and to prevent infection.

Tears are constantly produced to bathe, nourish, and protect the eye surface. They are also produced in response to emergencies, such as a particle of dust in the eye, an infection or irritation of the eye, or an onset of strong emotions. When the lacrimal glands fail to produce sufficient tears, dry eye can result.

Any disease process that alters the components of tears can make them unhealthy and result in dry eye.

Symptoms of Dry Eye

Dry eye symptoms may include any of the following:

*   stinging or burning of the eye

*   a sandy or gritty feeling as if something is in the eye

*   episodes of excess tears following very dry eye periods

*   a stringy discharge from the eye

*   pain and redness of the eye

*   episodes of blurred vision

*   heavy eyelids

*   inability to cry when emotionally stressed

*   uncomfortable contact lenses

*   decreased tolerance of reading, working on the computer, or any activity that requires sustained visual attention

*   eye fatigue

NOTE: If symptoms of dry eye persist, consult an eye care professional to get an accurate diagnosis of the condition and begin treatment to avoid permanent damage.

Causes and Risk Factors

What Are the Causes of Dry Eye?

Dry eye can be a temporary or chronic condition:

- Dry eye can be a side effect of some medications, including antihistamines, nasal decongestants, tranquilizers, certain blood pressure medicines, Parkinson disease medications, birth control pills and antidepressants.

- Skin disease on or around the eyelids can result in dry eye.

- Diseases of the glands in the eyelids, such as meibomian gland dysfunction, can cause dry eye.

- Dry eye can occur in women who are pregnant.

- Women who are on hormone replacement therapy may experience dry eye symptoms. Women taking only estrogen are 70 percent more likely to experience dry eye, whereas those taking estrogen and progesterone have a 30 percent increased risk of developing dry eye.

- Dry eye can also develop after the refractive surgery known as LASIK. These symptoms generally last three to six months, but may last longer in some cases.

- Dry eye can result from chemical and thermal burns that scar the membrane lining the eyelids and covering the eye.

- Allergies can be associated with dry eye.

- Infrequent blinking, associated with staring at computer or video screens, may also lead to dry eye symptoms.

- Both excessive and insufficient dosages of vitamins can contribute to dry eye.

- Homeopathic remedies may have an adverse impact on a dry eye condition.

- Loss of sensation in the cornea from long-term contact lens wear can lead to dry eye.

- Dry eye can be associated with immune system disorders such as Sjögren syndrome, lupus, and rheumatoid arthritis. Sjögren syndrome leads to inflammation and dryness of the mouth, eyes, and other mucous membranes. It can also affect other organs, including the kidneys, lungs and blood vessels.

- Dry eye can be a symptom of chronic inflammation of the conjunctiva, the membrane lining the eyelid and covering the front part of the eye, or the lacrimal gland. Chronic conjunctivitis can be caused by certain eye diseases, infection, exposure to irritants such as chemical fumes and tobacco smoke, or drafts from air conditioning or heating.

- If the surface area of the eye is increased, as in thyroid disease when the eye protrudes forward or after cosmetic surgery if the eyelids are opened too widely, dry eye can result.

- Dry eye may occur from exposure keratitis, in which the eyelids do not close completely during sleep.

Who Is Likely to Develop Dry Eye?

Elderly people frequently experience dryness of the eyes, but dry eye can occur at any age. Nearly five million Americans 50 years of age and older are estimated to have dry eye. Of these, more than three million are women and more than one and a half million are men. Tens of millions more have less severe symptoms. Dry eye is more common after menopause. Women who experience menopause prematurely are more likely to have eye surface damage from dry eye.

Treatment of Dry Eye

How Is Dry Eye Treated?

Depending on the causes of dry eye, your doctor may use various approaches to relieve the symptoms.

Dry eye can be managed as an ongoing condition. The first priority is to determine if a disease is the underlying cause of the dry eye (such as Sjögren syndrome or lacrimal and meibomian gland dysfunction). If it is, then the underlying disease needs to be treated.

Cyclosporine, an anti-inflammatory medication, is the only prescription drug available to treat dry eye. It decreases corneal damage, increases basic tear production, and reduces symptoms of dry eye. It may take three to six months of twice-a-day dosages for the medication to work. In some cases of severe dry eye, short-term use of corticosteroid eye drops that decrease inflammation is required.

If dry eye results from taking a medication, your doctor may recommend switching to a medication that does not cause the dry eye side effect.

If contact lens wear is the problem, your eye care practitioner may recommend another type of lens or reducing the number of hours you wear your lenses. In the case of severe dry eye, your eye care professional may advise you not to wear contact lenses at all.

Another option is to plug the drainage holes, small circular openings at the inner corners of the eyelids where tears drain from the eye into the nose. Lacrimal plugs, also called punctal plugs, can be inserted painlessly by an eye care professional. The patient usually does not feel them. These plugs are made of silicone or collagen, are reversible, and are a temporary measure. In severe cases, permanent plugs may be considered.

In some cases, a simple surgery, called **punctal cautery**, is recommended to permanently close the drainage holes. The procedure helps keep the limited volume of tears on the eye for a longer period of time.

In some patients with dry eye, supplements or dietary sources (such as tuna fish) of omega-3 fatty acids (especially DHA and EPA) may decrease symptoms of irritation. The use and dosage of nutritional supplements and vitamins should be discussed with your primary medical doctor.

What Can I Do to Help Myself?

- Use artificial tears, gels, gel inserts, and ointments—available over the counter—as the first line of therapy. They offer temporary relief and provide an important replacement of naturally produced tears in patients with aqueous tear deficiency. Avoid artificial tears with preservatives if you need to apply them more than four times a day or preparations with chemicals that cause blood vessels to constrict.

- Wearing glasses or sunglasses that fit close to the face (wrap around shades) or that have side shields can help slow tear evaporation from the eye surfaces. Indoors, an air cleaner to filter dust and other particles helps prevent dry eyes. A humidifier also may help by adding moisture to the air.

- Avoid dry conditions and allow your eyes to rest when performing activities that require you to use your eyes for long periods of time. Instill lubricating eye drops while performing these tasks.

Condition of Dry Eyes and Dry Mouth

If your eyes and mouth feel as dry as a desert, there are many possible causes, such as bad air quality and certain medications. But if you have long-lasting, uncomfortable dryness in your eyes and mouth, along with fatigue or pain and swelling in some of your joints, you may have a condition called **Sjögren syndrome**.

Sjögren syndrome affects as many as 4 million people nationwide. Men and women of all ages can develop the condition, but it most often shows up in women in their 50s and 60s. The disorder is 9 times more common in women than in men.

Sjögren syndrome arises when the body's immune system, which ordinarily attacks invading bacteria and viruses, starts killing off the body's own moisture-producing cells. The condition can occur on its own or alongside other diseases, such as lupus or rheumatoid arthritis, in which the immune system mistakenly attacks parts of the body.

In some cases of Sjögren syndrome, the immune system attacks several parts of the body, including the eyes, mouth, joints and internal organs. Because the disorder has such varying effects, diagnosing Sjögren syndrome can take a long time.

"The average time to diagnose Sjögren's is about 7 years from the first symptoms, because the symptoms can be very subtle," says Dr. Gabor Illei, head of the Sjögren's Clinic on the National Institutes of Health (NIH) campus in Bethesda, Maryland.

Physicians use several tests to make a diagnosis. These include measuring tear and saliva flow, blood tests, and biopsies. In the biopsy test, a surgeon removes a small saliva-producing gland from the lip and looks at it under a microscope. The blood tests and biopsies let physicians know if the body's immune system is attacking saliva-producing cells.

Since so many of the body's systems can be affected, people with Sjögren syndrome often need to see several specialists. These can include an ophthalmologist for the eyes, an oral disease specialist or a dentist who has experience with dry mouth, and a rheumatologist, who can manage and coordinate care.

Many treatments for Sjögren syndrome aim to relieve the symptoms of dryness. For patients with mild dryness, over-the-counter artificial tears can help with dry eye. Sips of water and sugar-free candies can help with dry mouth. Because saliva usually protects teeth from decay, people with dry mouth need to be careful to avoid sugary candies, and to take care of their teeth.

Section 21.3

Peters Anomaly

This section includes text excerpted from "Peters Anomaly,"
Genetics Home Reference (GHR), National Institutes
of Health (NIH), January 2014.

Peters anomaly is characterized by eye problems that occur in an area at the front part of the eye known as the anterior segment. The anterior segment consists of structures including the lens, the colored part (iris) of the eye, and the clear covering of the eye (cornea). During development of the eye, the elements of the anterior segment form separate structures. However, in Peters anomaly, development of the anterior segment is abnormal, leading to incomplete separation of the cornea from the iris or the lens. As a result, the cornea is cloudy (opaque), which causes blurred vision. The opaque area (opacity) of the cornea varies in size and intensity from a small, faint streak to a large, white cloudy area that covers the front surface of the eye. Additionally, the location of the opacity varies; the cloudiness may be at the center of the cornea or off-center. Large, centrally located opacities tend to cause poorer vision than smaller, off-center ones.

Nearly half of the individuals affected with Peters anomaly have low vision early in life and about a quarter are legally blind. Due to a lack of visual stimulation, some individuals develop "lazy eye" (amblyopia). Peters anomaly is often associated with other eye problems, such as increased pressure within the eye (glaucoma), clouding of the lens (cataract), and unusually small eyeballs (microphthalmia). In most cases, Peters anomaly is bilateral, which means that it affects both eyes, although the level of vision impairment may be different in each eye. These individuals may have eyes that do not point in the same direction (strabismus). In some people with Peters anomaly, corneal clouding improves over time leading to improved vision.

There are two types of Peters anomaly, which are distinguished by their signs and symptoms. Peters anomaly type I is characterized by an incomplete separation of the cornea and iris and mild to moderate corneal opacity. Type II is characterized by an incomplete separation of the cornea and lens and severe corneal opacity that may involve the entire cornea.

Frequency

The exact prevalence of Peters anomaly is unknown. This condition is one of a group of disorders known as congenital corneal opacities, which affect 3 to 6 individuals per 100,000.

Genetic Changes

Mutations in the *FOXC1, PAX6, PITX2,* or *CYP1B1* gene can cause Peters anomaly. The *FOXC1, PAX6,* and *PITX2* genes are all members of a family called homeobox genes that direct the formation of many parts of the body. These three genes are involved in the development of the anterior segment of the eye. The *CYP1B1* gene provides instructions for making an enzyme that is active in many tissues, including the eye. The enzyme's role in these tissues is unclear; it is likely involved in the development of the anterior segment.

Mutations in any of these four genes disrupt development of the anterior segment of the eye. These mutations can lead to severe developmental problems, such as incomplete separation of eye structures and complete corneal opacity, or they can result in minor eye abnormalities including small, faint opacities. It is likely that mutations that cause a complete absence of protein function result in the most severe eye problems. It is unknown why both eyes are affected in some cases and in others only one eye is abnormal.

In many cases of Peters anomaly, there is no mutation identified in any of these four genes. The cause of the condition in these cases is unknown.

Inheritance Pattern

Most cases of Peters anomaly are sporadic, which means that they occur in people with no apparent history of the disorder in their family. In many of these sporadic cases the genetic cause of the condition is unknown. However, some of these cases are caused by a new mutation in one of the previously mentioned genes or by the inheritance of a mutation from unaffected parents. In rare cases, the condition (or related eye disorders) has been reported to occur in multiple members of the same family.

Whether sporadic or inherited, when Peters anomaly is caused by mutations in the *CYP1B1* gene, it follows an autosomal recessive pattern of inheritance. Autosomal recessive inheritance means both copies of the gene in each cell have mutations. The parents of an individual with an autosomal recessive condition each carry one copy of the mutated gene, but they typically do not show signs and symptoms of the condition. When caused by mutations in the *FOXC1*, *PAX6*, or *PITX2* gene, the condition follows an autosomal dominant pattern of inheritance, which means one copy of the altered gene in each cell is sufficient to cause the disorder.

Other Names for This Condition

- Irido-corneo-trabecular dysgenesis

- Peters congenital glaucoma

Section 21.4

Leukocoria

Text in this section is excerpted from "Leukocoria," © 2017 American Association for Pediatric Ophthalmology and Strabismus (AAPOS). Reprinted with permission.

What Is Leukocoria?

Leukocoria literally means "white pupil." It occurs when the pupil (the round hole in the colored part of the eye) is white rather than the usual black.

How Is Leukocoria Detected?

In more obvious cases the pupil may appear white on casual observation. In other situations the pupil may appear white only in certain circumstances such as when the pupil becomes larger in a darkened room. Sometimes leukocoria is detected from photographs when one pupil has an abnormal or "white reflex" compared to the other eye having a normal "red reflex."

What Is a Red Reflex?

When light enters the eye through the pupil, the retina absorbs most of the light. A small amount of light, however, is reflected by the retina back out of the eye through the pupil. The light is reddish-orange, reflecting the color of normal retina. The red reflex is most easily seen when the observer's line of sight is very close to the direction of illumination into the eye. An example is a camera in which the flash is mounted very close to the lens resulting in photographs with red pupillary reflexes.

The red reflex is either absent or white with leukocoria. This occurs as a result of abnormal reflection of light coming out of the eye.

How Does an Ophthalmologist Detect Leukocoria?

Ophthalmologists utilize a retinoscope to examine the red reflex from the eye and an ophthalmoscope to directly visualize the interior of the eye. Dilating eye drops are generally used to enlarge the pupil which enables a more thorough examination.

What Conditions Cause Leukocoria?

Many conditions cause leukocoria including cataract, retinal detachment, retinopathy of prematurity, retinal malformation, intraocular infection endophthalmitis), retinal vascular abnormality, and intraocular tumor (retinoblastoma).

Are Any of These Conditions Serious?

All diseases which cause leukocoria represent a serious threat to vision and some pose a threat to life. Prompt evaluation of leukocoria by an ophthalmologist is always appropriate.

How Is Leukocoria Treated?

Management of leukocoria involves treatment of the underlying condition (cataract, retinal detachment, infection, etc.) responsible for the white appearing pupil.

Part Four

Understanding and Treating Disorders of the Macula, Optic Nerve, Retina, Vitreous, and Uvea

Chapter 22

Age-Related Macular Degeneration

What is Age-Related Macular Degeneration (AMD)?

AMD is a common eye condition and a leading cause of vision loss among people age 50 and older. It causes damage to the macula, a small spot near the center of the retina and the part of the eye needed for sharp, central vision, which lets us see objects that are straight ahead.

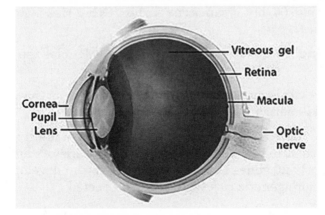

Figure 22.1. *Anatomy of the Eye*

This chapter includes text excerpted from "Facts about Age-Related Macular Degeneration," National Eye Institute (NEI), September 2015.

In some people, AMD advances so slowly that vision loss does not occur for a long time. In others, the disease progresses faster and may lead to a loss of vision in one or both eyes. As AMD progresses, a blurred area near the center of vision is a common symptom. Over time, the blurred area may grow larger or you may develop blank spots in your central vision. Objects also may not appear to be as bright as they used to be.

AMD by itself does not lead to complete blindness, with no ability to see. However, the loss of central vision in AMD can interfere with simple everyday activities, such as the ability to see faces, drive, read, write, or do close work, such as cooking or fixing things around the house.

The Macula

The macula is made up of millions of light-sensing cells that provide sharp, central vision. It is the most sensitive part of the retina, which is located at the back of the eye. The retina turns light into electrical signals and then sends these electrical signals through the optic nerve to the brain, where they are translated into the images we see. When the macula is damaged, the center of your field of view may appear blurry, distorted, or dark.

Who Is at Risk?

Age is a major risk factor for AMD. The disease is most likely to occur after age 60, but it can occur earlier. Other risk factors for AMD include:

- **Smoking.** Research shows that smoking doubles the risk of AMD.

- **Race.** AMD is more common among Caucasians than among African-Americans or Hispanics/Latinos.

- **Family history and genetics.** People with a family history of AMD are at higher risk. At last count, researchers had identified nearly 20 genes that can affect the risk of developing AMD. Many more genetic risk factors are suspected.

You may see offers for genetic testing for AMD. Because AMD is influenced by so many genes plus environmental factors such as smoking and nutrition, there are currently no genetic tests that can diagnose AMD, or predict with certainty who will develop it.

The American Academy of Ophthalmology (AAO) currently recommends against routine genetic testing for AMD, and insurance generally does not cover such testing.

Does Lifestyle Make a Difference?

Researchers have found links between AMD and some lifestyle choices, such as smoking. You might be able to reduce your risk of AMD or slow its progression by making these healthy choices:

- Avoid smoking.

- Exercise regularly.

- Maintain normal blood pressure and cholesterol levels.

- Eat a healthy diet rich in green, leafy vegetables and fish.

How Is AMD Detected?

The early and intermediate stages of AMD usually start without symptoms. Only a comprehensive dilated eye exam can detect AMD. The eye exam may include the following:

- **Visual acuity test.** This eye chart measures how well you see at distances.

- **Dilated eye exam.** Your eye care professional places drops in your eyes to widen or dilate the pupils. This provides a better view of the back of your eye. Using a special magnifying lens, he or she then looks at your retina and optic nerve for signs of AMD and other eye problems.

- **Amsler grid.** Your eye care professional also may ask you to look at an Amsler grid. Changes in your central vision may cause the lines in the grid to disappear or appear wavy, a sign of AMD.

- **Fluorescein angiogram.** In this test, which is performed by an ophthalmologist, a fluorescent dye is injected into your arm. Pictures are taken as the dye passes through the blood vessels in your eye. This makes it possible to see leaking blood vessels, which occur in a severe, rapidly progressive type of AMD. In rare cases, complications to the injection can arise, from nausea to more severe allergic reactions.

- **Optical coherence tomography (OCT).** You have probably heard of ultrasound, which uses sound waves to capture images of living tissues. OCT is similar except that it uses light waves, and can achieve very high-resolution images of any tissues that can be penetrated by light—such as the eyes. After your eyes are dilated, you'll be asked to place your head on a chin rest and hold still for several seconds while the images are obtained. The light beam is painless.

During the exam, your eye care professional will look for *drusen*, which are yellow deposits beneath the retina. Most people develop some very small *drusen* as a normal part of aging. The presence of medium-to-large drusen may indicate that you have AMD.

Another sign of AMD is the appearance of pigmentary changes under the retina. In addition to the pigmented cells in the iris (the colored part of the eye), there are pigmented cells beneath the retina. As these cells break down and release their pigment, your eye care professional may see dark clumps of released pigment and later, areas that are less pigmented. These changes will not affect your eye color.

Questions to Ask Your Eye Care Professional

Below are a few questions you may want to ask your eye care professional to help you understand your diagnosis and treatment. If you do not understand your eye care professional's responses, ask questions until you do understand.

- What is my diagnosis and how do you spell the name of the condition?

- Can my AMD be treated?

- How will this condition affect my vision now and in the future?

- What symptoms should I watch for and how should I notify you if they occur?

- Should I make lifestyle changes?

What Are the Stages of AMD?

There are three stages of AMD defined in part by the size and number of *drusen* under the retina. It is possible to have AMD in one eye only, or to have one eye with a later stage of AMD than the other.

- **Early AMD.** Early AMD is diagnosed by the presence of medium-sized *drusen*, which are about the width of an average human hair. People with early AMD typically do not have vision loss.

- **Intermediate AMD.** People with intermediate AMD typically have large *drusen*, pigment changes in the retina, or both. Again, these changes can only be detected during an eye exam. Intermediate AMD may cause some vision loss, but most people will not experience any symptoms.

- **Late AMD.** In addition to *drusen*, people with late AMD have vision loss from damage to the macula. There are two types of late AMD:

  - In geographic atrophy (also called dry AMD), there is a gradual breakdown of the light-sensitive cells in the macula that convey visual information to the brain, and of the supporting tissue beneath the macula. These changes cause vision loss.

  - In neovascular AMD (also called wet AMD), abnormal blood vessels grow underneath the retina. ("Neovascular" literally means "new vessels.") These vessels can leak fluid and blood, which may lead to swelling and damage of the macula. The damage may be rapid and severe, unlike the more gradual course of geographic atrophy. It is possible to have both geographic atrophy and neovascular AMD in the same eye, and either condition can appear first.

AMD has few symptoms in the early stages, so it is important to have your eyes examined regularly. If you are at risk for AMD because of age, family history, lifestyle, or some combination of these factors, you should not wait to experience changes in vision before getting checked for AMD.

Not everyone with early AMD will develop late AMD. For people who have early AMD in one eye and no signs of AMD in the other eye, about five percent will develop advanced AMD after 10 years. For people who have early AMD in both eyes, about 14 percent will develop late AMD in at least one eye after 10 years. With prompt detection of AMD, there are steps you can take to further reduce your risk of vision loss from late AMD.

If you have late AMD in one eye only, you may not notice any changes in your overall vision. With the other eye seeing clearly, you may still be able to drive, read, and see fine details. However, having late AMD in one eye means you are at increased risk for late AMD in your other eye. If you notice distortion or blurred vision, even if it doesn't have much effect on your daily life, consult an eye care professional.

How Is AMD Treated?

Early AMD

Currently, no treatment exists for early AMD, which in many people shows no symptoms or loss of vision. Your eye care professional may recommend that you get a comprehensive dilated eye exam at least once a year. The exam will help determine if your condition is advancing.

As for prevention, AMD occurs less often in people who exercise, avoid smoking, and eat nutritious foods including green leafy vegetables and fish. If you already have AMD, adopting some of these habits may help you keep your vision longer.

Intermediate and Late AMD

Researchers at the National Eye Institute (NEI) tested whether taking nutritional supplements could protect against AMD in the Age-Related Eye Disease Studies (AREDS and AREDS2). They found that daily intake of certain high-dose vitamins and minerals can slow progression of the disease in people who have intermediate AMD, and those who have late AMD in one eye.

The first AREDS trial showed that a combination of vitamin C, vitamin E, beta-carotene, zinc, and copper can reduce the risk of late AMD by 25 percent. The AREDS2 trial tested whether this formulation could be improved by adding lutein, zeaxanthin or omega-3 fatty acids. Omega-3 fatty acids are nutrients enriched in fish oils. Lutein, zeaxanthin, and beta-carotene all belong to the same family of vitamins, and are abundant in green leafy vegetables.

The AREDS2 trial found that adding lutein and zeaxanthin or omega-three fatty acids to the original AREDS formulation (with beta-carotene) had no overall effect on the risk of late AMD. However, the trial also found that replacing beta-carotene with a 5-to-1 mixture of lutein and zeaxanthin may help further reduce the risk of late AMD. Moreover, while beta-carotene has been linked to an increased risk of lung cancer in current and former smokers, lutein and zeaxanthin appear to be safe regardless of smoking status.

Here are the clinically effective doses tested in AREDS and AREDS2:

- 500 milligrams (mg) of vitamin C

- 400 international units of vitamin E

- 80 mg zinc as zinc oxide (25 mg in AREDS2)

- 2 mg copper as cupric oxide

- 15 mg beta-carotene, OR 10 mg lutein and 2 mg zeaxanthin

A number of manufacturers offer nutritional supplements that were formulated based on these studies. The label may refer to "AREDS" or "AREDS2."

If you have intermediate or late AMD, you might benefit from taking such supplements. But first, be sure to review and compare the labels. Many of the supplements have different ingredients, or different doses, from those tested in the AREDS trials. Also, consult your doctor or eye care professional about which supplement, if any, is right for you. For example, if you smoke regularly, or used to, your doctor may recommend that you avoid supplements containing beta-carotene.

Even if you take a daily multivitamin, you should consider taking an AREDS supplement if you are at risk for late AMD. The formulations tested in the AREDS trials contain much higher doses of vitamins and minerals than what is found in multivitamins. Tell your doctor or eye care professional about any multivitamins you are taking when you are discussing possible AREDS formulations.

You may see claims that your specific genetic makeup (genotype) can influence how you will respond to AREDS supplements. Some studies have claimed that, depending on genotype, some patients will benefit from AREDS supplements and others could be harmed. These claims are based on a portion of data from the AREDS research. NEI investigators have done comprehensive analyses of the complete AREDS data. Their findings to date indicate that AREDS supplements are beneficial for patients of all tested genotypes. Based on the overall data, the AAO does not support the use of genetic testing to guide treatment for AMD.

Finally, remember that the AREDS formulation is not a cure. It does not help people with early AMD, and will not restore vision already lost from AMD. But it may delay the onset of late AMD. It also may help slow vision loss in people who already have late AMD.

Advanced Neovascular AMD

Neovascular AMD typically results in severe vision loss. However, eye care professionals can try different therapies to stop further vision loss. You should remember that the therapies described below are not a cure. The condition may progress even with treatment.

- **Injections.** One option to slow the progression of neovascular AMD is to inject drugs into the eye. With neovascular AMD, abnormally high levels of vascular endothelial growth factor (VEGF) are secreted in your eyes. VEGF is a protein that promotes the growth of new abnormal blood vessels. Anti-VEGF injection therapy blocks this growth. If you get this treatment, you may need multiple monthly injections. Before each injection, your eye will be numbed and cleaned with antiseptics. To further reduce the risk of infection, you may be prescribed antibiotic drops. A few different anti-VEGF drugs are available. They vary in cost and in how often they need to be injected, so you may wish to discuss these issues with your eye care professional.

- **Photodynamic therapy.** This technique involves laser treatment of select areas of the retina. First, a drug called verteporfin will be injected into a vein in your arm. The drug travels through the blood vessels in your body, and is absorbed by new, growing blood vessels. Your eye care professional then shines a laser beam into your eye to activate the drug in the new abnormal blood vessels, while sparing normal ones. Once activated, the drug closes off the new blood vessels, slows their growth, and slows the rate of vision loss. This procedure is less common than anti-VEGF injections, and is often used in combination with them for specific types of neovascular AMD.

- **Laser surgery.** Eye care professionals treat certain cases of neovascular AMD with laser surgery, though this is less common than other treatments. It involves aiming an intense "hot" laser at the abnormal blood vessels in your eyes to destroy them. This laser is not the same one used in photodynamic therapy which may be referred to as a "cold" laser. This treatment is more likely to be used when blood vessel growth is limited to a compact area in your eye, away from the center of the macula, that can be easily targeted with the laser. Even so, laser treatment also may destroy some surrounding healthy tissue. This often results in a small blind spot where the laser has scarred the retina. In some cases, vision immediately after the surgery may be worse than it was before. But the surgery may also help prevent more severe vision loss from occurring years later.

Questions to Ask Your Eye Care Professional about Treatment

- What is the treatment for advanced neovascular AMD?

- When will treatment start and how long will it last?

- What are the benefits of this treatment and how successful is it?

- What are the risks and side effects associated with this treatment and how has this information been gathered?

- Should I avoid certain foods, drugs, or activities while I am undergoing treatment?

- Are other treatments available?

- When should I follow up after treatment?

Loss of Vision

Coping with AMD and vision loss can be a traumatic experience. This is especially true if you have just begun to lose your vision or have low vision. Having low vision means that even with regular glasses, contact lenses, medicine, or surgery, you find everyday tasks difficult to do. Reading the mail, shopping, cooking, and writing can all seem challenging.

However, help is available. You may not be able to restore your vision, but low vision services can help you make the most of what is remaining. You can continue enjoying friends, family, hobbies, and other interests just as you always have. The key is to not delay use of these services.

What Is Vision Rehabilitation?

To cope with vision loss, you must first have an excellent support team. This team should include you, your primary eye care professional, and an optometrist or ophthalmologist specializing in low vision. Occupational therapists, orientation and mobility specialists, certified low vision therapists, counselors, and social workers are also available to help. Together, the low vision team can help you make the most of your remaining vision and maintain your independence.

Second, talk with your eye care professional about your vision problems. Ask about vision rehabilitation, even if your eye care professional says that "nothing more can be done for your vision." Vision rehabilitation programs offer a wide range of services, including training for magnifying and adaptive devices, ways to complete daily living skills safely and independently, guidance on modifying your home, and information on where to locate resources and support to help you cope with your vision loss.

Medicare may cover part or all of a patient's occupational therapy, but the therapy must be ordered by a doctor and provided by a Medicare-approved healthcare provider. To see if you are eligible for Medicare-funded occupational therapy, call 800-MEDICARE or 800-633-4227.

Where to Go for Services

Low vision services can take place in different locations, including:

- ophthalmology or optometry offices that specialize in low vision
- hospital clinics
- state, nonprofit, or for-profit vision rehabilitation organizations
- independent-living centers

What Are Some Low Vision Devices?

Because low vision varies from person to person, specialists have different tools to help patients deal with vision loss. They include:

- reading glasses with high-powered lenses
- handheld magnifiers
- video magnifiers
- computers with large-print and speech-output systems
- large-print reading materials
- talking watches, clocks, and calculators
- computer aids and other technologies, such as a closed-circuit television, which uses a camera and television to enlarge printed text

For some patients with end-stage AMD, an Implantable Miniature Telescope (IMT) may be an option. This U.S. Food and Drug Administration (FDA)-approved device can help restore some lost vision by re-focusing images onto a healthier part of the retina. After the surgery to implant the IMT, patients participate in an extensive vision rehabilitation program.

Keep in mind that low vision aids without proper diagnosis, evaluation, and training may not work for you. It is important that you work closely with your low vision team to get the best device or combination of aids to help improve your ability to see.

Questions to Ask Your Eye Care Professional about Low Vision

- How can I continue my normal, routine activities?
- Are there resources to help me?
- Will any special devices help me with reading, cooking, or fixing things around the house?
- What training is available to me?
- Where can I find individual or group support to cope with my vision loss?

Charles Bonnet Syndrome (Visual Hallucinations)

People with impaired vision sometimes see things that are not there, called visual hallucinations. They may see simple patterns of colors or shapes, or detailed pictures of people, animals, buildings, or landscapes. Sometimes these images fit logically into a visual scene, but they often do not.

This condition can be alarming, but don't worry—it is not a sign of mental illness. It is called Charles Bonnet syndrome, and it is similar to what happens to some people who have lost an arm or leg. Even though the limb is gone, these people still feel their toes or fingers or experience itching. Similarly, when the brain loses input from the eyes, it may fill the void by generating visual images on its own.

Charles Bonnet syndrome is a common side effect of vision loss in people with AMD. However, it often goes away a year to 18 months after it begins. In the meantime, there are things you can do to reduce hallucinations. Many people find the hallucinations occur more frequently in evening or dim light. Turning on a light or television may help. It may also help to blink, close your eyes, or focus on a real object for a few moments.

Coping with AMD

AMD and vision loss can profoundly affect your life. This is especially true if you lose your vision rapidly.

Even if you experience gradual vision loss, you may not be able to live your life the way you used to. You may need to cut back on working, volunteering, and recreational activities. Your relationships may change, and you may need more help from family and friends than you are used to. These changes can lead to feelings of loss, lowered self-esteem, isolation, and depression.

In addition to getting medical treatment for AMD, there are things you can do to cope:

- Learn more about your vision loss.

- Visit a specialist in low vision and get devices and learning skills to help you with the tasks of everyday living.

- Try to stay positive. People who remain hopeful say they are better able to cope with AMD and vision loss.

- Stay engaged with family and friends.

- Seek a professional counselor or support group. Your doctor or eye care professional may be able to refer you to one.

Information for Family Members

Shock, disbelief, depression, and anger are common reactions among people who are diagnosed with AMD. These feelings can subside after a few days or weeks, or they may last longer. This can be upsetting to family members and caregivers who are trying to be as caring and supportive as possible.

Following are some ideas family members might consider:

- Obtain as much information as possible about AMD and how it affects sight. Share the information with the person who has AMD.

- Find support groups and other resources within the community.

- Encourage family and friends to visit and support the person with AMD.

- Allow for grieving. This is a natural process.

- Lend support by "being there."

Chapter 23

Other Macular Disorders

Chapter Contents

Section 23.1

Macular Hole

This section includes text excerpted from "Facts about
Macular Hole," National Eye Institute (NEI), April 2012;
Reviewed March 2017.

Macular Hole Basics

What Is a Macular Hole?

A macular hole is a small break in the macula, located in the center of the eye's light-sensitive tissue called the retina. The macula provides the sharp, central vision we need for reading, driving, and seeing fine detail.

A macular hole can cause blurred and distorted central vision. Macular holes are related to aging and usually occur in people over age 60.

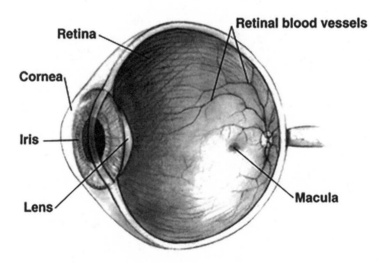

Figure 23.1. *Illustration of the Eye with Retina, Retinal Blood Vessels, Cornea, Iris, Lens, and Macula*

Are There Different Types of a Macular Hole?

Yes. There are three stages to a macular hole:

- Foveal detachments (Stage I). Without treatment, about half of Stage I macular holes will progress.
- Partial-thickness holes (Stage II). Without treatment, about 70 percent of Stage II macular holes will progress.
- Full-thickness holes (Stage III).

The size of the hole and its location on the retina determine how much it will affect a person's vision. When a Stage III macular hole develops, most central and detailed vision can be lost. If left untreated, a macular hole can lead to a detached retina, a sight-threatening condition that should receive immediate medical attention.

Is a Macular Hole the Same as Age-Related Macular Degeneration?

No. Macular holes and age-related macular degeneration are two separate and distinct conditions, although the symptoms for each are similar. Both conditions are common in people 60 and over. An eye care professional will know the difference.

Causes and Risk Factors

What Causes a Macular Hole?

Most of the eye's interior is filled with vitreous, a gel-like substance that fills about 80 percent of the eye and helps it maintain a round shape. The vitreous contains millions of fine fibers that are attached to the surface of the retina. As we age, the vitreous slowly shrinks and pulls away from the retinal surface. Natural fluids fill the area where the vitreous has contracted. This is normal. In most cases, there are no adverse effects. Some patients may experience a small increase in floaters, which are little "cobwebs" or specks that seem to float about in your field of vision.

However, if the vitreous is firmly attached to the retina when it pulls away, it can tear the retina and create a macular hole. Also, once the vitreous has pulled away from the surface of the retina, some of the fibers can remain on the retinal surface and can contract. This increases tension on the retina and can lead to a macular hole. In either case, the fluid that has replaced the shrunken vitreous can then seep through the hole onto the macula, blurring and distorting central vision.

Macular holes can also occur in other eye disorders, such as high myopia (nearsightedness), injury to the eye, retinal detachment, and, rarely, macular pucker.

Is My Other Eye at Risk?

If a macular hole exists in one eye, there is a 10–15 percent chance that a macular hole will develop in your other eye over your lifetime. Your doctor can discuss this with you.

Symptoms of Macular Hole

Macular holes often begin gradually. In the early stage of a macular hole, people may notice a slight distortion or blurriness in their straight-ahead vision. Straight lines or objects can begin to look bent or wavy. Reading and performing other routine tasks with the affected eye become difficult.

Treatment of Macular Hole

How Is a Macular Hole Treated?

Although some macular holes can seal themselves and require no treatment, surgery is necessary in many cases to help improve vision. In this surgical procedure—called a vitrectomy—the vitreous gel is removed to prevent it from pulling on the retina and replaced with a bubble containing a mixture of air and gas. The bubble acts as an internal, temporary bandage that holds the edge of the macular hole in place as it heals. Surgery is performed under local anesthesia and often on an outpatient basis.

Following surgery, patients must remain in a face-down position, normally for a day or two but sometimes for as long as two-to-three weeks. This position allows the bubble to press against the macula and be gradually reabsorbed by the eye, sealing the hole. As the bubble is reabsorbed, the vitreous cavity refills with natural eye fluids.

Maintaining a face-down position is crucial to the success of the surgery. Because this position can be difficult for many people, it is important to discuss this with your doctor before surgery.

What Are the Risks of Surgery?

The most common risk following macular hole surgery is an increase in the rate of cataract development. In most patients, a cataract can progress rapidly, and often becomes severe enough to require removal. Other less common complications include infection and retinal detachment either during surgery or afterward, both of which can be immediately treated.

For a few months after surgery, patients are not permitted to travel by air. Changes in air pressure may cause the bubble in the eye to expand, increasing pressure inside the eye.

How Successful Is This Surgery?

Vision improvement varies from patient to patient. People that have had a macular hole for less than six months have a better chance of recovering vision than those who have had one for a longer period. Discuss vision recovery with your doctor before your surgery. Vision recovery can continue for as long as three months after surgery.

What If I Cannot Remain in a Face-Down Position after the Surgery?

If you cannot remain in a face-down position for the required period after surgery, vision recovery may not be successful. People who are unable to remain in a face-down position for this length of time may not be good candidates for a vitrectomy. However, there are a number of devices that can make the "face-down" recovery period easier on you. There are also some approaches that can decrease the amount of "face-down" time. Discuss these with your doctor.

Section 23.2

Macular Pucker

This section includes text excerpted from "Macular Pucker," National
Eye Institute (NEI), April 2012; Reviewed March 2017.

Macular Pucker Defined

A macular pucker is scar tissue that has formed on the eye's macula, located in the center of the light-sensitive tissue called the retina. The macula provides the sharp, central vision we need for reading, driving, and seeing fine detail. A macular pucker can cause blurred and distorted central vision.

Macular pucker is also known as epiretinal membrane, preretinal membrane, cellophane maculopathy, retina wrinkle, surface wrinkling retinopathy, premacular fibrosis, and internal limiting membrane disease.

Frequently Asked Questions about Macular Pucker

Is a Macular Pucker the Same as Age-Related Macular Degeneration?

No. A macular pucker and age-related macular degeneration are two separate and distinct conditions, although the symptoms for each are similar. An eye care professional will know the difference.

Can Macular Pucker Get Worse?

For most people, vision remains stable and does not get progressively worse. Usually macular pucker affects one eye, although it may affect the other eye later.

Is a Macular Pucker Similar to a Macular Hole?

Although both have similar symptoms—distorted and blurred vision—macular pucker and a macular hole are different conditions. They both result from tugging on the retina from a shrinking vitreous. When the vitreous separates from the retina, usually as part of the aging process, it can cause microscopic damage to the retina. As the retina heals itself, the resulting scar tissue can cause a macular pucker. Rarely, a macular pucker will develop into a macular hole. An eye care professional can readily tell the difference between macular pucker and macular hole.

Cause of Macular Pucker

Most of the eye's interior is filled with vitreous, a gel-like substance that fills about 80 percent of the eye and helps it maintain a round shape. The vitreous contains millions of fine fibers that are attached to the surface of the retina. As we age, the vitreous slowly shrinks and pulls away from the retinal surface. This is called a vitreous detachment, and is normal. In most cases, there are no adverse effects, except for a small increase in floaters, which are little "cobwebs" or specks that seem to float about in your field of vision.

However, sometimes when the vitreous pulls away from the retina, there is microscopic damage to the retina's surface (Note: This is not a macular hole). When this happens, the retina begins a healing process to the damaged area and forms scar tissue, or an epiretinal membrane, on the surface of the retina. This scar tissue is firmly attached to the retina surface. When the scar tissue contracts, it causes the retina to wrinkle, or pucker, usually without any effect on central vision. However, if the scar tissue has formed over the macula, our sharp, central vision becomes blurred and distorted.

Symptoms of Macular Pucker

Vision loss from a macular pucker can vary from no loss to severe loss, although severe vision loss is uncommon. People with a macular pucker may notice that their vision is blurry or mildly distorted, and straight lines can appear wavy. They may have difficulty in seeing fine detail and reading small print. There may be a gray area in the center of your vision, or perhaps even a blind spot.

Treatment of Macular Pucker

How Is a Macular Pucker Treated?

A macular pucker usually requires no treatment. In many cases, the symptoms of vision distortion and blurriness are mild, and no treatment is necessary. People usually adjust to the mild visual distortion, since it does not affect activities of daily life, such as reading and driving. Neither eye drops, medications, nor nutritional supplements will improve vision distorted from macular pucker. Sometimes the scar tissue—which causes a macular pucker—separates from the retina, and the macular pucker clears up.

Rarely, vision deteriorates to the point where it affects daily routine activities. However, when this happens, surgery may be recommended. This procedure is called a vitrectomy, in which the vitreous gel is removed to prevent it from pulling on the retina and replaced with a salt solution (Because the vitreous is mostly water, you will notice no change between the salt solution and the normal vitreous). Also, the scar tissue which causes the wrinkling is removed. A vitrectomy is usually performed under local anesthesia.

After the operation, you will need to wear an eye patch for a few days or weeks to protect the eye. You will also need to use medicated eye drops to protect against infection.

How Successful Is This Surgery?

Surgery to repair a macular pucker is very delicate, and while vision improves in most cases, it does not usually return to normal. On average, about half of the vision lost from a macular pucker is restored; some people have significantly more vision restored, some less. In most cases, vision distortion is significantly reduced. Recovery of vision can take up to three months. Patients should talk with their eye care professional about whether treatment is appropriate.

What Are the Risks of Surgery?

The most common complication of a vitrectomy is an increase in the rate of cataract development. Cataract surgery may be needed within a few years after the vitrectomy. Other, less common complications are retinal detachment either during or after surgery, and infection after surgery. Also, the macular pucker may grow back, but this is rare.

Chapter 24

Glaucoma

Glaucoma Basics

What Is Glaucoma?

Glaucoma is a group of diseases that damage the eye's optic nerve and can result in vision loss and blindness. However, with early detection and treatment, you can often protect your eyes against serious vision loss.

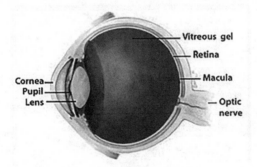

Figure 24.1. *The Optic Nerve*

The optic nerve is a bundle of more than 1 million nerve fibers. It connects the retina to the brain. The retina is the light-sensitive tissue at the back of the eye. A healthy optic nerve is necessary for good vision.

This chapter includes text excerpted from "Facts about Glaucoma," National Eye Institute (NEI), November 14, 2014.

How Does the Optic Nerve Get Damaged by Open-Angle Glaucoma?

Several large studies have shown that eye pressure is a major risk factor for optic nerve damage. In the front of the eye is a space called the anterior chamber. A clear fluid flows continuously in and out of the chamber and nourishes nearby tissues. The fluid leaves the chamber at the open angle where the cornea and iris meet. (See Figure 24.2.) When the fluid reaches the angle, it flows through a spongy meshwork, like a drain, and leaves the eye.

In open-angle glaucoma, even though the drainage angle is "open," the fluid passes too slowly through the meshwork drain. Since the fluid builds up, the pressure inside the eye rises to a level that may damage the optic nerve. When the optic nerve is damaged from increased pressure, open-angle glaucoma—and vision loss—may result. That's why controlling pressure inside the eye is important.

Another risk factor for optic nerve damage relates to blood pressure. Thus, it is important to also make sure that your blood pressure is at a proper level for your body by working with your medical doctor.

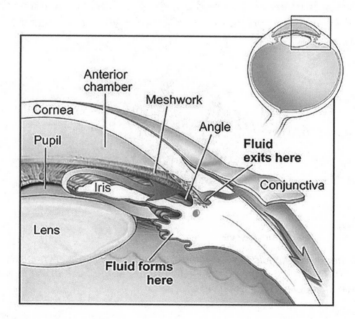

Figure 24.2. *Fluid Pathway*

Can I Develop Glaucoma If I Have Increased Eye Pressure?

Not necessarily. Not every person with increased eye pressure will develop glaucoma. Some people can tolerate higher levels of eye pressure better than others. Also, a certain level of eye pressure may be high for one person but normal for another.

Whether you develop glaucoma depends on the level of pressure your optic nerve can tolerate without being damaged. This level is different for each person. That's why a comprehensive dilated eye exam is very important. It can help your eye care professional determine what level of eye pressure is normal for you.

Can I Develop Glaucoma without an Increase in My Eye Pressure?

Yes. Glaucoma can develop without increased eye pressure. This form of glaucoma is called low-tension or normal-tension glaucoma. It is a type of open-angle glaucoma.

Who Is at Risk for Open-Angle Glaucoma?

Anyone can develop glaucoma. Some people, listed below, are at higher risk than others:

• African Americans over age 40

• everyone over age 60, especially Mexican Americans

• people with a family history of glaucoma

A comprehensive dilated eye exam can reveal more risk factors, such as high eye pressure, thinness of the cornea, and abnormal optic nerve anatomy. In some people with certain combinations of these high-risk factors, medicines in the form of eye drops reduce the risk of developing glaucoma by about half.

Symptoms of Glaucoma

At first, open-angle glaucoma has no symptoms. It causes no pain. Vision stays normal. Glaucoma can develop in one or both eyes.

Without treatment, people with glaucoma will slowly lose their peripheral (side) vision. As glaucoma remains untreated, people may miss objects to the side and out of the corner of their eye. They seem to be looking through a tunnel. Over time, straight-ahead (central) vision may decrease until no vision remains.

How Is Glaucoma Detected?

Glaucoma is detected through a comprehensive dilated eye exam that includes the following:

- **Visual acuity test.** This eye chart test measures how well you see at various distances.

- **Visual field test.** This test measures your peripheral vision. It helps your eye care professional tell if you have lost peripheral vision, a sign of glaucoma.

- **Dilated eye exam.** In this exam, drops are placed in your eyes to widen, or dilate, the pupils. Your eye care professional uses a special magnifying lens to examine your retina and optic nerve for signs of damage and other eye problems. After the exam, your close-up vision may remain blurred for several hours.

- **Tonometry** is the measurement of pressure inside the eye by using an instrument called a tonometer. Numbing drops may be applied to your eye for this test. A tonometer measures pressure inside the eye to detect glaucoma.

- **Pachymetry** is the measurement of the thickness of your cornea. Your eye care professional applies a numbing drop to your eye and uses an ultrasonic wave instrument to measure the thickness of your cornea.

Can Glaucoma Be Cured?

No. There is no cure for glaucoma. Vision lost from the disease cannot be restored.

Treatments of Glaucoma

Immediate treatment for early-stage, open-angle glaucoma can delay progression of the disease. That's why early diagnosis is very important.

Glaucoma treatments include medicines, laser trabeculoplasty, conventional surgery, or a combination of any of these. While these treatments may save remaining vision, they do not improve sight already lost from glaucoma.

Medicines. Medicines, in the form of eye drops or pills, are the most common early treatment for glaucoma. Taken regularly, these eye-drops lower eye pressure. Some medicines cause the eye to make less fluid. Others lower pressure by helping fluid drain from the eye.

Before you begin glaucoma treatment, tell your eye care professional about other medicines and supplements that you are taking. Sometimes the drops can interfere with the way other medicines work.

Glaucoma medicines need to be taken regularly as directed by your eye care professional. Most people have no problems. However, some medicines can cause headaches or other side effects. For example, drops may cause stinging, burning, and redness in the eyes.

Many medicines are available to treat glaucoma. If you have problems with one medicine, tell your eye care professional. Treatment with a different dose or a new medicine may be possible.

Because glaucoma often has no symptoms, people may be tempted to stop taking, or may forget to take, their medicine. You need to use the drops or pills as long as they help control your eye pressure. Regular use is very important.

Make sure your eye care professional shows you how to put the drops into your eye.

Laser trabeculoplasty. Laser trabeculoplasty helps fluid drain out of the eye. Your doctor may suggest this step at any time. In many cases, you will need to keep taking glaucoma medicines after this procedure.

Laser trabeculoplasty is performed in your doctor's office or eye clinic. Before the surgery, numbing drops are applied to your eye. As you sit facing the laser machine, your doctor holds a special lens to your eye. A high-intensity beam of light is aimed through the lens and reflected onto the meshwork inside your eye. You may see flashes of bright green or red light. The laser makes several evenly spaced burns that stretch the drainage holes in the meshwork. This allows the fluid to drain better.

Like any surgery, laser surgery can cause side effects, such as inflammation. Your doctor may give you some drops to take home for any soreness or inflammation inside the eye. You will need to make several follow-up visits to have your eye pressure and eye monitored.

If you have glaucoma in both eyes, usually only one eye will be treated at a time. Laser treatments for each eye will be scheduled several days to several weeks apart.

Studies show that laser surgery can be very good at reducing the pressure in some patients. However, its effects can wear off over time. Your doctor may suggest further treatment.

Conventional surgery. Conventional surgery makes a new opening for the fluid to leave the eye. (See Figure 24.3.) Your doctor may suggest this treatment at any time. Conventional surgery often is done after medicines and laser surgery have failed to control pressure.

Conventional surgery, called trabeculectomy, is performed in an operating room. Before the surgery, you are given medicine to help you relax. Your doctor makes small injections around the eye to numb it. A small piece of tissue is removed to create a new channel for the fluid to drain from the eye. This fluid will drain between the eye tissue layers and create a blister-like "filtration bleb."

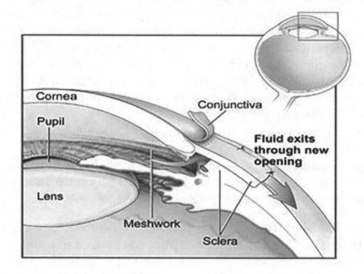

Figure 24.3. *Conventional Surgery*

Conventional surgery makes a new opening for the fluid to leave the eye.

For several weeks after the surgery, you must put drops in the eye to fight infection and inflammation. These drops will be different from those you may have been using before surgery.

Conventional surgery is performed on one eye at a time. Usually the operations are four to six weeks apart.

Conventional surgery is about 60 to 80 percent effective at lowering eye pressure. If the new drainage opening narrows, a second operation may be needed. Conventional surgery works best if you have not had previous eye surgery, such as a cataract operation.

Sometimes after conventional surgery, your vision may not be as good as it was before conventional surgery. Conventional surgery can cause side effects, including cataract, problems with the cornea, inflammation, infection inside the eye, or low eye pressure problems. If you have any of these problems, tell your doctor so a treatment plan can be developed.

What Are Some Other Forms of Glaucoma and How Are They Treated?

Open-angle glaucoma is the most common form. Some people have other types of the disease.

In **low-tension** or **normal-tension glaucoma**, optic nerve damage and narrowed side vision occur in people with normal eye pressure. Lowering eye pressure at least 30 percent through medicines slows the disease in some people. Glaucoma may worsen in others despite low pressures.

A comprehensive medical history is important to identify other potential risk factors, such as low blood pressure, that contribute to low-tension glaucoma. If no risk factors are identified, the treatment options for low-tension glaucoma are the same as for open-angle glaucoma.

In **angle-closure glaucoma**, the fluid at the front of the eye cannot drain through the angle and leave the eye. The angle gets blocked by part of the iris. People with this type of glaucoma may have a sudden increase in eye pressure. Symptoms include severe pain and nausea, as well as redness of the eye and blurred vision. If you have these symptoms, you need to seek treatment immediately. **This is a medical emergency**. If your doctor is unavailable, go to the nearest hospital or clinic. Without treatment to restore the flow of fluid, the eye can become blind. Usually, prompt laser surgery and medicines can clear the blockage, lower eye pressure, and protect vision.

In **congenital glaucoma**, children are born with a defect in the angle of the eye that slows the normal drainage of fluid. These children usually have obvious symptoms, such as cloudy eyes, sensitivity to light, and excessive tearing. Conventional surgery typically is the suggested treatment, because medicines are not effective and can cause more serious side effects in infants and be difficult to administer. Surgery is safe and effective. If surgery is done promptly, these children usually have an excellent chance of having good vision.

Secondary glaucomas can develop as complications of other medical conditions. For example, a severe form of glaucoma is called neovascular glaucoma, and can be a result from poorly controlled diabetes or high blood pressure. Other types of glaucoma sometimes occur with cataract, certain eye tumors, or when the eye is inflamed or irritated by a condition called uveitis. Sometimes glaucoma develops after other eye surgeries or serious eye injuries. Steroid drugs used to treat eye inflammations and other diseases can trigger glaucoma in some people. There are two eye conditions known to cause secondary forms of glaucoma.

Pigmentary glaucoma occurs when pigment from the iris sheds off and blocks the meshwork, slowing fluid drainage.

Pseudoexfoliation glaucoma occurs when extra material is produced and shed off internal eye structures and blocks the meshwork, again slowing fluid drainage.

Depending on the cause of these secondary glaucomas, treatment includes medicines, laser surgery, or conventional or other glaucoma surgery.

What You Can Do

If you are being treated for glaucoma, be sure to take your glaucoma medicine every day. See your eye care professional regularly.

You also can help protect the vision of family members and friends who may be at high risk for glaucoma—African Americans over age 40; everyone over age 60, especially Mexican Americans; and people with a family history of the disease. Encourage them to have a comprehensive dilated eye exam at least once every two years. Remember that lowering eye pressure in the early stages of glaucoma slows progression of the disease and helps save vision.

Medicare covers an annual comprehensive dilated eye exam for some people at high risk for glaucoma. These people include those with diabetes, those with a family history of glaucoma, and African Americans age 50 and older.

What Should I Ask My Eye Care Professional?

You can protect yourself against vision loss by working in partnership with your eye care professional. Ask questions and get the information you need to take care of yourself and your family.

What Are Some Questions to Ask?

About my eye disease or disorder...

- What is my diagnosis?
- What caused my condition?

- Can my condition be treated?

- How will this condition affect my vision now and in the future?

- Should I watch for any particular symptoms and notify you if they occur?

- Should I make any lifestyle changes?

About my treatment...

- What is the treatment for my condition?

- When will the treatment start and how long will it last?

- What are the benefits of this treatment and how successful is it?

- What are the risks and side effects associated with this treatment?

- Are there foods, medicines, or activities I should avoid while I'm on this treatment?

- If my treatment includes taking medicine, what should I do if I miss a dose?

- Are other treatments available?

About my tests...

- What kinds of tests will I have?

- What can I expect to find out from these tests?

- When will I know the results?

- Do I have to do anything special to prepare for any of the tests?

- Do these tests have any side effects or risks?

- Will I need more tests later?

Other suggestions

- If you don't understand your eye care professional's responses, ask questions until you do understand.

- Take notes or get a friend or family member to take notes for you. Or, bring a tape recorder to help you remember the discussion.

- Ask your eye care professional to write down his or her instructions to you.

- Ask your eye care professional for printed material about your condition.

- If you still have trouble understanding your eye care professional's answers, ask where you can go for more information.

- Other members of your healthcare team, such as nurses and pharmacists, can be good sources of information. Talk to them, too.

Today, patients take an active role in their healthcare. Be an active patient about your eye care.

Chapter 25

Other Disorders of the Optic Nerve

Chapter Contents

Section 25.1

Neuromyelitis Optica

This section contains text excerpted from the following sources: Text
in this section begins with excerpts from "Neuromyelitis Optica,"
Genetics Home Reference (GHR), National Institutes of Health
(NIH), March 2015; Text beginning with the heading "Treatment" is
excerpted from "Neuromyelitis Optica Information Page,"
National Institute of Neurological Disorders and Stroke
(NINDS), February 27, 2016.

Neuromyelitis optica (NMO) is an autoimmune disorder that affects
the nerves of the eyes and the central nervous system, which includes
the brain and spinal cord. Autoimmune disorders occur when the
immune system malfunctions and attacks the body's own tissues and
organs. In NMO, the autoimmune attack causes inflammation of the
nerves, and the resulting damage leads to the signs and symptoms of
the condition.

NMO is characterized by optic neuritis, which is inflammation of
the nerve that carries information from the eye to the brain (optic
nerve). Optic neuritis causes eye pain and vision loss, which can occur
in one or both eyes.

NMO is also characterized by transverse myelitis, which is inflammation of the spinal cord. The inflammation associated with transverse
myelitis damages the spinal cord, causing a lesion that often extends
the length of three or more bones of the spine (vertebrae). In addition,
myelin, which is the covering that protects nerves and promotes the
efficient transmission of nerve impulses, can be damaged. Transverse
myelitis causes weakness, numbness, and paralysis of the arms and
legs. Other effects of spinal cord damage can include disturbances in
sensations, loss of bladder and bowel control, uncontrollable hiccup-
ping, and nausea. In addition, muscle weakness may make breathing
difficult and can cause life-threatening respiratory failure in people
with NMO.

There are two forms of NMO, the relapsing form and the monophasic
form. The relapsing form is most common. This form is characterized
by recurrent episodes of optic neuritis and transverse myelitis. These
episodes can be months or years apart, and there is usually partial

recovery between episodes. However, most affected individuals eventually develop permanent muscle weakness and vision impairment that persist even between episodes. For unknown reasons, approximately nine times more women than men have the relapsing form. The monophasic form, which is less common, causes a single episode of NMO that can last several months. People with this form of the condition can also have lasting muscle weakness or paralysis and vision loss. This form affects men and women equally. The onset of either form of NMO can occur anytime from childhood to adulthood, although the condition most frequently begins in a person's forties.

Approximately one-quarter of individuals with NMO have signs or symptoms of another autoimmune disorder such as myasthenia gravis, systemic lupus erythematosus, or Sjögren syndrome. Some scientists believe that a condition described in Japanese patients as optic-spinal multiple sclerosis (or opticospinal multiple sclerosis (MS)) that affects the nerves of the eyes and central nervous system is the same as NMO.

Other Names for This Condition

- Devic disease
- Devic neuromyelitis optica
- Devic syndrome
- Devic's disease
- Optic-spinal MS
- Opticospinal MS

Frequency

NMO affects approximately 1 to 2 per 100,000 people worldwide. Women are affected by this condition more frequently than men.

Genetic Changes

No genes associated with NMO have been identified. However, a small percentage of people with this condition have a family member who is also affected, which indicates that there may be one or more genetic changes that increase susceptibility. It is thought that the inheritance of this condition is complex and that many environmental and genetic factors are involved in the development of the condition.

The aquaporin-4 protein (AQP4), a normal protein in the body, plays a role in NMO. The AQP4 protein is found in several body systems but is most abundant in tissues of the central nervous system. Approximately 70 percent of people with this disorder produce an immune protein called an antibody that attaches (binds) to the AQP4 protein. Antibodies normally bind to specific foreign particles and germs, marking them for destruction, but the antibody in people with NMO attacks a normal human protein; this type of antibody is called an autoantibody. The autoantibody in this condition is called NMO-IgG or anti-AQP4.

The binding of the NMO-IgG autoantibody to the AQP4 protein turns on (activates) the complement system, which is a group of immune system proteins that work together to destroy pathogens, trigger inflammation, and remove debris from cells and tissues. Complement activation leads to the inflammation of the optic nerve and spinal cord that is characteristic of NMO, resulting in the signs and symptoms of the condition.

The levels of the NMO-IgG autoantibody are high during episodes of NMO, and the levels decrease between episodes with treatment of the disorder. However, it is unclear what triggers episodes to begin or end.

Inheritance Pattern

NMO is usually not inherited. Rarely, this condition is passed through generations in families, but the inheritance pattern is unknown.

Treatment

There is no cure for NMO and no U.S. Food and Drug Administration (FDA)-approved therapies, but there are therapies to treat an attack while it is happening, to reduce symptoms, and to prevent relapses. NMO relapses and attacks are often treated with corticosteroid drugs and plasma exchange (also called plasmapheresis, a process used to remove harmful antibodies from the bloodstream). Immunosuppressive drugs used to prevent attacks include mycophenolate mofetil, rituximab, and azathioprine. Pain, stiffness, muscle spasms, and bladder and bowel control problems can be managed with medications and therapies. Individuals with major disability will require the combined efforts to physical and occupational therapists, along with social services professionals to address complex rehabilitation needs.

Prognosis

Most individuals with NMO have an unpredictable, relapsing course of disease with attacks occurring months or years apart.

Disability is cumulative, the result of each attack damaging new areas of the central nervous system. Some individuals are severely affected by NMO and can lose vision in both eyes and the use of their arms and legs. Most individuals experience some degree of permanent limb weakness or vision loss from NMO. However, reducing the number of attacks with immunosuppressive medications may help prevent with accumulation of disability. Rarely, muscle weakness can be severe enough to cause breathing difficulties and may require the use of artificial ventilation.

Section 25.2

Optic Nerve Drusen

Text in this section is excerpted from "Optic Nerve Drusen,"
© 2017 American Association for Pediatric Ophthalmology
and Strabismus (AAPOS). Reprinted with permission.

What Are Optic Nerve Drusen?

The optic nerve is the physical connection between the eye and the brain. All the visual information taken in by the eye is transmitted to the brain along the optic nerve.

Optic nerve drusen are abnormal globular collections of protein and calcium salts which accumulate in the optic nerve. Drusen usually become visible after the first decade of life, but can be seen before age ten in some children. Often they are present in both eyes (bilateral), but sometimes occur in only one eye (unilateral).

How Common Are Optic Nerve Drusen?

Optic nerve drusen are relatively common and estimated to occur in about 1–2 percent of the population. However, many cases are never diagnosed because most patients with this condition have no problems with their vision.

How Are Optic Nerve Drusen Diagnosed?

Your doctor will do a full (dilated) eye exam and can often diagnose this condition based on the appearance of the optic nerve. Ocular ultrasound, CT scan and/or fundus photography can also aid in the diagnosis. Drusen can be inherited, so it may be helpful to examine other family members.

How Can Optic Nerve Drusen Affect Vision?

Optic nerve drusen usually do not affect vision. However, peripheral vision loss may occur slowly and be so minimal that the abnormality is never noticed. Less commonly there may be an abrupt, painless loss of part of the peripheral vision. Visual field exams may be performed to monitor for decreased peripheral vision in older children.

A rare complication from optic nerve drusen is choroidal neovascular membrane. This is a collection of abnormal blood vessels which grow beneath the retina near the optic nerve. If these abnormal vessels bleed, they can cause a sudden decrease in central or "straight ahead" vision.

Do Optic Nerve Drusen Resemble Any Other Optic Nerve Abnormalities?

Sometimes when the margins of the optic nerve are blurred by drusen it can appear as though the nerve is swollen. Swelling of the optic nerves is called "papilledema," and is a serious condition which indicates the pressure in the brain is too high.

These two conditions – optic nerve drusen and papilldema – may look similar but are very different. As mentioned before, ocular ultrasound and other tests may be used to help make the correct diagnosis and differentiate these two conditions. It is important to be aware of drusen so that unnecessary tests for papilledema are not performed.

What Are "Buried" Optic Nerve Drusen?

In many individuals, particularly children, drusen are not visible on the optic disc surface but are instead buried deeper within the nerve tissue. The optic disc appears swollen despite the drusen not being visible on the surface. As the drusen enlarge and the overlying tissue (nerve fiber layer) thins with age, the disc drusen become more apparent.

How Are Optic Disc Drusen Treated?

There is no treatment for drusen. In the rare cases (with choroidal neovascularization) laser treatment may be indicated.

Section 25.3

Optic Nerve Hypoplasia

Text in this section is excerpted from "Optic Nerve Hypoplasia," © 2017 American Association for Pediatric Ophthalmology and Strabismus (AAPOS). Reprinted with permission.

What Is the Optic Nerve?

The optic nerve is a collection of more than a million nerve fibers that transmit visual signals from the eye to the brain. The optic nerve develops the first trimester of intrauterine life.

What Is Optic Nerve Hypoplasia?

Optic nerve hypoplasia (ONH) is a congenital condition in which the optic nerve is underdeveloped (small).

How Is Optic Nerve Hypoplasia Diagnosed?

The diagnosis of ONH is typically made by the appearance of small/pale optic nerve on ophthalmoscopic examination of the eye. It is difficult to predict visual acuity potential on the basis of optic nerve appearance.

What Causes Optic Nerve Hypoplasia?

Most cases of ONH have no clearly identifiable cause. There are no known racial or socioeconomic factors in the development of ONH, nor is there a known association with exposure to pesticides.

What Visual Problems Are Associated with Optic Nerve Hypoplasia?

Vision impairment from ONH ranges from mild to severe and may affect one or both eyes. Nystagmus (shaking of the eyes) may be seen with both unilateral and bilateral cases. The incidence of strabismus is increased with ONH.

Is Optic Nerve Hypoplasia Associated with Non-Visual Problems?

Optic nerve hypoplasia can be associated with central nervous system (CNS) malformations which put the patient at risk for other problems, including seizure disorder and developmental delay. Hormone deficiencies occur in most children, regardless of associated midline brain abnormalities or pituitary gland abnormalities on MRI. In fact, most children with growth hormone deficiency have a normal MRI.

What Tests Should Be Done for Children with Optic Nerve Hypoplasia?

An MRI scan is indicated for all children with optic nerve hypoplasia. Evaluation by an endocrinologist should be mandatory for all patients under five years of age.

Does Optic Nerve Hypoplasia Get Worse over Time?

In general, ONH is a stable and nonprogressive condition which does not deteriorate. Vision may improve slightly and nystagmus may decrease over time.

Is There Any Treatment for Optic Nerve Hypoplasia?

There is no medical or surgical treatment for ONH. However, occlusion of the better seeing eye may improve vision in the other eye. Children with significant vision loss in both eyes may benefit from early supportive attention by low vision specialists. Stem cell treatment has not been shown to be effective for ONH.

Section 25.4

Optic Neuritis

Text in this section is excerpted from "Optic Neuritis,"
© 2017 American Association for Pediatric Ophthalmology
and Strabismus (AAPOS). Reprinted with permission.

What Is Optic Neuritis?

Optic neuritis is inflammation of the optic nerve. The optic nerve becomes swollen and the blood vessels become larger. This inflammation can cause loss of vision because the optic nerve is crucial for vision. It is the structure that carries visual information from the eye to the brain to produce visual images.

What Are the Symptoms of Optic Neuritis?

The first symptom of optic neuritis in a child is most commonly a rapid, often profound decrease in vision (visual acuity less than 20/400). It can occur in both eyes and it may be worse in one eye than another. Patients may also have headaches and pain with eye movement. Many children with optic neuritis have a history of a fever, flu-like illness, or immunizations 1–2 weeks prior to the onset of the decreased vision.

What Causes Optic Neuritis?

Optic neuritis is thought to be an autoimmune disorder, in which the immune system mistakenly attacks the body's own optic nerve tissue. The attack of the immune system causes inflammation, swelling and impaired function of the optic nerve. The trigger for this immune reaction may be a viral illness, infection around the optic nerve, multiple sclerosis, or other neurological problems.

How Is Optic Neuritis Diagnosed?

A careful history including inquiring about recent illness, fever, neurological symptoms, or recent immunizations is helpful. The Eye

MD checks vision (which is usually markedly decreased) and evaluates optic nerve function including the pupil reactions, color vision, and peripheral vision. The Eye MD also examines the optic nerve with ophthalmoscopy for swelling and dilated blood vessels. Other tests performed may include an MRI, a spinal tap (lumbar puncture), and blood tests.

What Is the Prognosis and Treatment for Optic Neuritis?

Fortunately, most children with optic neuritis recover much of their vision. This usually occurs spontaneously and treatment may not be necessary. Recovery usually begins within a few weeks, and can continue for several months. Intravenous corticosteroids may speed the recovery of vision, but probably do not improve the final visual outcome. Unfortunately, a small percentage of children do not recover vision.

What Are the Differences between Optic Neuritis in Children and Adults?

Both eyes are usually affected in children, while adults usually have only one eye affected. Children with optic neuritis usually have a history of recent illness or immunization and adults do not. Both adults and children have an increased risk of multiple sclerosis if they develop optic neuritis, but children have much less risk.

Chapter 26

Disorders of the Retina

Chapter Contents

Section 26.1

Retinal Detachment

This section includes text excerpted from "Facts about
Retinal Detachment," National Eye Institute (NEI),
October 2009. Reviewed March 2017.

What Is Retinal Detachment?

The retina is the light-sensitive layer of tissue that lines the inside
of the eye and sends visual messages through the optic nerve to the
brain. When the retina detaches, it is lifted or pulled from its normal
position. If not promptly treated, retinal detachment can cause permanent vision loss.

In some cases there may be small areas of the retina that are torn.
These areas, called retinal tears or retinal breaks, can lead to retinal
detachment.

What Are the Different Types of Retinal Detachment?

There are three different types of retinal detachment:

- **Rhegmatogenous**—A tear or break in the retina allows fluid
  to get under the retina and separate it from the retinal pigment
  epithelium (RPE), the pigmented cell layer that nourishes the
  retina. These types of retinal detachments are the most common.

- **Tractional**—In this type of detachment, scar tissue on the retina's surface contracts and causes the retina to separate from the
  RPE. This type of detachment is less common.

- **Exudative**—Frequently caused by retinal diseases, including
  inflammatory disorders and injury/trauma to the eye. In this
  type, fluid leaks into the area underneath the retina, but there
  are no tears or breaks in the retina.

Who Is at Risk for Retinal Detachment?

A retinal detachment can occur at any age, but it is more common
in people over age 40.

It affects men more than women, and Whites more than African Americans.

A retinal detachment is also more likely to occur in people who:

- are extremely nearsighted
- have had a retinal detachment in the other eye
- have a family history of retinal detachment
- have had cataract surgery
- have other eye diseases or disorders, such as retinoschisis, uveitis, degenerative myopia, or lattice degeneration
- have had an eye injury

What Are the Symptoms of Retinal Detachment?

Symptoms include a sudden or gradual increase in either the number of floaters, which are little "cobwebs" or specks that float about in your field of vision, and/or light flashes in the eye. Another symptom is the appearance of a curtain over the field of vision. **A retinal detachment is a medical emergency.** Anyone experiencing the symptoms of a retinal detachment should see an eye care professional immediately.

How Is Retinal Detachment Treated?

Small holes and tears are treated with laser surgery or a freeze treatment called cryopexy. These procedures are usually performed in the doctor's office. During laser surgery tiny burns are made around the hole to "weld" the retina back into place. Cryopexy freezes the area around the hole and helps reattach the retina.

Retinal detachments are treated with surgery that may require the patient to stay in the hospital. In some cases a scleral buckle, a tiny synthetic band, is attached to the outside of the eyeball to gently push the wall of the eye against the detached retina. If necessary, a vitrectomy may also be performed. During a vitrectomy, the doctor makes a tiny incision in the sclera (white of the eye). Next, a small instrument is placed into the eye to remove the vitreous, a gel-like substance that fills the center of the eye and helps the eye maintain a round shape. Gas is often injected to into the eye to replace the vitreous and reattach the retina; the gas pushes the retina back against the wall of the eye. During the healing process, the eye makes fluid that gradually replaces the gas and fills the eye. With all of these procedures, either laser or cryopexy is used to "weld" the retina back in place.

With modern therapy, over 90 percent of those with a retinal detachment can be successfully treated, although sometimes a second treatment is needed. However, the visual outcome is not always predictable. The final visual result may not be known for up to several months following surgery. Even under the best of circumstances, and even after multiple attempts at repair, treatment sometimes fails and vision may eventually be lost. Visual results are best if the retinal detachment is repaired before the macula (the center region of the retina responsible for fine, detailed vision) detaches. That is why it is important to contact an eye care professional immediately if you see a sudden or gradual increase in the number of floaters and/or light flashes, or a dark curtain over the field of vision.

Section 26.2

Retinitis Pigmentosa

This section includes text excerpted from "Facts about Retinitis Pigmentosa," National Eye Institute (NEI), May 2014.

What Is Retinitis Pigmentosa?

Retinitis pigmentosa (RP) is a group of rare, genetic disorders that involve a breakdown and loss of cells in the retina—which is the light sensitive tissue that lines the back of the eye. Common symptoms include difficulty seeing at night and a loss of side (peripheral) vision.

What Causes Retinitis Pigmentosa?

RP is an inherited disorder that results from harmful changes in any one of more than 50 genes. These genes carry the instructions for making proteins that are needed in cells within the retina, called photoreceptors. Some of the changes, or mutations, within genes are so severe that the gene cannot make the required protein, limiting the cell's function. Other mutations produce a protein that is toxic to the cell. Still other mutations lead to an abnormal protein that doesn't function properly. In all three cases, the result is damage to the photoreceptors.

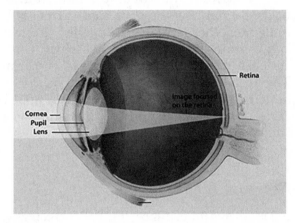

Figure 26.1. *Retina*

The retina is the light-sensitive tissue at the back of the eye that contains photoreceptors and other cell types

What Are Photoreceptors?

Photoreceptors are cells in the retina that begin the process of seeing. They absorb and convert light into electrical signals. These signals are sent to other cells in the retina and ultimately through the optic nerve to the brain where they are processed into the images we see. There are two general types of photoreceptors, called rods and cones. Rods are in the outer regions of the retina, and allow us to see in dim and dark light. Cones reside mostly in the central portion of the retina, and allow us to perceive fine visual detail and color.

How Does Retinitis Pigmentosa Affect Vision?

In the early stages of RP, rods are more severely affected than cones. As the rods die, people experience night blindness and a progressive loss of the visual field, the area of space that is visible at a given instant without moving the eyes. The loss of rods eventually leads to a breakdown and loss of cones. In the late stages of RP, as cones die, people tend to lose more of the visual field, developing "tunnel vision." They may have difficulty performing essential tasks of daily living such as reading, driving, walking without assistance, or recognizing faces and objects.

How Is Retinitis Pigmentosa Inherited?

To understand how RP is inherited, it is important to know a little more about genes and how they are passed from parent to child. Genes are bundled together on structures called chromosomes. Each cell in your body contains 23 pairs of chromosomes. One copy of each chromosome is passed by a parent at conception through egg and sperm cells. The X and Y chromosomes, known as sex chromosomes, determine whether a person is born female (XX) or male (XY). The 22 other paired chromosomes, called autosomes, contain the vast majority of genes that determine non-sex traits. RP can be inherited in one of three ways:

Autosomal Recessive Inheritance

In autosomal recessive inheritance, it takes two copies of the mutant gene to give rise to the disorder. An individual with a recessive gene mutation is known as a carrier. When two carriers have a child, there is a:

- 1 in 4 chance the child will have the disorder

- 1 in 2 chance the child will be a carrier

- 1 in 4 chance the child will neither have the disorder nor be a carrier

Autosomal Dominant Inheritance

In this inheritance pattern, it takes just one copy of the gene with a disorder-causing mutation to bring about the disorder. When a parent has a dominant gene mutation, there is a 1 in 2 chance that any children will inherit this mutation and the disorder.

X-Linked Inheritance

In this form of inheritance, mothers carry the mutated gene on one of their X chromosomes and pass it to their sons. Because females have two X chromosomes, the effect of a mutation on one X chromosome is offset by the normal gene on the other X chromosome. If a mother is a carrier of an X-linked disorder there is a:

- 1 in 2 chance of having a son with the disorder

- 1 in 2 chance of having a daughter who is a carrier

How Common Is Retinitis Pigmentosa?

RP is considered a rare disorder. Although current statistics are not available, it is generally estimated that the disorder affects roughly 1 in 4,000 people, both in the United States and worldwide.

How Does Retinitis Pigmentosa Progress?

The symptoms of RP typically appear in childhood. Children often have difficulty getting around in the dark. It can also take abnormally long periods of time to adjust to changes in lighting. As their visual field becomes restricted, patients often trip over things and appear clumsy. People with RP often find bright lights uncomfortable, a condition known as photophobia. Because there are many gene mutations that cause the disorder, its progression can differ greatly from person to person. Some people retain central vision and a restricted visual field into their 50s, while others experience significant vision loss in early adulthood. Eventually, most individuals with RP will lose most of their sight.

How Is Retinitis Pigmentosa Diagnosed?

RP is diagnosed in part through an examination of the retina. An eye care professional will use an ophthalmoscope, a tool that allows for a wider, clear view of the retina. This typically reveals abnormal, dark pigment deposits that streak the retina. These pigment deposits are in part why the disorder was named retinitis pigmentosa. Other tests for RP include:

- **Electroretinogram (ERG).** An ERG measures the electrical activity of photoreceptor cells. This test uses gold foil or a contact lens with electrodes attached. A flash of light is sent to the retina and the electrodes measure rod and cone cell responses. People with RP have a decreased electrical activity, reflecting the declining function of photoreceptors.

- **Visual field testing.** To determine the extent of vision loss, a clinician will give a visual field test. The person watches as a dot of light moves around the half-circle (180 degrees) of space directly in front of the head and to either side. The patient pushes a button to indicate that he or she can see the light. This process results in a map of their visual field and their central vision.

- **Genetic testing.** In some cases, a clinician takes a deoxyribonucleic acid (DNA) sample from the person to give a genetic diagnosis. In this way a person can learn about the progression of their particular form of the disorder. Genetic testing is available for a limited number of patients with RP through National Eye Institute's (NEI) National Ophthalmic Disorder Genotyping and Phenotyping Network (eyeGENE). Participants in this program agree to make their DNA sample and clinical information available to researchers in exchange for genetic testing. They also agree to join a patient registry for possible recruitment into clinical trials.

Are There Treatments for Retinitis Pigmentosa?

Living with Vision Loss

A number of services and devices are available to help people with vision loss carry out daily activities and maintain their independence. In addition to an eye care professional, it is important to have help from a team of experts, which may include occupational therapists, orientation and mobility specialists, certified low vision therapists, and others.

Children with RP may benefit from low vision aids that maximize existing vision. For example, there are special lenses that magnify central vision to expand visual field and eliminate glare. Computer programs that read text are readily available. Closed circuit televisions with a camera can adjust text to suit one's vision. Portable lighting devices can adjust a dark or dim environment. Mobility training can teach people to use a cane or a guide dog, and eye scanning techniques can help people to optimize remaining vision. Once a child is diagnosed, he or she will be referred to a low vision specialist for a comprehensive evaluation. Parents may also want to meet with the child's school administrators and teachers to make sure that necessary accommodations are put in place.

For parents of children with RP, one challenge is to determine when a child might need to learn to use a cane or a guide dog. Having regular eye examinations to measure the progress of the disorder will help parents make informed decisions regarding low vision services and rehabilitation.

Targeted Therapies for Retinitis Pigmentosa

An NEI-sponsored clinical trial found that a daily dose of 15,000 international units of vitamin A palmitate modestly slowed the progression of the disorder in adults. Because there are so many forms of RP, it is difficult to predict how any one patient will respond to this treatment. Talk to an eye care professional to determine if taking vitamin A is right for you or your child.

An artificial vision device called the Argus II has also shown promise for restoring some vision to people with late-stage RP. The Argus II, developed by Second Sight with NEI support, is a prosthetic device that functions in place of lost photoreceptor cells. It consists of a light-sensitive electrode that is surgically implanted on the retina. A pair of glasses with a camera wirelessly transmits signals to the electrode that are then relayed to the brain. Although it does not restore normal vision, in clinical studies, the Argus II enabled people with RP to read large letters and navigate environments without the use of a cane or guide dog. In 2012, the U.S. Food and Drug Administration (FDA) granted a humanitarian device exemption for use of the Argus II to treat late-stage RP. This means the device has not proven effective, but the FDA has determined that its probable benefits outweigh its risks to health. The Argus II is eligible for Medicare payment.

Section 26.3

Retinoblastoma

This section includes text excerpted from "Retinoblastoma Treatment (PDQ®)—Patient Version," National Cancer Institute (NCI), November 4, 2016.

Retinoblastoma is a disease in which malignant (cancer) cells form in the tissues of the retina.

The retina is the nerve tissue that lines the inside of the back of the eye. The retina senses light and sends images to the brain by way of the optic nerve.

Although retinoblastoma may occur at any age, it occurs most often in children younger than 2 years. The cancer may be in one eye (unilateral) or in both eyes (bilateral). Retinoblastoma rarely spreads from the eye to nearby tissue or other parts of the body.

Cavitary retinoblastoma is a rare type of retinoblastoma in which cavities (hollow spaces) form within the tumor.

Retinoblastoma occurs in heritable and nonheritable forms.

A child is thought to have the heritable form of retinoblastoma when one of the following is true:

- There is a family history of retinoblastoma.

- There is a certain mutation (change) in the *RB1* gene. The mutation in the *RB1* gene may be passed from the parent to the child or it may occur in the egg or sperm before conception or soon after conception.

- There is more than one tumor in the eye or there is a tumor in both eyes.

- There is a tumor in one eye and the child is younger than 1 year.

After heritable retinoblastoma has been diagnosed and treated, new tumors may continue to form for a few years. Regular eye exams to check for new tumors are usually done every 2 to 4 months for at least 28 months.

Nonheritable retinoblastoma is retinoblastoma that is not the heritable form. Most cases of retinoblastoma are the nonheritable form.

Genetic Counseling

Parents should receive genetic counseling (a discussion with a trained professional about the risk of genetic diseases) to discuss genetic testing to check for a mutation (change) in the *RB1* gene. Genetic counseling also includes a discussion of the risk of retinoblastoma for the child and the child's brothers or sisters.

Eye Exams

A child with a family history of retinoblastoma should have regular eye exams beginning early in life to check for retinoblastoma, unless it is known that the child does not have the *RB1* gene change. Early diagnosis of retinoblastoma may mean the child will need less intense treatment.

Brothers or sisters of a child with retinoblastoma should have regular eye exams by an ophthalmologist until age 3 to 5 years, unless it is known that the brother or sister does not have the *RB1* gene change.

Risk of Other Cancers

A child with heritable retinoblastoma has an increased risk of a pineal tumor in the brain. When retinoblastoma and a brain tumor occur at the same time, it is called trilateral retinoblastoma. The brain tumor is usually diagnosed between 20 and 36 months of age. Regular screening using MRI (magnetic resonance imaging) may be done for a child thought to have heritable retinoblastoma or for a child with retinoblastoma in one eye and a family history of the disease. CT (computerized tomography) scans are usually not used for routine screening in order to avoid exposing the child to ionizing radiation.

Heritable retinoblastoma also increases the child's risk of other types of cancer such as lung cancer, bladder cancer, or melanoma in later years. Regular follow-up exams are important.

Signs and Symptoms of Retinoblastoma

Check with a doctor if your child has any of the following:

- Pupil of the eye appears white instead of red when light shines into it. This may be seen in flash photographs of the child.
- Eyes appear to be looking in different directions (lazy eye).
- Pain or redness in the eye.
- Infection around the eye.
- Eyeball is larger than normal.
- Colored part of the eye and pupil look cloudy.

Diagnostic Tests for Retinoblastoma

The following tests and procedures may be used:

- **Physical exam and history:** An exam of the body to check general signs of health, including checking for signs of disease, such as lumps or anything else that seems unusual. A history of the patient's health habits and past illnesses and treatments will also be taken. The doctor will ask if there is a family history of retinoblastoma.

- **Eye exam with dilated pupil:** An exam of the eye in which the pupil is dilated (opened wider) with medicated eye drops to allow the doctor to look through the lens and pupil to the retina.

The inside of the eye, including the retina and the optic nerve, is examined with a light. Depending on the age of the child, this exam may be done under anesthesia.

There are several types of eye exams that are done with the pupil dilated:

- **Ophthalmoscopy:** An exam of the inside of the back of the eye to check the retina and optic nerve using a small magnifying lens and a light.

- **Slit-lamp biomicroscopy:** An exam of the inside of the eye to check the retina, optic nerve, and other parts of the eye using a strong beam of light and a microscope.

- **Fluorescein angiography:** A procedure to look at blood vessels and the flow of blood inside the eye. An orange fluorescent dye called fluorescein is injected into a blood vessel in the arm and goes into the bloodstream. As the dye travels through blood vessels of the eye, a special camera takes pictures of the retina and choroid to find any blood vessels that are blocked or leaking.

- *RB1* **gene test:** A laboratory test in which a sample of blood or tissue is tested for a change in the *RB1* gene.

- **Ultrasound exam of the eye:** A procedure in which high-energy sound waves (ultrasound) are bounced off the internal tissues of the eye to make echoes. Eye drops are used to numb the eye and a small probe that sends and receives sound waves is placed gently on the surface of the eye. The echoes make a picture of the inside of the eye and the distance from the cornea to the retina is measured. The picture, called a sonogram, shows on the screen of the ultrasound monitor. The picture can be printed to be looked at later.

- **MRI:** A procedure that uses a magnet, radio waves, and a computer to make a series of detailed pictures of areas inside the body, such as the eye. This procedure is also called nuclear magnetic resonance imaging (NMRI).

- **CT scan (CAT scan):** A procedure that makes a series of detailed pictures of areas inside the body, such as the eye, taken from different angles. The pictures are made by a computer linked to an X-ray machine. A dye may be injected into a vein or swallowed to help the organs or tissues show up more clearly. This procedure is also called computed tomography, computerized tomography, or computerized axial tomography (CAT).

Retinoblastoma can usually be diagnosed without a biopsy.
When retinoblastoma is in one eye, it sometimes forms in the other eye. Exams of the unaffected eye are done until it is known if the retinoblastoma is the heritable form.

Factors That Affect Prognosis, and Treatment Options

The prognosis (chance of recovery) and treatment options depend on the following:

- whether the cancer is in one or both eyes
- the size and number of tumors
- whether the tumor has spread to the area around the eye, to the brain, or to other parts of the body
- whether there are symptoms at the time of diagnosis, for trilateral retinoblastoma
- the age of the child
- how likely it is that vision can be saved in one or both eyes
- whether a second type of cancer has formed

Stages of Retinoblastoma

Staging

After retinoblastoma has been diagnosed, tests are done to find out if cancer cells have spread within the eye or to other parts of the body.

The process used to find out if cancer has spread within the eye or to other parts of the body is called staging. The information gathered from the staging process determines whether retinoblastoma is only in the eye (intraocular) or has spread outside the eye (extraocular). It is important to know the stage in order to plan treatment. The results of the tests used to diagnose cancer are often also used to stage the disease.

The following tests and procedures may be used in the staging process:

- **Bone scan:** A procedure to check if there are rapidly dividing cells, such as cancer cells, in the bone. A very small amount of radioactive material is injected into a vein and travels through the bloodstream. The radioactive material collects in the bones and is detected by a scanner that also takes a picture of the body. Areas of bone with cancer show up brighter in the picture because they take up more radioactive material than normal bone cells do.

- **Bone marrow aspiration and biopsy:** The removal of bone marrow and a small piece of bone by inserting a hollow needle into the hipbone or breastbone. A pathologist views the bone marrow under a microscope to look for signs of cancer. A bone marrow aspiration and biopsy is done if the doctor thinks the cancer has spread outside of the eye.

- **Lumbar puncture (LP):** A procedure used to collect cerebrospinal fluid (CSF) from the spinal column. This is done by placing a needle between two bones in the spine and into the CSF around the spinal cord and removing a sample of the fluid. The sample of CSF is checked under a microscope for signs that the cancer has spread to the brain and spinal cord. This procedure is also called an LP or spinal tap.

International Retinoblastoma Staging System (IRSS)

There are several staging systems for retinoblastoma. The IRSS stages are based on how much cancer remains after surgery to remove the tumor and whether the cancer has spread.

Stage 0: The tumor is in the eye only. The eye has not been removed and the tumor was treated without surgery.

Stage I: The tumor is in the eye only. The eye has been removed and no cancer cells remain.

Stage II: The tumor is in the eye only. The eye has been removed and there are cancer cells left that can be seen only with a microscope.

Stage III: Stage III is divided into stages IIIa and IIIb:

- In stage IIIa, cancer has spread from the eye to tissues around the eye socket.

- In stage IIIb, cancer has spread from the eye to lymph nodes near the ear or in the neck.

Stage IV: Stage IV is divided into stages IVa and IVb:

- In stage IVa, cancer has spread to the blood but not to the brain or spinal cord. One or more tumors may have spread to other parts of the body such as the bone or liver.

- In stage IVb, cancer has spread to the brain or spinal cord. It also may have spread to other parts of the body.

Spread of Cancer

There are three ways that cancer spreads in the body. Cancer can spread through tissue, the lymph system, and the blood:

- **Tissue.** The cancer spreads from where it began by growing into nearby areas.

- **Lymph system.** The cancer spreads from where it began by getting into the lymph system. The cancer travels through the lymph vessels to other parts of the body.

- **Blood.** The cancer spreads from where it began by getting into the blood. The cancer travels through the blood vessels to other parts of the body.

Cancer may spread from where it began to other parts of the body. When cancer spreads to another part of the body, it is called metastasis. Cancer cells break away from where they began (the primary tumor) and travel through the lymph system or blood.

- **Lymph system.** The cancer gets into the lymph system, travels through the lymph vessels, and forms a tumor (metastatic tumor) in another part of the body.

- **Blood.** The cancer gets into the blood, travels through the blood vessels, and forms a tumor (metastatic tumor) in another part of the body.

The metastatic tumor is the same type of cancer as the primary tumor. For example, if retinoblastoma spreads to the bone, the cancer cells in the bone are actually retinoblastoma cells. The disease is metastatic retinoblastoma, not bone cancer.

Treatment for retinoblastoma depends on whether it is intraocular (within the eye) or extraocular (outside the eye).

- **Intraocular retinoblastoma:** In intraocular retinoblastoma, cancer is found in one or both eyes and may be in the retina only or may also be in other parts of the eye such as the choroid, ciliary body, or part of the optic nerve. Cancer has not spread to tissues around the outside of the eye or to other parts of the body.

- **Extraocular retinoblastoma (metastatic):** In extraocular retinoblastoma, cancer has spread beyond the eye. It may be found in tissues around the eye (orbital retinoblastoma) or it may have spread to the central nervous system (brain and spinal cord) or to other parts of the body such as the liver, bones, bone marrow, or lymph nodes.

Progressive and Recurrent Retinoblastoma

Progressive retinoblastoma is retinoblastoma that does not respond to treatment. Instead, the cancer grows, spreads, or gets worse.

Recurrent retinoblastoma is cancer that has recurred (come back) after it has been treated. The cancer may recur in the eye, in tissues around the eye, or in other places in the body.

Treatment Options for Retinoblastoma

Different types of treatment are available for patients with retinoblastoma. Some treatments are standard (the currently used treatment), and some are being tested in clinical trials. A treatment clinical trial is a research study meant to help improve current treatments or obtain information on new treatments for patients with cancer. When clinical trials show that a new treatment is better than the standard treatment, the new treatment may become the standard treatment.

Because cancer in children is rare, taking part in a clinical trial should be considered. Some clinical trials are open only to patients who have not started treatment.

Children with retinoblastoma should have their treatment planned by a team of healthcare providers who are experts in treating cancer in children.

The goals of treatment are to save the child's life, to save vision and the eye, and to prevent serious side effects. Treatment will be overseen by a pediatric oncologist, a doctor who specializes in treating children with cancer. The pediatric oncologist works with other healthcare providers who are experts in treating children with eye cancer and who specialize in certain areas of medicine. These may include a pediatric ophthalmologist (children's eye doctor) who has a lot of experience in treating retinoblastoma and the following specialists:

- Pediatric surgeon

- Radiation oncologist

- Pediatrician

- Pediatric nurse specialist

- Rehabilitation specialist

- Social worker

- Geneticist or genetic counselor

Late Effects

Side effects from cancer treatment that begin during or after treatment and continue for months or years are called late effects. Late effects of treatment for retinoblastoma may include the following:

- physical problems such as seeing or hearing problems or, if the eye is removed, a change in the shape and size of the bone around the eye

- changes in mood, feelings, thinking, learning, or memory

- second cancers (new types of cancer), such as lung and bladder cancers, osteosarcoma, soft tissue sarcoma, or melanoma

The following risk factors may increase the risk of having another cancer:

- having the heritable form of retinoblastoma

- past treatment with radiation therapy, especially before age 1 year

- having already had a previous second cancer

It is important to talk with your child's doctors about the effects cancer treatment can have on your child. Regular follow-up by health professionals who are experts in diagnosing and treating late effects is important.

Standard Treatment Types

Six types of standard treatment are used:

1. **Cryotherapy:** Cryotherapy is a treatment that uses an instrument to freeze and destroy abnormal tissue. This type of treatment is also called cryosurgery.

2. **Thermotherapy:** Thermotherapy is the use of heat to destroy cancer cells. Thermotherapy may be given using a laser beam aimed through the dilated pupil or onto the outside of the eyeball. Thermotherapy may be used alone for small tumors or combined with chemotherapy for larger tumors. This treatment is a type of laser therapy.

3. **Chemotherapy:** Chemotherapy is a cancer treatment that uses drugs to stop the growth of cancer cells, either by killing the cells or by stopping them from dividing. The way the chemotherapy is given depends on the stage of the cancer and where the cancer is in the body.

   There are different types of chemotherapy:

   • **Systemic chemotherapy:** When chemotherapy is taken by mouth or injected into a vein or muscle, the drugs enter the bloodstream and can reach cancer cells throughout the body. Systemic chemotherapy is given to shrink the tumor (chemoreduction) and avoid surgery to remove the eye. After chemoreduction, other treatments may include radiation therapy, cryotherapy, laser therapy, or regional chemotherapy.

   Systemic chemotherapy may also be given to kill any cancer cells that are left after the initial treatment or to patients with retinoblastoma that occurs outside the eye. Treatment given after the initial treatment, to lower the risk that the cancer will come back, is called adjuvant therapy.

   • **Regional chemotherapy:** When chemotherapy is placed directly into the cerebrospinal fluid (intrathecal chemotherapy), an organ (such as the eye), or a body cavity, the drugs mainly affect cancer cells in those areas. Several types of regional chemotherapy are used to treat retinoblastoma.

   • **Ophthalmic artery infusion chemotherapy:** Ophthalmic artery infusion chemotherapy carries anticancer drugs directly to the eye. A catheter is put into an artery that leads to the eye and the anticancer drug is given through the catheter. After the drug is given, a small balloon may be inserted into the artery to block it and keep most of the anticancer drug trapped near the tumor. This type of chemotherapy may be given as the initial treatment when the tumor is in the eye only or when the tumor has not responded to other types of treatment. Ophthalmic artery infusion chemotherapy is given at special retinoblastoma treatment centers.

- **Intravitreal chemotherapy:** Intravitreal chemotherapy is the injection of anticancer drugs directly into the vitreous humor (jelly-like substance) inside in the eye. It is used to treat cancer that has spread to the vitreous humor and has not responded to treatment or has come back after treatment.

4. **Radiation therapy:** Radiation therapy is a cancer treatment that uses high-energy X-rays or other types of radiation to kill cancer cells or keep them from growing. There are two types of radiation therapy:

- **External-beam radiation therapy** uses a machine outside the body to send radiation toward the cancer. Certain ways of giving radiation therapy can help keep radiation from damaging nearby healthy tissue. These types of radiation therapy include the following:

  - **Intensity-modulated radiation therapy (IMRT):** IMRT is a type of 3-dimensional (3-D) external radiation therapy that uses a computer to make pictures of the size and shape of the tumor. Thin beams of radiation of different intensities (strengths) are aimed at the tumor from many angles.

  - **Proton-beam radiation therapy:** Proton-beam therapy is a type of high-energy, external radiation therapy. A radiation therapy machine aims streams of protons (tiny, invisible, positively-charged particles) at the cancer cells to kill them.

- **Internal radiation therapy** uses a radioactive substance sealed in needles, seeds, wires, or catheters that are placed directly into or near the cancer. Certain ways of giving radiation therapy can help keep radiation from damaging nearby healthy tissue. This type of internal radiation therapy may include the following:

  - **Plaque radiotherapy:** Radioactive seeds are attached to one side of a disk, called a plaque, and placed directly on the outside wall of the eye near the tumor. The side of the plaque with the seeds on it faces the eyeball, aiming radiation at the tumor. The plaque helps protect other nearby tissue from the radiation.

The way the radiation therapy is given depends on the type and stage of the cancer being treated and how the cancer responded to other treatments. External and internal radiation therapy are used to treat retinoblastoma.

5. **High-dose chemotherapy with stem cell rescue:** High-dose chemotherapy with stem cell rescue is a way of giving high doses of chemotherapy and replacing blood-forming cells destroyed by the cancer treatment. Stem cells (immature blood cells) are removed from the blood or bone marrow of the patient and are frozen and stored. After the chemotherapy is completed, the stored stem cells are thawed and given back to the patient through an infusion. These reinfused stem cells grow into (and restore) the body's blood cells.

6. **Surgery (enucleation):** Enucleation is surgery to remove the eye and part of the optic nerve. A sample of the eye tissue that is removed will be checked under a microscope to see if there are any signs that the cancer is likely to spread to other parts of the body. This should be done by an experienced pathologist, who is familiar with retinoblastoma and other diseases of the eye. Enucleation is done if there is little or no chance that vision can be saved and when the tumor is large, did not respond to treatment, or comes back after treatment. The patient will be fitted for an artificial eye.

Close follow-up is needed for 2 years or more to check for signs of recurrence in the area around the affected eye and to check the other eye.

Clinical Trials

New types of treatment are being tested in clinical trials. Patients may want to think about taking part in a clinical trial.

For some patients, taking part in a clinical trial may be the best treatment choice. Clinical trials are part of the cancer research process. Clinical trials are done to find out if new cancer treatments are safe and effective or better than the standard treatment.

Many of today's standard treatments for cancer are based on earlier clinical trials. Patients who take part in a clinical trial may receive the standard treatment or be among the first to receive a new treatment.

Patients who take part in clinical trials also help improve the way cancer will be treated in the future. Even when clinical trials do not lead to effective new treatments, they often answer important questions and help move research forward.

Patients can enter clinical trials before, during, or after starting their cancer treatment.

Some clinical trials only include patients who have not yet received treatment. Other trials test treatments for patients whose cancer has not gotten better. There are also clinical trials that test new ways to stop cancer from recurring (coming back) or reduce the side effects of cancer treatment.

Clinical trials are taking place in many parts of the country.

Follow-up Tests

Some of the tests that were done to diagnose the cancer or to find out the stage of the cancer may be repeated. Some tests will be repeated in order to see how well the treatment is working. Decisions about whether to continue, change, or stop treatment may be based on the results of these tests.

Some of the tests will continue to be done from time to time after treatment has ended. The results of these tests can show if your child's condition has changed or if the cancer has recurred (come back). These tests are sometimes called follow-up tests or check-ups.

Section 26.4

Retinopathy of Prematurity

This section includes text excerpted from "Facts about Retinopathy of Prematurity (ROP)," National Eye Institute (NEI), June 2014.

What Is Retinopathy of Prematurity?

Retinopathy of Prematurity (ROP) is a potentially blinding eye disorder that primarily affects premature infants weighing about 2¾ pounds (1250 grams) or less that are born before 31 weeks of gestation (A full-term pregnancy has a gestation of 38–42 weeks). The smaller a baby is at birth, the more likely that baby is to develop ROP. This disorder—which usually develops in both eyes—is one of the most common causes of visual loss in childhood and can lead to lifelong vision impairment and blindness. ROP was first diagnosed in 1942.

Frequently Asked Questions about Retinopathy of Prematurity

How Many Infants Have Retinopathy of Prematurity?

Today, with advances in neonatal care, smaller and more premature infants are being saved. These infants are at a much higher risk for ROP. Not all babies who are premature develop ROP. There are approximately 3.9 million infants born in the United States each year; of those, about 28,000 weigh 2¾ pounds or less. About 14,000–16,000 of these infants are affected by some degree of ROP. The disease improves and leaves no permanent damage in milder cases of ROP. About 90 percent of all infants with ROP are in the milder category and do not need treatment. However, infants with more severe disease can develop impaired vision or even blindness. About 1,100–1,500 infants annually develop ROP that is severe enough to require medical treatment. About 400–600 infants each year in the United States become legally blind from ROP.

Are There Different Stages of Retinopathy of Prematurity?

Yes. ROP is classified in five stages, ranging from mild (stage I) to severe (stage V):

Stage I—Mildly abnormal blood vessel growth. Many children who develop stage I improve with no treatment and eventually develop normal vision. The disease resolves on its own without further progression.

Stage II—Moderately abnormal blood vessel growth. Many children who develop stage II improve with no treatment and eventually develop normal vision. The disease resolves on its own without further progression.

Stage III—Severely abnormal blood vessel growth. The abnormal blood vessels grow toward the center of the eye instead of following their normal growth pattern along the surface of the retina. Some infants who develop stage III improve with no treatment and eventually develop normal vision. However, when infants have a certain degree of Stage III and "plus disease" develops, treatment is considered.

300

"Plus disease" means that the blood vessels of the retina have become enlarged and twisted, indicating a worsening of the disease. Treatment at this point has a good chance of preventing retinal detachment.

Stage IV—Partially detached retina. Traction from the scar produced by bleeding, abnormal vessels pulls the retina away from the wall of the eye.

Stage V—Completely detached retina and the end stage of the disease. If the eye is left alone at this stage, the baby can have severe visual impairment and even blindness.

Most babies who develop ROP have stages I or II. However, in a small number of babies, ROP worsens, sometimes very rapidly. Untreated ROP threatens to destroy vision.

Can Retinopathy of Prematurity Cause Other Complications?

Yes. Infants with ROP are considered to be at higher risk for developing certain eye problems later in life, such as retinal detachment, myopia (nearsightedness), strabismus (crossed eyes), amblyopia (lazy eye), and glaucoma. In many cases, these eye problems can be treated or controlled.

Causes and Risk Factors

What Causes Retinopathy of Prematurity?

ROP occurs when abnormal blood vessels grow and spread throughout the retina, the tissue that lines the back of the eye. These abnormal blood vessels are fragile and can leak, scarring the retina and pulling it out of position. This causes a retinal detachment. Retinal detachment is the main cause of visual impairment and blindness in ROP.

Several complex factors may be responsible for the development of ROP. The eye starts to develop at about 16 weeks of pregnancy, when the blood vessels of the retina begin to form at the optic nerve in the back of the eye. The blood vessels grow gradually toward the edges of the developing retina, supplying oxygen and nutrients. During the last 12 weeks of a pregnancy, the eye develops rapidly. When a baby is born full-term, the retinal blood vessel growth is mostly complete (The retina usually finishes growing a few weeks to a month after birth). But if a baby is born prematurely, before these blood vessels have reached the edges of the retina, normal vessel growth may stop. The edges of the retina (the periphery) may not get enough oxygen and nutrients.

Scientists believe that the periphery of the retina then sends out signals to other areas of the retina for nourishment. As a result, new abnormal vessels begin to grow. These new blood vessels are fragile and weak and can bleed, leading to retinal scarring. When these scars shrink, they pull on the retina, causing it to detach from the back of the eye.

Are There Other Risk Factors for Retinopathy of Prematurity?

In addition to birth weight and how early a baby is born, other factors contributing to the risk of ROP include anemia, blood transfusions, respiratory distress, breathing difficulties, and the overall health of the infant.

An ROP epidemic occurred in the 1940s and early 1950s when hospital nurseries began using excessively high levels of oxygen in incubators to save the lives of premature infants. During this time, ROP was the leading cause of blindness in children in the United States. In 1954, scientists funded by the National Institutes of Health (NIH) determined that the relatively high levels of oxygen routinely given to premature infants at that time were an important risk factor, and that reducing the level of oxygen given to premature babies reduced the incidence of ROP. With newer technology and methods to monitor the oxygen levels of infants, oxygen use as a risk factor has diminished in importance.

Although it had been suggested as a factor in the development of ROP, researchers supported by the NIH determined that lighting levels in hospital nurseries has no effect on the development of ROP.

Treatment of Retinopathy of Prematurity

How Is Retinopathy of Prematurity Treated?

The most effective proven treatments for ROP are laser therapy or cryotherapy. Laser therapy "burns away" the periphery of the retina, which has no normal blood vessels. With cryotherapy, physicians use an instrument that generates freezing temperatures to briefly touch spots on the surface of the eye that overlie the periphery of the retina. Both laser treatment and cryotherapy destroy the peripheral areas of the retina, slowing or reversing the abnormal growth of blood vessels. Unfortunately, the treatments also destroy some side vision. This is done to save the most important part of our sight—the sharp, central vision we need for "straight ahead" activities such as reading, sewing, and driving.

Both laser treatments and cryotherapy are performed only on infants with advanced ROP, particularly stage III with "plus disease." Both treatments are considered invasive surgeries on the eye, and doctors don't know the long-term side effects of each.

In the later stages of ROP, other treatment options include:

- **Scleral buckle.** This involves placing a silicone band around the eye and tightening it. This keeps the vitreous gel from pulling on the scar tissue and allows the retina to flatten back down onto the wall of the eye. Infants who have had a scleral buckle need to have the band removed months or years later, since the eye continues to grow; otherwise they will become nearsighted. Sclera buckles are usually performed on infants with stage IV or V.

- **Vitrectomy.** Vitrectomy involves removing the vitreous and replacing it with a saline solution. After the vitreous has been removed, the scar tissue on the retina can be peeled back or cut away, allowing the retina to relax and lay back down against the eye wall. Vitrectomy is performed only at stage V.

What Happens If Treatment Does Not Work?

While ROP treatment decreases the chances for vision loss, it does not always prevent it. Not all babies respond to ROP treatment, and the disease may get worse. If treatment for ROP does not work, a retinal detachment may develop. Often, only part of the retina detaches (stage IV). When this happens, no further treatments may be needed, since a partial detachment may remain the same or go away without treatment. However, in some instances, physicians may recommend treatment to try to prevent further advancement of the retinal detachment (stage V). If the center of the retina or the entire retina detaches, central vision is threatened, and surgery may be recommended to reattach the retina.

Section 26.5

X-Linked Juvenile Retinoschisis

This section includes text excerpted from "X-Linked Juvenile Retinoschisis," Genetics Home Reference (GHR), National Institutes of Health (NIH), March 2015.

X-linked juvenile retinoschisis is a condition characterized by impaired vision that begins in childhood and occurs almost exclusively in males. This disorder affects the retina, which is a specialized light-sensitive tissue that lines the back of the eye. Damage to the retina impairs the sharpness of vision (visual acuity) in both eyes. Typically, X-linked juvenile retinoschisis affects cells in the central area of the retina called the macula. The macula is responsible for sharp central vision, which is needed for detailed tasks such as reading, driving, and recognizing faces. X-linked juvenile retinoschisis is one type of a broader disorder called macular degeneration, which disrupts the normal functioning of the macula. Occasionally, side (peripheral) vision is affected in people with X-linked juvenile retinoschisis.

X-linked juvenile retinoschisis is usually diagnosed when affected boys start school and poor vision and difficulty with reading become apparent. In more severe cases, eye squinting and involuntary movement of the eyes (nystagmus) begin in infancy. Other early features of X-linked juvenile retinoschisis include eyes that do not look in the same direction (strabismus) and farsightedness (hyperopia). Visual acuity often declines in childhood and adolescence but then stabilizes throughout adulthood until a significant decline in visual acuity typically occurs in a man's fifties or sixties. Sometimes, severe complications develop, such as separation of the retinal layers (retinal detachment) or leakage of blood vessels in the retina (vitreous hemorrhage). These eye abnormalities can further impair vision or cause blindness.

Frequency

The prevalence of X-linked juvenile retinoschisis is estimated to be 1 in 5,000 to 25,000 men worldwide.

Genetic Changes

Mutations in the *RS1* gene cause most cases of X-linked juvenile retinoschisis. The *RS1* gene provides instructions for making a protein called retinoschisin, which is found in the retina. Studies suggest that retinoschisin plays a role in the development and maintenance of the retina. The protein is probably involved in the organization of cells in the retina by attaching cells together (cell adhesion).

RS1 gene mutations result in a decrease in or complete loss of functional retinoschisin, which disrupts the maintenance and organization of cells in the retina. As a result, tiny splits (schisis) or tears form in the retina. This damage often forms a "spoke-wheel" pattern in the macula, which can be seen during an eye examination. In half of affected individuals, these abnormalities can occur in the area of the macula, affecting visual acuity, in the other half of cases the schisis occurs in the sides of the retina, resulting in impaired peripheral vision.

Some individuals with X-linked juvenile retinoschisis do not have a mutation in the *RS1* gene. In these individuals, the cause of the disorder is unknown.

Inheritance Pattern

This condition is inherited in an X-linked recessive pattern. The gene associated with this condition is located on the X chromosome, which is one of the two sex chromosomes. In males (who have only one X chromosome), one altered copy of the gene in each cell is sufficient to cause the condition. In females (who have two X chromosomes), a mutation would have to occur in both copies of the gene to cause the disorder. Because it is unlikely that females will have two altered copies of this gene, males are affected by X-linked recessive disorders much more frequently than females. A characteristic of X-linked inheritance is that fathers cannot pass X-linked traits to their sons.

Other Names for This Condition

- Congenital X-linked retinoschisis
- Degenerative retinoschisis
- Juvenile retinoschisis
- X-linked retinoschisis
- XJR

Chapter 27

Disorders of the Vitreous

Chapter Contents

Section 27.1

Floaters

This section includes text excerpted from "Facts about Floaters," National Eye Institute (NEI), October 2009. Reviewed March 2017.

What Are Floaters?

Floaters are little "cobwebs" or specks that float about in your field of vision. They are small, dark, shadowy shapes that can look like spots, thread-like strands, or squiggly lines. They move as your eyes move and seem to dart away when you try to look at them directly. They do not follow your eye movements precisely, and usually drift when your eyes stop moving.

Most people have floaters and learn to ignore them; they are usually not noticed until they become numerous or more prominent. Floaters can become apparent when looking at something bright, such as white paper or a blue sky.

Floaters and Retinal Detachment

Sometimes a section of the vitreous pulls the fine fibers away from the retina all at once, rather than gradually, causing many new floaters to appear suddenly. This is called a vitreous detachment, which in most cases is not sight-threatening and requires no treatment.

However, a sudden increase in floaters, possibly accompanied by light flashes or peripheral (side) vision loss, could indicate a retinal detachment. A retinal detachment occurs when any part of the retina, the eye's light-sensitive tissue, is lifted or pulled from its normal position at the back wall of the eye.

A retinal detachment is a serious condition and should always be considered an emergency. If left untreated, it can lead to permanent visual impairment within two or three days or even blindness in the eye.

Those who experience a sudden increase in floaters, flashes of light in peripheral vision, or a loss of peripheral vision should have an eye care professional examine their eyes as soon as possible.

Causes and Risk Factors

What Causes Floaters?

Floaters occur when the vitreous, a gel-like substance that fills about 80 percent of the eye and helps it maintain a round shape, slowly shrinks.

As the vitreous shrinks, it becomes somewhat stringy, and the strands can cast tiny shadows on the retina. These are floaters.

In most cases, floaters are part of the natural aging process and simply an annoyance. They can be distracting at first, but eventually tend to "settle" at the bottom of the eye, becoming less bothersome. They usually settle below the line of sight and do not go away completely.

However, there are other, more serious causes of floaters, including infection, inflammation (uveitis), hemorrhaging, retinal tears, and injury to the eye.

Who Is at Risk for Floaters?

Floaters are more likely to develop as we age and are more common in people who are very nearsighted, have diabetes, or who have had a cataract operation.

How Are Floaters Treated?

For people who have floaters that are simply annoying, no treatment is recommended.

On rare occasions, floaters can be so dense and numerous that they significantly affect vision. In these cases, a vitrectomy, a surgical procedure that removes floaters from the vitreous, may be needed.

A vitrectomy removes the vitreous gel, along with its floating debris, from the eye. The vitreous is replaced with a salt solution. Because the vitreous is mostly water, you will not notice any change between the salt solution and the original vitreous.

This operation carries significant risks to sight because of possible complications, which include retinal detachment, retinal tears, and cataract. Most eye surgeons are reluctant to recommend this surgery unless the floaters seriously interfere with vision.

Section 27.2

Posterior Vitreous Detachment

"Posterior Vitreous Detachment,"
© 2017 Omnigraphics. Reviewed March 2017.

Posterior vitreous detachment (PVD) occurs when the vitreous—a clear, jelly-like substance that fills rear portion of the eye—shrinks and pulls away from the back of the eye. As it detaches from the retina—a layer of light-sensitive cells that transmit visual images to the brain in the form of nerve impulses—it causes "floaters" and flashes of light to appear in the field of vision. PVD is a very common, naturally occurring, age-related change that affects more than 75 percent of people over the age of 65. It ordinarily does not cause any pain or result in long-term vision changes or sight loss. In rare instances, however, PVD symptoms are associated with holes or tears in the retina, which can result in vision loss without prompt medical treatment.

Symptoms

The main symptoms of PVD are the appearance of floaters and flashes in the field of vision. Floaters may look like dots, dust, rings, amoebas, cobwebs, or shadows that move around in the eye and float randomly across the field of vision. Although having some floaters is normal, a sudden increase in floaters—especially after the age of 60—may indicate PVD. In many cases people also notice flashes of light or tiny lightning streaks along the sides of their field of vision.

The symptoms of PVD usually appear somewhat suddenly and then gradually become less intense or noticeable over several weeks or months. People who experience a PVD in one eye will typically have it in the other eye within a year. If the normal floaters and flashes are accompanied by decreased, distorted, or blurry vision—and especially the appearance of a dark "curtain" extending into the field of vision—it can indicate a potentially serious complication, such as vitreous hemorrhage, retinal detachment, or macular hole.

Causes

PVD is caused by normal age-related changes to the eyes. The vitreous gel that fills the rear portion of the eye is made up of 99 percent water and 1 percent collagen fibers and other proteins. The collagen fibers give the vitreous a stiff, jelly-like consistency that enables it to hold its shape and remain attached to the retina at the back of the eye. As the eye ages, however, the vitreous condenses, becomes more watery, and loses its shape. When it can no longer fill the vitreous cavity in the eye, it begins to pull away from the retina and move toward the center of the eye.

As the vitreous tugs on the photoreceptive nerve endings of the retina, many people see flashes of light at the edges of their vision. At the same time, the collagen fibers clump together and float around within the vitreous, creating more numerous or noticeable floaters of various shapes and sizes. The symptoms typically resolve within 1 to 3 months, once the PVD is complete. At this point the vitreous is detached from the retina except at its base, and clear vitreous fluid has filled in the empty space.

Potential Complications

For 85 percent to 95 percent of people, PVD is a harmless, normal part of the aging process. The symptoms may be mildly annoying, but they will dissipate within a few months, leaving the vision unaffected. In rare cases, however, the vitreous can make a hole or tear in the retina as it pulls away and separates. Tearing of the retina or retinal blood vessels creates an increased risk of retinal detachment, a serious health condition that can result in permanent vision loss without urgent medical treatment.

The symptoms are likely to be similar for a harmless PVD and a PVD that causes a retinal tear, vitreous hemorrhage, or other serious complication. As a result, experts recommend that people who experience a sudden increase in floaters or flashes—especially if they are accompanied by decreased or distorted vision or a black curtain extending into the field of vision—get a professional eye examination as soon as possible.

Diagnosis and Treatment

PVD can be diagnosed through a dilated eye examination. The eye doctor puts drops into the patient's eyes to dilate the pupils, then

311

examines the interior structure of the eyes using an instrument called a slit lamp microscope. If necessary, such additional tests as optical coherence tomography (OCT) or ocular ultrasound can be used to confirm the diagnosis. In most cases, the symptoms of PVD subside within a few weeks or months without treatment. It is important to get an eye examination at the onset of symptoms, however, to rule out retinal tearing or take steps to prevent retinal detachment.

References

1. Esmaili, Daniel D. "Posterior Vitreous Detachment," Discovery Eye Foundation, October 30, 2014.

2. "Posterior Vitreous Detachment," American Society of Retina Specialists, 2017.

3. "Understanding Posterior Vitreous Detachment," Royal National Institute for Blind People, 2016.

Chapter 28

Disorders of the Uvea

Chapter Contents

Section 28.1

Uveal Coloboma

This section includes text excerpted from "Facts
about Uveal Coloboma," National Eye Institute (NEI),
June 2012. Reviewed March 2017.

Coloboma Basics

What Is a Coloboma?

Coloboma comes from a Greek word which means "curtailed." It is
used to describe conditions where normal tissue in or around the eye
is missing from birth.

To understand coloboma, it is useful to be familiar with the normal
structure and appearance of the eye, and the terms related to the
different parts of the eye.

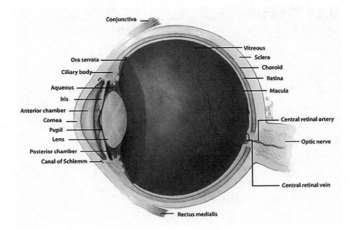

Figure 28.1. *Diagram of the Eye*

Uveal Coloboma

This coloboma can present as an iris coloboma (the iris is the colored
part of the eye), with the traditional "keyhole" or "cat-eye" appearance

to the iris, and/or as a chorio-retinal coloboma where the retina in the lower inside corner of the eye is missing.

How Common Is Uveal Coloboma?

Uveal coloboma is a rare condition that is not always well documented. Depending on the study and where the study was conducted, estimates range from 0.5 to 2.2 cases per 10,000 births. Some cases may go unnoticed because uveal coloboma does not always affect vision or the outside appearance of the eye.

Uveal coloboma is a significant cause of blindness. Studies estimate that 5 to 10 percent of blind European children have uveal coloboma or uveal coloboma-related malformations.

Frequently Asked Questions about Coloboma

What Are the Different Kinds of Coloboma?

There are different kinds of coloboma, depending on which part of the eye is missing. Coloboma can affect the:

- eyelid
- lens
- macula
- optic nerve
- uvea

Eyelid Coloboma

In eyelid coloboma a piece of either the upper or lower eyelid is absent. Eyelid coloboma may be part of a genetic syndrome, or happen as a result of a disruption of eyelid development in a baby. A syndrome is a specific grouping of birth defects or symptoms present in one person.

Lens Coloboma

In this type of coloboma, a piece of the lens is absent. The lens, which helps focus light on the retina, will typically appear with a notch.

Macular Coloboma

This happens when the center of the retina, called the macula, does not develop normally. The macula is responsible for daylight, fine and color vision. Macular coloboma may be caused when normal eye development is interrupted or following an inflammation of the retina during development of the baby.

Optic Nerve Coloboma

Optic nerve coloboma refers to one of two distinct things:

1. An abnormal optic nerve that is deeply "excavated" or hollowed out. In some cases it can also be referred to as an optic nerve pit. The optic nerve is the bundle of nerve fibers that relays the light signals from the eye to the brain.

2. A uveal coloboma that is large enough to involve the optic nerve, either the inferior portion or the entire optic disc.

Are There Other Diseases or Conditions Associated with Coloboma?

In the Eye

Coloboma is sometimes found in association with other eye features. These may include:

• Difference in eye color between the two eyes (heterochromia)

• Small eye (microphthalmia)

• Increased thickness of the cornea. The cornea is the clear front part of the eye.

• Clouding of the lens (cataract)

• Elevated pressure in the eye (glaucoma)

• Retinal malformation (retinal dysplasia)

• Nearsightedness (myopia) or farsightedness (hyperopia)

• Involuntary eye movements (nystagmus)

• Protrusion of the back of the eyeball (posterior staphyloma)

In Other Parts of the Body

Coloboma may be an isolated feature, or may be found with other features. Sometimes these other features may be few and minor, such as skin tags near the ear. Sometimes they may be more numerous and severe, such as a heart or a kidney defect. A few of these associations may be genetic syndromes. These include (but are not limited to):

- CHARGE syndrome
- Cat-Eye syndrome
- Kabuki syndrome
- 13q deletion syndrome
- Wolf-Hirshhorn syndrome

Causes of Coloboma

What Causes Uveal Coloboma?

It is believed that uveal coloboma is primarily genetic in origin. "Genetic" means that the coloboma was caused by a gene that was not working properly when the eye was forming. Sometimes coloboma is part of a specific genetic syndrome, for which the genetics are known. For instance, coloboma is one feature of CHARGE syndrome, which is associated with a change in, or a complete deletion of a gene called *CHD7*.

Researchers have found genes associated with coloboma in a few cases. To date, however, we still do not know which genes explain most cases of coloboma.

Some researchers have proposed that certain environmental factors may contribute to developing coloboma, either in humans or in animals. These findings have been published over time in the research literature, but there have been no systematic analysis of possible links. For instance, it is known that babies exposed to alcohol during pregnancy can develop coloboma—but they also have other anomalies. There are no known strong links between environmental exposures and isolated coloboma.

It is always possible that coloboma happens strictly by chance. In summary, there is little data to presently say why coloboma happened to a person in a family where no one else is affected.

How Does Uveal Coloboma Happen?

To understand how uveal coloboma happens, we first have to understand how the eye forms in the developing baby. The eyes start as stalks coming out of the brain. The tip of each stalk will become the eye itself, while the rest of the stalk will become the optic nerve linking the eye to the brain. There is a seam at the bottom of each stalk, where blood vessels originally run. This seam is known as the optic fissure, or the choroidal fissure, or the embryonic fissure. Starting at the fifth week of gestation (pregnancy), this seam must close. The closure starts roughly in the middle of the developing eye, and runs in both directions. This process is finished by the seventh week of gestation. If, for some reason, the closure does not happen, a uveal coloboma is formed.

Depending on where the closure did not happen, the baby can have an iris coloboma (front of the fissure), a chorio-retinal coloboma (back of the fissure), or any combination of these. Uveal coloboma can affect one eye (unilateral) or both eyes (bilateral). The condition can be the same in both eyes (symmetric) or different in both eyes (asymmetric). A uveal coloboma may go from front to back (continuous) or have "skip lesions." The fact that the seam runs at the bottom of the stalk is the reason why uveal coloboma is always located in the lower inside corner of the eye.

How Can Uveal Coloboma Be Inherited?

Isolated coloboma can follow all possible patterns of single gene inheritance, namely autosomal dominant, autosomal recessive and X-linked. In one family, however, coloboma will follow only one pattern. For instance, in case of an autosomal dominant pattern, a person with coloboma would have a one in two chance of passing on the coloboma to each of his or her offspring. In families with a single case of coloboma, it is not possible to say what pattern of inheritance is involved; therefore it is not possible to give an exact recurrence risk number. The recurrence risk of coloboma computed from averaging data across many families (empiric risk) is about 10 percent. This is an imperfect number, as it mixes information from families where this risk may be close to 0 percent with information from families where the actual risk may be 25 percent or even 50 percent.

The topic of inheritance of coloboma is complicated by several factors:

- Sometimes a person who is at risk for developing coloboma may not develop the condition, or it may be so minor that it goes unnoticed. This may appear in the family history as an inconsistent, non-interpretable pattern of inheritance.

- Knowing the pattern of inheritance of coloboma in a family does not give information on how severely an at-risk person will be affected (e.g., how good their visual acuity will be).

- There may be more than one gene involved in being at risk for coloboma, which makes predicting inheritance even more difficult.

For coloboma due to a known syndrome, such as CHARGE syndrome, inheritance is based on what is known about that particular syndrome. However, it is rarely, if ever, possible to say whether coloboma will be a feature of the syndrome in a person inheriting the genetic background responsible for this syndrome.

Symptoms of Coloboma

There may or may not be any symptoms related to coloboma; it all depends on the amount and location of the missing tissue. People with a coloboma affecting the macula and the optic nerve will likely have reduced vision. In general, it is difficult to exactly predict what level of vision a baby will have only by looking at how much of the retina is missing.

People with a coloboma affecting any part of the retina will have what is called a "field defect." A field defect means that a person is missing vision in a specific location. Because coloboma is located in the lower part of the retina, vision in the upper part of the field of vision will be missing. This may or may not be noticeable to the affected person.

A person with a coloboma affecting the front of the eye only will not have any decreased vision from it. Some people, however, have reported being more sensitive to light.

Treatment of Coloboma

Can Uveal Coloboma Be Treated?

Patients with uveal coloboma should have yearly follow-up exams by an eye care professional. However, there is currently no medication or surgery that can cure or reverse coloboma and make the eye whole again. Treatment consists of helping patients adjust to vision problems and make the most of the vision they have by:

- Correcting any refractive error with glasses or contact lenses.

- Maximizing the vision of the most affected eye in asymmetric cases. This may involve patching or using drops to temporarily blur vision in the stronger eye for a limited period of time.

- Ensuring that amblyopia (lazy eye) does not develop in childhood in case of asymmetry. Sometimes amblyopia treatment (patching, glasses and/or drops) can improve vision in eyes even with severe colobomas.

- Treating any other eye condition that may be present with coloboma, such as cataracts.

- Treating any complications that might arise from a retinal coloboma later in life, such as the growth of new blood vessels at the back of the eye (neovascularization) and/or retinal detachment.

- Using low vision devices, as needed.

- Making use of rehabilitation services, such as early intervention programs.

- Offering genetic counseling to the patient and family members.

If the eye with the coloboma is very small (microphthalmia), other follow-ups may be needed. Conformers and expanders may be used to help support the face and encourage the eye socket to grow. Children may also be fitted for a prosthetic (artificial) eye to improve appearance. As the face develops, new conformers will need to be made.

For people who wish to alter the appearance of a coloboma affecting the front of the eye, two options are currently available:

- Colored contact lenses that make the black part of the eye (pupil) round.

- Surgery to make the pupil rounder. This procedure pulls and sutures together the lower edges of the iris.

Is Genetic Testing Available for Uveal Coloboma?

Testing may be available in cases where the coloboma is part of a specific genetic syndrome. This testing would look for the gene(s) causing whole syndrome and not just the coloboma. Genetic testing is done on a blood sample and may involve looking at the patient's chromosomes, or looking at a specific gene on one of the chromosomes.

There is no specific recommended testing for isolated coloboma. Testing for some of the genes that were reported in the medical literature might be performed as part of research projects. However, results from such testing will likely be negative, since these genes explain very few cases of uveal coloboma.

Section 28.2

Uveal Melanoma

This section includes text excerpted from "Intraocular
(Uveal) Melanoma Treatment (PDQ®)—Patient Version,"
National Cancer Institute (NCI), July 19, 2016.

Intraocular melanoma is a disease in which malignant (cancer) cells
form in the tissues of the eye.

Intraocular melanoma begins in the middle of three layers of the
wall of the eye. The outer layer includes the white sclera (the "white of
the eye") and the clear cornea at the front of the eye. The inner layer
has a lining of nerve tissue, called the retina, which senses light and
sends images along the optic nerve to the brain.

The middle layer, where intraocular melanoma forms, is called the
uvea or uveal tract, and has three main parts:

- **Iris:** The iris is the colored area at the front of the eye (the "eye
  color"). It can be seen through the clear cornea. The pupil is in
  the center of the iris and it changes size to let more or less light
  into the eye. Intraocular melanoma of the iris is usually a small
  tumor that grows slowly and rarely spreads to other parts of the
  body.

- **Ciliary body:** The ciliary body is a ring of tissue with muscle
  fibers that change the size of the pupil and the shape of the
  lens. It is found behind the iris. Changes in the shape of the
  lens help the eye focus. The ciliary body also makes the clear
  fluid that fills the space between the cornea and the iris. Intraocular melanoma of the ciliary body is often larger and more
  likely to spread to other parts of the body than intraocular melanoma of the iris.

- **Choroid:** The choroid is a layer of blood vessels that bring oxygen and nutrients to the eye. Most intraocular melanomas begin
  in the choroid. Intraocular melanoma of the choroid is often
  larger and more likely to spread to other parts of the body than
  intraocular melanoma of the iris.

Intraocular melanoma is a rare cancer that forms from cells that make melanin in the iris, ciliary body, and choroid. It is the most common eye cancer in adults.

Risk Factors for Uveal Melanoma

Anything that increases your risk of getting a disease is called a risk factor. Having a risk factor does not mean that you will get cancer; not having risk factors doesn't mean that you will not get cancer. Talk with your doctor if you think you may be at risk.

Risk factors for intraocular melanoma include the following:

- having a fair complexion, which includes the following:

- fair skin that freckles and burns easily, does not tan, or tans poorly

- blue or green or other light-colored eyes

- older age

- being white

Signs and Symptoms of Uveal Melanoma

Intraocular melanoma may not cause early signs or symptoms. It is sometimes found during a regular eye exam when the doctor dilates the pupil and looks into the eye. Signs and symptoms may be caused by intraocular melanoma or by other conditions. Check with your doctor if you have any of the following:

- blurred vision or other change in vision

- floaters (spots that drift in your field of vision) or flashes of light

- a dark spot on the iris

- a change in the size or shape of the pupil

- a change in the position of the eyeball in the eye socket

Diagnostic Tests for Uveal Melanoma

The following tests and procedures may be used:

- **Physical exam and history:** An exam of the body to check general signs of health, including checking for signs of disease, such as lumps or anything else that seems unusual. A history of the patient's health habits and past illnesses and treatments will also be taken.

- **Eye exam with dilated pupil:** An exam of the eye in which the pupil is dilated (enlarged) with medicated eye drops to allow the doctor to look through the lens and pupil to the retina. The inside of the eye, including the retina and the optic nerve, is checked. Pictures may be taken over time to keep track of changes in the size of the tumor. There are several types of eye exams:

- **Ophthalmoscopy:** An exam of the inside of the back of the eye to check the retina and optic nerve using a small magnifying lens and a light.

- **Slit-lamp biomicroscopy:** An exam of the inside of the eye to check the retina, optic nerve, and other parts of the eye using a strong beam of light and a microscope.

- **Gonioscopy:** An exam of the front part of the eye between the cornea and iris. A special instrument is used to see if the area where fluid drains out of the eye is blocked.

- **Ultrasound exam of the eye:** A procedure in which high-energy sound waves (ultrasound) are bounced off the internal tissues of the eye to make echoes. Eye drops are used to numb the eye and a small probe that sends and receives sound waves is placed gently on the surface of the eye. The echoes make a picture of the inside of the eye and the distance from the cornea to the retina is measured. The picture, called a sonogram, shows on the screen of the ultrasound monitor.

- **High-resolution ultrasound biomicroscopy:** A procedure in which high-energy sound waves (ultrasound) are bounced off the internal tissues of the eye to make echoes. Eye drops are used to numb the eye and a small probe that sends and receives sound waves is placed gently on the surface of the eye. The echoes make a more detailed picture of the inside of the eye than a regular ultrasound. The tumor is checked for its size, shape, and thickness, and for signs that the tumor has spread to nearby tissue.

- **Transillumination of the globe and iris:** An exam of the iris, cornea, lens, and ciliary body with a light placed on either the upper or lower lid.

- **Fluorescein angiography:** A procedure to look at blood vessels and the flow of blood inside the eye. An orange fluorescent dye (fluorescein) is injected into a blood vessel in the arm and goes into the bloodstream. As the dye travels through blood vessels of the eye, a special camera takes pictures of the retina and choroid to find any areas that are blocked or leaking.

- **Indocyanine green angiography:** A procedure to look at blood vessels in the choroid layer of the eye. A green dye (indocyanine green) is injected into a blood vessel in the arm and goes into the bloodstream. As the dye travels through blood vessels of the eye, a special camera takes pictures of the retina and choroid to find any areas that are blocked or leaking.

- **Ocular coherence tomography:** An imaging test that uses light waves to take cross-section pictures of the retina, and sometimes the choroid, to see if there is swelling or fluid beneath the retina.

Uveal Melanoma Biopsy

A biopsy is the removal of cells or tissues so they can be viewed under a microscope to check for signs of cancer. Rarely, a biopsy of the tumor is needed to diagnose intraocular melanoma. Tissue that is removed during a biopsy or surgery to remove the tumor may be tested to get more information about prognosis and which treatment options are best.

The following tests may be done on the sample of tissue:

- **Cytogenetic analysis:** A laboratory test in which cells in a sample of tissue are viewed under a microscope to look for certain changes in the chromosomes.

- **Gene expression profiling:** A laboratory test in which cells in a sample of tissue are checked for certain types of ribonucleic acid (RNA).

A biopsy may result in retinal detachment (the retina separates from other tissues in the eye). This can be repaired by surgery.

Certain factors affect prognosis (chance of recovery) and treatment options.

The prognosis (chance of recovery) and treatment options depend on the following:

- How the melanoma cells look under a microscope.

- The size and thickness of the tumor.
- The part of the eye the tumor is in (the iris, ciliary body, or choroid).
- Whether the tumor has spread within the eye or to other places in the body.
- Whether there are certain changes in the genes linked to intra-ocular melanoma.
- The patient's age and general health.
- Whether the tumor has recurred (come back) after treatment.

Stages of Uveal Melanoma

Staging

The process used to find out if cancer has spread to other parts of the body is called staging. The information gathered from the staging process determines the stage of the disease. It is important to know the stage in order to plan treatment.

The following tests and procedures may be used in the staging process:

- Blood chemistry studies
- Liver function tests
- Ultrasound exam
- Chest X-ray
- Magnetic resonance imaging (MRI)
- Computerized tomography (CT) scan or computerized axial tomography (CAT) scan
- Positron emission tomography (PET) scan

Spread of Cancer

There are three ways that cancer spreads in the body. Cancer can spread through tissue, the lymph system, and the blood:

- **Tissue.** The cancer spreads from where it began by growing into nearby areas.
- **Lymph system.** The cancer spreads from where it began by getting into the lymph system. The cancer travels through the lymph vessels to other parts of the body.

- **Blood.** The cancer spreads from where it began by getting into the blood. The cancer travels through the blood vessels to other parts of the body.

Cancer may spread from where it began to other parts of the body.

When cancer spreads to another part of the body, it is called metastasis. Cancer cells break away from where they began (the primary tumor) and travel through the lymph system or blood.

- **Lymph system.** The cancer gets into the lymph system, travels through the lymph vessels, and forms a tumor (metastatic tumor) in another part of the body.

- **Blood.** The cancer gets into the blood, travels through the blood vessels, and forms a tumor (metastatic tumor) in another part of the body.

The metastatic tumor is the same type of cancer as the primary tumor. For example, if intraocular melanoma spreads to the liver, the cancer cells in the liver are actually intraocular melanoma cells. The disease is metastatic intraocular melanoma, not liver cancer.

Recurrent Uveal Melanoma

Recurrent intraocular melanoma is cancer that has recurred (come back) after it has been treated. The melanoma may come back in the eye or in other parts of the body.

Treatment of Uveal Melanoma

Different types of treatments are available for patients with intraocular melanoma. Some treatments are standard (the currently used treatment), and some are being tested in clinical trials. A treatment clinical trial is a research study meant to help improve current treatments or obtain information on new treatments for patients with cancer. When clinical trials show that a new treatment is better than the standard treatment, the new treatment may become the standard treatment. Patients may want to think about taking part in a clinical trial. Some clinical trials are open only to patients who have not started treatment.

Five Types of Standard Treatment

Surgery

Surgery is the most common treatment for intraocular melanoma. The following types of surgery may be used:

- **Resection:** Surgery to remove the tumor and a small amount of healthy tissue around it.

- **Enucleation:** Surgery to remove the eye and part of the optic nerve. This is done if vision cannot be saved and the tumor is large, has spread to the optic nerve, or causes high pressure inside the eye. After surgery, the patient is usually fitted for an artificial eye to match the size and color of the other eye.

- **Exenteration:** Surgery to remove the eye and eyelid, and muscles, nerves, and fat in the eye socket. After surgery, the patient may be fitted for an artificial eye to match the size and color of the other eye or a facial prosthesis.

Watchful Waiting

Watchful waiting is closely monitoring a patient's condition without giving any treatment until signs or symptoms appear or change. Pictures are taken over time to keep track of changes in the size of the tumor and how fast it is growing.

Watchful waiting is used for patients who do not have signs or symptoms and the tumor is not growing. It is also used when the tumor is in the only eye with useful vision.

Radiation Therapy

Radiation therapy is a cancer treatment that uses high-energy X-rays or other types of radiation to kill cancer cells or keep them from growing. There are two types of radiation therapy:

- **External radiation therapy** uses a machine outside the body to send radiation toward the cancer. Certain ways of giving radiation therapy can help keep radiation from damaging nearby healthy tissue. These types of external radiation therapy include the following:

  - **Charged-particle external beam radiation therapy**
  - **Gamma Knife therapy**

- **Internal radiation therapy** uses a radioactive substance sealed in needles, seeds, wires, or catheters that are placed directly into or near the cancer. Certain ways of giving radiation therapy can help keep radiation from damaging healthy tissue. This type of internal radiation therapy may include the following:

  - **Localized plaque radiation therapy**

The way the radiation therapy is given depends on the type and stage of the cancer being treated. External and internal radiation therapy are used to treat intraocular melanoma.

Photocoagulation

Photocoagulation is a procedure that uses laser light to destroy blood vessels that bring nutrients to the tumor, causing the tumor cells to die. Photocoagulation may be used to treat small tumors. This is also called light coagulation.

Thermotherapy

Thermotherapy is the use of heat from a laser to destroy cancer cells and shrink the tumor.

Section 28.3

Uveitis

This section includes text excerpted from "Facts about Uveitis," National Eye Institute (NEI), August 2011. Reviewed March 2017.

Uveitis Basics

What Is Uveitis?

Uveitis is a general term describing a group of inflammatory diseases that produces swelling and destroys eye tissues. These diseases can slightly reduce vision or lead to severe vision loss.

The term "uveitis" is used because the diseases often affect a part of the eye called the uvea. Nevertheless, uveitis is not limited to the uvea. These diseases also affect the lens, retina, optic nerve, and vitreous, producing reduced vision or blindness.

Uveitis may be caused by problems or diseases occurring in the eye or it can be part of an inflammatory disease affecting other parts of the body.

It can happen at all ages and primarily affects people between 20−60 years old.

Uveitis can last for a short (acute) or a long (chronic) time. The severest forms of uveitis reoccur many times.

Eye care professionals may describe the disease more specifically as:

- anterior uveitis

- intermediate uveitis

- posterior uveitis

- panuveitis uveitis

Eye care professionals may also describe the disease as infectious or noninfectious uveitis.

What Is the Uvea and What Parts of the Eye Are Most Affected by Uveitis?

The uvea is the middle layer of the eye which contains much of the eye's blood vessels (see Figure 28.2). This is one way that inflammatory cells can enter the eye. Located between the sclera, the eye's white outer coat, and the inner layer of the eye, called the retina, the uvea consists of the iris, ciliary body, and choroid:

- **Iris:** The colored circle at the front of the eye. It defines eye color, secretes nutrients to keep the lens healthy, and controls the amount of light that enters the eye by adjusting the size of the pupil.

- **Ciliary Body:** It is located between the iris and the choroid. It helps the eye focus by controlling the shape of the lens and it provides nutrients to keep the lens healthy.

- **Choroid:** A thin, spongy network of blood vessels, which primarily provides nutrients to the retina.

Uveitis disrupts vision by primarily causing problems with the lens, retina, optic nerve, and vitreous (see Figure 28.2):

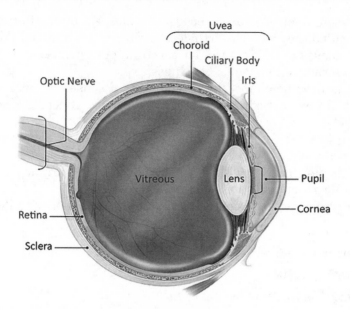

Figure 28.2. *Eye Diagram Showing the Uvea, Optic Nerve, Retina, Sclera, Cornea and Pupil*

Lens: *Transparent tissue that allows light into the eye.*
Retina: *The layer of cells on the back, inside part of the eye that converts light into electrical signals sent to the brain*
Optic Nerve: *A bundle of nerve fibers that transmits electrical signals from the retina to the brain*
Vitreous: *The fluid filled space inside the eye*

Causes and Risk Factors

What Causes Uveitis?

Uveitis is caused by inflammatory responses inside the eye.

Inflammation is the body's natural response to tissue damage, germs, or toxins. It produces swelling, redness, heat, and destroys tissues as certain white blood cells rush to the affected part of the body to contain or eliminate the insult.

Uveitis may be caused by:

- an attack from the body's own immune system (autoimmunity)

- infections or tumors occurring within the eye or in other parts of the body

- bruises to the eye

330

- toxins that may penetrate the eye

The disease will cause symptoms, such as decreased vision, pain, light sensitivity, and increased floaters. In many cases the cause is unknown.

Uveitis is usually classified by where it occurs in the eye.

What Is Anterior Uveitis?

Anterior uveitis occurs in the front of the eye. It is the most common form of uveitis, predominantly occurring in young and middle-aged people. Many cases occur in healthy people and may only affect one eye but some are associated with rheumatologic, skin, gastrointestinal, lung and infectious diseases.

What Is Intermediate Uveitis?

Intermediate uveitis is commonly seen in young adults. The center of the inflammation often appears in the vitreous. It has been linked to several disorders including, sarcoidosis and multiple sclerosis.

What Is Posterior Uveitis?

Posterior uveitis is the least common form of uveitis. It primarily occurs in the back of the eye, often involving both the retina and the choroid. It is often called choroditis or chorioretinitis. There are many infectious and noninfectious causes to posterior uveitis.

What Is Pan-Uveitis?

Pan-uveitis is a term used when all three major parts of the eye are affected by inflammation. Behcet disease is one of the most well-known forms of pan-uveitis and it greatly damages the retina.

Intermediate, posterior, and pan-uveitis are the most severe and highly recurrent forms of uveitis. They often cause blindness if left untreated.

Diseases Associated with Uveitis

Uveitis can be associated with many diseases including:

- AIDS
- Ankylosing spondylitis
- Behcet syndrome

- CMV retinitis
- Herpes zoster infection
- Histoplasmosis
- Kawasaki disease
- Multiple sclerosis
- Psoriasis
- Reactive arthritis
- Rheumatoid arthritis
- Sarcoidosis
- Syphilis
- Toxoplasmosis
- Tuberculosis
- Ulcerative colitis
- Vogt Koyanagi Harada disease

Symptoms and Detection of Uveitis

What Are the Symptoms?

Uveitis can affect one or both eyes. Symptoms may develop rapidly and can include:

- blurred vision
- dark, floating spots in the vision (floaters)
- eye pain
- redness of the eye
- sensitivity to light (photophobia)

Anyone suffering eye pain, severe light sensitivity, and any change in vision should immediately be examined by an ophthalmologist.

The signs and symptoms of uveitis depend on the type of inflammation.

Acute anterior uveitis may occur in one or both eyes and in adults is characterized by eye pain, blurred vision, sensitivity to light, a small pupil, and redness.

Intermediate uveitis causes blurred vision and floaters. Usually it is not associated with pain.

Posterior uveitis can produce vision loss. This type of uveitis can only be detected during an eye examination.

How Is Uveitis Detected?

Diagnosis of uveitis includes a thorough examination and the recording of the patient's complete medical history. Laboratory tests may be done to rule out an infection or an autoimmune disorder.

A central nervous system evaluation will often be performed on patients with a subgroup of intermediate uveitis, called pars planitis, to determine whether they have multiple sclerosis which is often associated with pars planitis.

The eye exams used, include:

- **An Eye Chart or Visual Acuity Test:** This test measures whether a patient's vision has decreased.

- **A Funduscopic Exam:** The pupil is widened (dilated) with eye drops and then a light is shown through with an instrument called an ophthalmoscope to noninvasively inspect the back, inside part of the eye.

- **Ocular Pressure:** An instrument, such a tonometer or a tonopen, measures the pressure inside the eye. Drops that numb the eye may be used for this test.

- **A Slit Lamp Exam:** A slit lamp noninvasively inspects much of the eye. It can inspect the front and back parts of the eye and some lamps may be equipped with a tonometer to measure eye pressure. A dye called fluorescein, which makes blood vessels easier to see, may be added to the eye during the examination. The dye only temporarily stains the eye.

Treatment of Uveitis

How Is Uveitis Treated?

Uveitis treatments primarily try to eliminate inflammation, alleviate pain, prevent further tissue damage, and restore any loss of vision. Treatments depend on the type of uveitis a patient displays. Some, such as using corticosteroid eye drops and injections around the eye or inside the eye, may exclusively target the eye whereas other treatments, such immunosuppressive agents taken by mouth, may be used when the disease is occurring in both eyes, particularly in the back of both eyes.

An eye care professional will usually prescribe steroidal anti-inflammatory medication that can be taken as eye drops, swallowed as a pill, injected around or into the eye, infused into the blood intravenously, or, released into the eye via a capsule that is surgically implanted inside the eye. Long-term steroid use may produce side effects such as stomach ulcers, osteoporosis (bone thinning), diabetes, cataracts, glaucoma, cardiovascular disease, weight gain, fluid retention, and Cushing's syndrome. Usually other agents are started if it appears that patients need moderate or high doses of oral steroids for more than 3 months.

Other immunosuppressive agents that are commonly used include medications such as methotrexate, mycophenolate, azathioprine, and cyclosporine. These treatments require regular blood tests to monitor for possible side effects. In some cases, biologic response modifiers (BRM), or biologics, such as, adalimumab, infliximab, daclizumab, abatacept, and rituximab are used. These drugs target specific elements of the immune system. Some of these drugs may increase the risk of having cancer.

Anterior Uveitis Treatments

Anterior uveitis may be treated by:

- Taking eye drops that dilate the pupil to prevent muscle spasms in the iris and ciliary body.

- Taking eye drops containing steroids, such as prednisone, to reduce inflammation.

Intermediate, Posterior, and Pan-Uveitis Treatments

Intermediate, posterior, and pan-uveitis are often treated with injections around the eye, medications given by mouth, or, in some instances, time-release capsules that are surgically implanted inside the eye. Other immunosuppressive agents may be given. A doctor must make sure a patient is not fighting an infection before proceeding with these therapies.

A National Eye Institute (NEI)-funded study, called the Multicenter Uveitis Treatment Trial (MUST), compared the safety and effectiveness of conventional treatment for these forms of uveitis, which suppresses a patient's entire immune system, with a new local treatment that exclusively suppressed inflammation in the affected eye. Conventionally-treated patients were initially given high doses of prednisone, a corticosteroid medication, for 1 to 4 weeks which were then reduced gradually to low doses whereas locally-treated patients had a capsule that slowly released fluocinolone, another corticosteroid medication, surgically inserted in their affected eyes. Both treatments improved vision to a similar degree, with patients gaining almost one line on an eye chart. Conventional treatment produced few side effects. In contrast, the implant produced more eye problems, such as abnormally high eye pressure, glaucoma, and cataracts. Although both treatments decreased inflammation in the eye, the implant did so faster and to a greater degree. Nevertheless, visual improvements were similar to those of patients given conventional treatment.

Section 28.4

Choroideremia

This section includes text excerpted from "Choroideremia," Genetics Home Reference (GHR), National Institutes of Health (NIH), July 2013. Reviewed March 2017.

Choroideremia is a condition characterized by progressive vision loss that mainly affects males. The first symptom of this condition is usually an impairment of night vision (night blindness), which can occur in early childhood. A progressive narrowing of the field of vision (tunnel vision) follows, as well as a decrease in the ability to see details (visual acuity). These vision problems are due to an ongoing loss of cells (atrophy) in the specialized light-sensitive tissue that lines the back of the eye (retina) and a nearby network of blood vessels (the choroid). The vision impairment in choroideremia worsens over time, but the progression varies among affected individuals. However, all individuals with this condition will develop blindness, most commonly in late adulthood.

Frequency

The prevalence of choroideremia is estimated to be 1 in 50,000 to 100,000 people. However, it is likely that this condition is underdiagnosed because of its similarities to other eye disorders. Choroideremia is thought to account for approximately 4 percent of all blindness.

Genetic Changes

Mutations in the CHM gene cause choroideremia. The CHM gene provides instructions for producing the Rab escort protein-1 (REP-1). As an escort protein, REP-1 attaches to molecules called Rab proteins within the cell and directs them to the membranes of various cell compartments (organelles). Rab proteins are involved in the movement of proteins and organelles within cells (intracellular trafficking). Mutations in the CHM gene lead to an absence of REP-1 protein or the production of a REP-1 protein that cannot carry out its protein escort function. This lack of functional REP-1 prevents Rab proteins from reaching and attaching (binding) to the organelle membranes. Without the aid of Rab proteins in intracellular trafficking, cells die prematurely.

The REP-1 protein is active (expressed) throughout the body, as is a similar protein, REP-2. Research suggests that when REP-1 is absent or nonfunctional, REP-2 can perform the protein escort duties of REP-1 in many of the body's tissues. Very little REP-2 protein is present in the retina, however, so it cannot compensate for the loss of REP-1 in this tissue. Loss of REP-1 function and subsequent misplacement of Rab proteins within the cells of the retina causes the progressive vision loss characteristic of choroideremia.

Inheritance Pattern

Choroideremia is inherited in an X-linked recessive pattern. The CHM gene is located on the X chromosome, which is one of the two sex chromosomes. In males (who have only one X chromosome), one altered copy of the gene in each cell is sufficient to cause the condition. In females (who have two X chromosomes), a mutation must be present in both copies of the gene to cause the disorder. Males are affected by X-linked recessive disorders much more frequently than females. A characteristic of X-linked inheritance is that fathers cannot pass X-linked traits to their sons.

In X-linked recessive inheritance, a female with one mutated copy of the gene in each cell is called a carrier. She can pass on the altered gene, but usually does not experience signs and symptoms of the disorder. Females who carry a CHM mutation may show small areas of cell loss within the retina that can be observed during a thorough eye examination. These changes can impair vision later in life.

Other Names for This Condition

- Choroidal sclerosis
- Progressive tapetochoroidal dystrophy
- TCD

Part Five

Eye Injuries and Disorders of the Surrounding Structures

Chapter 29

Eye Injury Prevention

Preventing Injuries to the Eye[1]

According to the American Academy of Ophthalmology (AAO), an estimated 90 percent of eye injuries are preventable with the use of proper safety eyewear. Even a minor injury to the cornea—like that from a small particle of dust or debris—can be painful and become a lifelong issue, so take the extra precaution and always protect the eyes. If the eye is injured, seek emergency medical help immediately.

Dangers at Home[1]

When we think of eye protection, we tend to think of people wearing hardhats and lab coats. We often forget that even at home, we might find ourselves dealing with similar threats to our eyes. Dangerous chemicals that could burn or splash the eyes aren't restricted to chemical laboratories. They're also in our garages and under our kitchen sinks. Debris and other air-borne irritants are present at home, too,

---

This chapter includes text excerpted from documents published by three public domain sources. Text under headings marked 1 are excerpted from "Eye Injury Prevention," Federal Occupational Health (FOH), U.S. Department of Health and Human Services (HHS), March 20, 2012. Reviewed March 2017; text under heading marked 2 is excerpted from "Eye Safety at Work Is Everyone's Business," National Eye Institute (NEI), February 8, 2017; and text under heading marked 3 is excerpted from "Workplace Safety and Health Topics: Eye Safety," National Institute for Occupational Safety and Health (NIOSH), Centers for Disease Control and Prevention (CDC), July 29, 2013. Reviewed March 2017.

whether one is doing a home construction project or working in the yard. The debris from a lawnmower or "weed wacker," for example, can be moving at high speeds and provide no time to react. Some sports also put the eyes at risk of injury from foreign objects moving at high speeds.

Dangers at Work[2]

Each day, about 2,000 U.S. workers receive medical treatment because of eye injuries sustained at work. Workplace injury is a leading cause of eye trauma, vision loss, disability, and blindness, and can interfere with your ability to perform your job and carry out normal activities.

Employers and workers need to be aware of the risks to sight, especially if they work in high-risk occupations. High-risk occupations include construction, manufacturing, mining, carpentry, auto repair, electrical work, plumbing, welding, and maintenance. The combination of removing or minimizing eye safety hazards and wearing proper eye safety protection can prevent many eye injuries.

Personal protective eyewear such as safety glasses with side shields, goggles, face shields, and/or welding helmets can protect you from common hazards, including flying fragments, large chips, hot sparks, optical radiation, splashes from molten metals, objects, particles, and glare. The risk of eye injury and the need for preventive measures depend on your job and the conditions in your workplace.

Effective Eyewear[1]

The best ways to prevent injury to the eye is to always wear the appropriate eye protection. The Bureau of Labor Statistics (BLS) reports that approximately three out of every five workers injured were either not wearing eye protection at the time of the accident or wearing the wrong kind of eye protection for the job. To be effective, eyewear must fit properly and be effectively designed to protect the eyes based on the activity being performed. The Occupational Safety Health Administration (OSHA) has standards that require employers to provide their workers with the appropriate eye protection.

When to Wear Protective Eyewear[1]

According to these standards, you (or anyone who is watching you work) should always wear properly fitted eye protective gear, such as safety glasses with side protection/shields, when:

- doing work that may produce particles, slivers, or dust from materials like wood, metal, plastic, cement, and drywall

- hammering, sanding, grinding, or doing masonry work

- working with power tools

- working with chemicals, including common household chemicals like ammonia, oven cleaners, and bleach

- using a lawnmower, riding mower, or other motorized gardening devices like string trimmers (also called "weed wacker" or "weed whip")

- working with wet or powdered cement

- welding (which requires extra protection like a welding mask or helmet from sparks and ultraviolet (UV) radiation)

- "jumping" the battery of a motor vehicle

- being a bystander to any of the above

Sports

It's also recommended that you protect your eyes from injury when participating in certain sports, including:

- indoor racket sports
- paintball
- baseball
- basketball
- hockey
- cycling
- riding or being a passenger on a motorcycle

Sun Exposure

The eyes also need to be protected from prolonged sun exposure, so have sunglasses with UV protection at hand. If you're putting on sunscreen, you should also be wearing sunglasses with UV protection.

Vision is a gift. Make the extra effort to protect it.

First Aid[3]

Specks in the Eye

- Do not rub the eye.

- Flush the eye with large amounts of water.

- See a doctor if the speck does not wash out or if pain or redness continues.

Cuts, Punctures, and Foreign Objects in the Eye

- Do not wash out the eye.

- Do not try to remove a foreign object stuck in the eye.

- Seek immediate medical attention.

Chemical Burns

- Immediately flush the eye with water or any drinkable liquid. Open the eye as wide as possible. Continue flushing for at least 15 minutes. For caustic or basic solutions, continue

- flushing while on the way to medical care.

- If a contact lens is in the eye, begin flushing over the lens immediately. Flushing may dislodge the lens.

- Seek immediate medical attention.

Blows to the Eye

- Apply a cold compress without pressure, or tape crushed ice in a plastic bag to the forehead and allow it to rest gently on the injured eye.

- Seek immediate medical attention if pain continues, if vision is reduced, or if blood or discoloration appears in the eye.

Chapter 30

Protecting Eyes from Workplace Injuries

Chapter Contents

Section 30.1

Workplace Eye Injuries and Diseases

This section includes text excerpted from "Eye Safety,"
National Institute for Occupational Safety and Health (NIOSH),
Centers for Disease Control and Prevention (CDC),
July 29, 2013. Reviewed March 2017.

Eye Safety

Each day about 2000 U.S. workers sustain a job-related eye injury that requires medical treatment. About one third of the injuries are treated in hospital emergency departments, and more than 100 of these injuries result in one or more days away from work.

How Do Eye Injuries Happen to Workers?

- **Striking or scraping:** The majority of eye injuries result from small particles or objects striking or scraping the eye, such as: dust, cement chips, metal slivers, and wood chips. These materials are often ejected by tools, windblown, or fall from above a worker. Large objects may also strike the eye or face, or a worker may run into an object causing blunt-force trauma to the eyeball or eye socket.

- **Penetration:** Objects like nails, staples, or slivers of wood or metal can go through the eyeball and result in a permanent loss of vision.

- **Chemical and thermal burns:** Industrial chemicals or cleaning products are common causes of chemical burns to one or both eyes. Thermal burns to the eye also occur, often among welders. These burns routinely damage workers' eyes and surrounding tissue.

How Do Workers Acquire Eye Diseases?

Eye diseases are often transmitted through the mucous membranes of the eye as a result of direct exposure to things like blood splashes, and droplets from coughing or sneezing or from touching the eyes with a contaminated finger or object. Eye diseases can result in minor reddening or soreness of the eye or in a life threatening disease such as human immunodeficiency virus (HIV), hepatitis B virus, or avian influenza.

What Can Workers Do to Prevent Eye Injury and Disease?

Wear personal protective eyewear, such as goggles, face shields, safety glasses, or full face respirators.

The eye protection chosen for specific work situations depends upon the nature and extent of the hazard, the circumstances of exposure, other protective equipment used, and personal vision needs. Eye protection should be fit to an individual or adjustable to provide appropriate coverage. It should be comfortable and allow for sufficient peripheral vision.

What Can Employers Do to Prevent Worker Eye Injury and Disease?

Employers can ensure engineering controls are used to reduce eye injuries and to protect against ocular infection exposures. Employers can also conduct a hazard assessment to determine the appropriate type of protective eyewear appropriate for a given task.

Eye Safety Checklist

1. **Create a safe work environment.**

    *   Minimize hazards from falling or unstable debris.
    *   Make sure that tools work and safety features (machine guards) are in place.
    *   Make sure that workers (particularly volunteers) know how to use tools properly.
    *   Keep bystanders out of the hazard area.

2. **Evaluate safety hazards.**

    *   Identify the primary hazards at the site.
    *   Identify hazards posed by nearby workers, large machinery, and falling/shifting debris.

3. **Wear the proper eye and face protection.**

- Select the appropriate Z87 eye protection for the hazard.

- Make sure the eye protection is in good condition.

- Make sure the eye protection fits properly and will stay in place.

4. **Use good work practices.**

  - Caution—brush, shake, or vacuum dust and debris from hard hats, hair, forehead, or the top of the eye protection before removing the protection.

  - Do not rub eyes with dirty hands or clothing.

  - Clean eyewear regularly.

5. **Prepare for eye injuries and first aid needs. Have an eye wash or sterile solution on hand.**

Section 30.2

Preventing Eye Injuries in the Workplace

This section includes text excerpted from "Eye and Face Protection eTool: Selecting Personal Protective Equipment (PPE) for the Workplace," Occupational Safety and Health Administration (OSHA), December 20, 2016.

Selecting Personal Protective Equipment (PPE) for the Workplace

Personal protective equipment (PPE) for the eyes and face is designed to prevent or lessen the severity of injuries to workers. The employer must assess the workplace and determine if hazards that necessitate the use of eye and face protection are present or are likely to be present before assigning PPE to workers.

A hazard assessment should determine the risk of exposure to eye and face hazards, including those which may be encountered in an emergency. Employers should be aware of the possibility of multiple and simultaneous hazard exposures and be prepared to protect against the highest level of each hazard.

Table 30.1. Workplace Hazard Assessment

Hazard type	Examples of Hazard	Common Related Tasks
Impact	Flying objects such as large chips, fragments, particles, sand, and dirt	Chipping, grinding, machining, masonry work, wood working, sawing, drilling, chiseling, powered fastening, riveting, and sanding
Heat	Anything emitting extreme heat	Furnace operations, pouring, casting, hot dipping, and welding
Chemicals	Splash, fumes, vapors, and irritating mists	Acid and chemical handling, degreasing, plating, and working with blood
Dust	Harmful dust	Woodworking, buffing, and general dusty conditions
Optical Radiation	Radiant energy, glare, and intense light	Welding, torch-cutting, brazing, soldering, and laser work

Impact Hazards

The majority of impact injuries result from flying or falling objects, or sparks striking the eye. Most of these objects are smaller than a pinhead and can cause serious injury such as punctures, abrasions, and contusions.

While working in a hazardous area where the worker is exposed to flying objects, fragments, and particles, primary protective devices such as safety spectacles with side shields or goggles must be worn. Secondary protective devices such as face shields are required in conjunction with primary protective devices during severe exposure to impact hazards.

PPE devices for impact hazards:

- **Safety Spectacles:** Primary protectors intended to shield the eyes from a variety of impact hazards.

- **Safety Goggles:** Primary protectors intended to shield the eyes against flying fragments, objects, large chips, and particles.

- **Face Shields:** Secondary protectors intended to protect the entire face against exposure to impact hazards.

Safety Spectacles

Safety spectacles are intended to shield the wearer's eyes from impact hazards such as flying fragments, objects, large chips, and particles. Workers are required to use eye safety spectacles with side shields when there is a hazard from flying objects. Non-side shield spectacles are not acceptable eye protection for impact hazards.

The frames of safety spectacles are constructed of metal and/or plastic and can be fitted with either corrective or plano impact-resistant lenses. Side shields may be incorporated into the frames of safety spectacles when needed. Consider each component of safety spectacles when selecting the appropriate device for your workplace.

Safety Goggles

Safety goggles are intended to shield the wearer's eyes from impact hazards such as flying fragments, objects, large chips, and particles. Goggles fit the face immediately surrounding the eyes and form a protective seal around the eyes. This prevents objects from entering under or around the goggles.

Safety goggles may incorporate prescription lenses mounted behind protective lenses for individuals requiring vision correction. Take time to consider specific lens, frame, and ventilation options when selecting safety goggles.

Face Shields

Face shields are intended to protect the entire face or portions of it from impact hazards such as flying fragments, objects, large chips, and particles. When worn alone, face shields do not protect employees from impact hazards. Use face shields in combination with safety spectacles or goggles, even in the absence of dust or potential splashes, for additional protection beyond that offered by spectacles or goggles alone.

Face shield windows are made with different transparent materials and in varying degrees or levels of thickness. These levels should correspond with specific tasks. Window and headgear devices are available in various combinations to enable the worker to select the appropriate equipment.

Heat Hazards

Heat injuries may occur to the eye and face when workers are exposed to high temperatures, splashes of molten metal, or hot sparks.

Protect your eyes from heat when workplace operations involve pouring, casting, hot dipping, furnace operations, and other similar activities. Burns to eye and face tissue are the main concern when working with heat hazards.

Working with heat hazards requires eye protection such as goggles or safety spectacles with special-purpose lenses and side shields. However, many heat hazard exposures require the use of a face shield in addition to safety spectacles or goggles. When selecting PPE, consider the source and intensity of the heat and the type of splashes that may occur in the workplace.

PPE devices for heat hazards:

- **Safety Spectacles:** Primary protectors intended to shield the eyes from a variety of heat hazards.

- **Safety Goggles:** Primary protectors intended to shield the eyes from a variety of heat hazards.

- **Face Shields:** Secondary protectors intended to protect the entire face from a variety of heat hazards.

Safety Spectacles

Safety spectacles with side shields are used as primary protection to shield the eyes from heat hazards. To adequately protect the eyes and face from high temperature exposure, use safety spectacles in combination with a heat-reflective face shield.

The frames of safety spectacles are constructed out of metal and/or plastic and can be fitted with either corrective or plano impact-resistant lenses. Side shields are incorporated into the frames of safety spectacles when workplace operations expose workers to angular impact hazards. Consider each component of safety spectacles when selecting the appropriate device for your workplace.

Safety Goggles

Safety goggles are used as primary protection to shield the eyes from heat hazards. Goggles form a protective seal around the eyes, preventing objects or liquids from entering under or around the goggles. This is especially important when working with or around molten metals that may splash.

When employees are exposed to high temperatures, additional protection beyond that offered by primary protectors may be required. Use safety goggles in combination with a heat-reflective face shield

351

for severe temperatures exposure. Consider specific lens, frame, and ventilation options when selecting safety goggles.

Face Shields

Heat-reflective and wire-screen face shields are intended to shield the entire face from a range of heat hazards. Specific hazards associated with heat include high temperatures, splash from molten metal, and hot sparks. Face shields are considered secondary protectors to be used in addition to primary protection such as safety spectacles or goggles.

Face shield windows are made with different transparent materials and in varying degrees or levels of thickness. The thickness of the face shield window should be matched to the task. Window and headgear devices come in various styles in order to enable the worker to select the appropriate equipment.

Chemical Hazards

A large percentage of eye injuries are caused by direct contact with chemicals. These injuries often result from an inappropriate choice of PPE, that allows a chemical substance to enter from around or under protective eye equipment. Serious and irreversible damage can occur when chemical substances contact the eyes in the form of splash, mists, vapors, or fumes. When working with or around chemicals, it is important to know the location of emergency eyewash stations and how to access them with restricted vision.

When fitted and worn correctly, goggles protect your eyes from hazardous substances. A face shield may be required in areas where workers are exposed to severe chemical hazards.

PPE devices for chemical hazards:

- **Safety Goggles:** Primary protectors intended to shield the eyes against liquid or chemical splash, irritating mists, vapors, and fumes.

- **Face Shields:** Secondary protectors intended to protect the entire face against exposure to chemical hazards.

Safety Goggles

Safety goggles protect the eyes, eye sockets, and the facial area immediately surrounding the eyes from a variety of chemical hazards.

Goggles form a protective seal around the eyes, preventing objects or liquids from entering under or around the goggles. This is especially important when working with or around liquids that may splash, spray, or mist.

Safety goggles may incorporate prescription lenses mounted behind protective lenses for individuals requiring vision correction. Take time to consider specific lens, frame, and ventilation options when selecting safety goggles.

Face Shields

Heat-reflective and wire-screen face shields are intended to shield the entire face from a range of heat hazards. Specific hazards associated with heat include high temperatures, splash from molten metal, and hot sparks. Face shields are considered secondary protectors to be used in addition to primary protection such as safety spectacles or goggles.

Face shield windows are made with different transparent materials and in varying degrees or levels of thickness. The thickness of the face shield window should be matched to the task. Window and headgear devices come in various styles in order to enable the worker to select the appropriate equipment.

Dust Hazards

Dust is present in the workplace during operations such as woodworking and buffing. Working in a dusty environment can causes eye injuries and presents additional hazards to contact lens wearers.

Either eyecup or cover-type safety goggles should be worn when dust is present. Safety goggles are the only effective type of eye protection from nuisance dust because they create a protective seal around the eyes.

PPE devices for dust hazards:

- **Safety Goggles:** Primary protectors intended to protect the eyes against a variety of airborne particles and harmful dust.

Safety Goggles

Safety goggles are intended to protect the eyes against dust hazards. Goggles form a protective seal around the eyes, preventing nuisance dust from entering under or around the goggles. Ventilation should be adequate, but well protected from dust entry.

Safety goggles may incorporate prescription lenses mounted behind protective lenses for individuals requiring vision correction. Take time to consider specific lens, frame, and ventilation options when selecting safety goggles.

Optical Radiation Hazards

Laser work and similar operations create intense concentrations of heat, ultraviolet, infrared, and reflected light radiation. A laser beam, of sufficient power, can produce intensities greater than those experienced when looking directly at the sun. Unprotected laser exposure may result in eye injuries including retinal burns, cataracts, and permanent blindness. When lasers produce invisible ultraviolet, or other radiation, both employees and visitors should use appropriate eye protection at all times.

Determine the maximum power density, or intensity, lasers produce when workers are exposed to laser beams. Based on this knowledge, select lenses that protect against the maximum intensity. The selection of laser protection should depend upon the lasers in use and the operating conditions. Workers with exposure to laser beams must be furnished suitable laser protection.

PPE devices for optical radiation hazards:

- Lens Requirements
- Welding Protection
- Lasers
- Glare Protection

Lens Requirements

When selecting filter lenses, begin with a shade too dark to see the welding zone. Then try lighter shades until one allows a sufficient view of the welding zone without going below the minimum protective shade.

Welding Protection

The intensity of visible light and radiant energy produced by welding operations varies depending on the task, the electrode size, and the arc current. Workers involved in welding, cutting, and brazing operations must use appropriate welding protection depending on specific welding operations.

Only filter lenses with the appropriate shade number will provide protection against optical radiation. Filter lenses must coincide to specific radiant energy exposure. Welding protectors are constructed of heat resistant material such as vulcanized fiber or fiberglass and fitted with a filtered lens to protect workers eyes from burns caused by infrared or other intense radiant energy. These devices protect the eyes and face from flying sparks, metal spatter, and slag chips produced during welding, brazing, soldering, and cutting.

Welding helmets are secondary protectors intended to shield the eyes and face from optical radiation, heat, and impact. Use welding helmets in addition to primary protection such as safety spectacles or goggles to provide adequate protection.

Lasers

Laser work and similar operations create intense concentrations of heat, ultraviolet, infrared, and reflected light radiation. A laser beam, of sufficient power, can produce intensities greater than those experienced when looking directly at the sun. Unprotected laser exposure may result in eye injuries including retinal burns, cataracts, and permanent blindness. When lasers produce invisible ultraviolet, or other radiation, both employees and visitors should use appropriate eye protection at all times.

Determine the maximum power density, or intensity, lasers produce when workers are exposed to laser beams. Based on this knowledge, select lenses that protect against the maximum intensity. The selection of laser protection should depend upon the lasers in use and the operating conditions. Workers with exposure to laser beams must be furnished suitable laser protection.

Glare Protection

Control Glare with:

- Special-purpose spectacles that include filter or special-purpose lenses to provide protection against eye strain.

- Changes in your work area or lighting.

- Tinted eyeglass lenses or visor-type shade.

Section 30.3

Eye Protection for Infection Control

This section includes text excerpted from "Eye Safety," National
Institute for Occupational Safety and Health (NIOSH), Centers
for Disease Control and Prevention (CDC), July 29, 2013.
Reviewed March 2017.

The Centers for Disease Control and Prevention (CDC) recommends
eye protection for a variety of potential exposure settings where workers may be at risk of acquiring infectious diseases via ocular exposure.
This section provides background information and specific details on
eye protection that can be used to supplement eye protection recommendations provided in current CDC infection control guidance documents. It is intended to familiarize workers with the various types
of eye protection available, their characteristics, and their applicable
use. Workers should understand that regular prescription eyeglasses
and contact lenses are not considered eye protection.

Infectious diseases can be transmitted through various mechanisms,
among which are infections that can be introduced through the mucous
membranes of the eye (conjunctiva). These include viruses and bacteria than can cause conjunctivitis (e.g., adenovirus, herpes simplex,
Staphylococcus aureus) and viruses that can cause systemic infections,
including blood borne viruses (e.g., hepatitis B and C viruses, human
immunodeficiency virus (HIV)), herpes viruses, and rhinoviruses.
Infectious agents are introduced to the eye either directly (e.g., blood
splashes, respiratory droplets generated during coughing or suctioning)
or from touching the eyes with contaminated fingers or other objects.

Eye protection provides a barrier to infectious materials entering
the eye and is often used in conjunction with other personal protective
equipment (PPE) such as gloves, gowns, masks or respirators.

Infection Control FAQs

What Types of Eye Protection Should Be Worn?

The eye protection chosen for specific work situations depends upon
the circumstances of exposure, other PPE used, and personal vision

needs. There is wide variety in the types of protective eyewear, and appropriate selection should be based on a number of factors, the most important of which is the nature and extent of the hazard. Eye protection must be comfortable and allow for sufficient peripheral vision and must be adjustable to ensure a secure fit. It may be necessary to provide several different types, styles, and sizes. Selection of protective eyewear appropriate for a given task should be made from an evaluation of each activity, including regulatory requirements when applicable. These hazard assessments require a clear understanding of the work tasks, including knowledge of the potential routes of exposure and the opportunities for exposure in the task assessed (nature and extent of worker contact). Exposure incident reports should be reviewed to identify those incidents (whether or not infection occurred) that could have been prevented by the proper use of protective eyewear.

What Are Common Types of Eye Protection?

Goggles

Appropriately fitted, indirectly-vented goggles* with a manufacturer's anti-fog coating provide the most reliable practical eye protection from splashes, sprays, and respiratory droplets. Newer styles of goggles may provide better indirect airflow properties to reduce fogging, as well as better peripheral vision and more size options for fitting goggles to different workers. Many styles of goggles fit adequately over prescription glasses with minimal gaps. However, to be efficacious, goggles must fit snugly, particularly from the corners of the eye across the brow. While highly effective as eye protection, goggles do not provide splash or spray protection to other parts of the face.

* Directly-vented goggles may allow penetration by splashes or sprays; therefore, indirectly-vented or non-vented goggles are preferred for infection control.

Face Shields

Face shields are commonly used as an infection control alternative to goggles.† As opposed to goggles, a face shield can also provide protection to other facial areas. To provide better face and eye protection from splashes and sprays, a face shield should have crown and chin protection and wrap around the face to the point of the ear, which reduces the likelihood that a splash could go around the edge of the shield and reach the eyes. Disposable face shields for medical personnel made of lightweight films that are attached to a surgical mask or fit loosely around the face should not be relied upon as optimal protection.

† *In a chemical exposure or industrial setting, faceshields should be used in addition to goggles, not as a substitute for goggles* (ANSI Z87.1-2003 Practice for Occupational and Educational Eye and Face Protection*).*

Safety Glasses

Safety glasses provide impact protection but do not provide the same level of splash or droplet protection as goggles and generally should not be used for infection control purposes.

Full-Face Respirators

Full facepiece elastomeric respirators and powered air-purifying respirators (PAPRs) are designed and used for respiratory protection, but because of their design incidentally provide highly effective eye protection as well. Selection of this type of PPE should be based on an assessment of the respiratory hazard in an infection control situation, but will also provide, as an additional benefit, optimal eye protection.

Why Eye Protection Is Available for Prescription Lenses Users?

Many safety goggles or plano (non-prescription) safety glasses fit comfortably over street eyewear and can provide satisfactory protection without impairing the fit of the prescription eyewear. Prescription safety glasses with side protection are available, but do not protect against splashes or droplets as well as goggles. Special prescription inserts are available for goggles. When full facepiece elastomeric negative pressure (i.e., non-powered) respirators or tight-fitting powered air purifying respirators (PAPRs) are indicated for respiratory protection, these devices require appropriate prescription inserts to avoid compromising the seal around the face; PAPRs designed with loose-fitting facepieces or with hoods that completely cover the head and neck may be more accommodating to prescription lens wearers.

Contact lenses, by themselves, offer no infection control protection. However, contact lenses may be worn with any of the recommended eye protection devices, including full-face respirators. Contact lens users should rigorously adhere to hand washing guidelines when inserting, adjusting, or removing contact lenses.

What Combination of Eye Protection and Other PPE Should Be Used?

Eye protection should be selected in the context of other PPE use requirements. Safety goggles may not fit properly when used with certain half-face respirators, and similarly, face shields may not fit properly over some respirators. Once PPE requirements have been established for a specific infection control situation, the selected PPE should be pre-tested to assure suitable fit and protection when used as an ensemble. Elastomeric, full facepiece respirators and PAPRs have the advantage of incidentally providing optimal eye protection. In situations where all combinations of PPE may not be readily available to workers, judicious selection of complementary PPE is important to allow for appropriate protection.

How Should Potentially Contaminated Eye Protection Be Removed?

Eye protection should be removed by handling only the portion of this equipment that secures the device to the head (i.e., plastic temples, elasticized band, ties), as this is considered relatively "clean." The front and sides of the device (i.e., goggles, face shield) should not be touched, as these are the surfaces most likely to become contaminated by sprays, splashes, or droplets during patient care. Non-disposable eye protection should be placed in a designated receptacle for subsequent cleaning and disinfection. The sequence of PPE removal should follow a defined regimen that should be developed by infection control staff and take into consideration the need to remove other PPE.

Is It Safe for Others to Reuse My Eye Protection?

The eyewear described above is generally not disposable and must be disinfected before reuse. Where possible, each individual worker should be assigned his/her own eye protection to insure appropriate fit and to minimize the potential of exposing the next wearer. A labeled container for used (potentially contaminated) eye protection should be available in the healthcare worker (HCW) change-out / locker room. Eye protection deposited here can be collected, disinfected, washed, and then reused.

How Should Eye Protection Be Disinfected?

Healthcare setting-specific procedures for cleaning and disinfecting used patient care equipment should be followed for reprocessing reusable eye protection devices. Manufacturers may be consulted for their guidance and experience in disinfecting their respective products. Contaminated eye protection devices should be reprocessed in an area where other soiled equipment is handled. Eye protection should be physically cleaned and disinfected with the designated hospital disinfectant, rinsed, and allowed to air dry. Gloves should be worn when cleaning and disinfecting these devices.

Chapter 31

Protecting Eyes from Sports Injuries

Most athletes think of knee and shoulder problems when we talk about sports-related injuries. It is important to remember that eye injuries in sports are not only common, but they are potentially very serious.

According to the American Academy of Ophthalmology (AAO), sports account for approximately 100,000 eye injuries each year. Roughly 42,000 of those injuries require evaluation in emergency departments. In fact, a patient with a sports-related eye injury presents to a United States emergency room every 13 minutes. It is estimated that sports-related eye injuries cost between $175 million and $200 million per year.

Generally baseball, basketball and racquet sports cause the highest numbers of eye injuries. One of every three of these eye injuries in sports occurs in children. In kids between the ages of five and 14,

This section contains text excerpted from the following sources: Text in this section begins with excerpts from "Simple Steps to Prevent Eye Injuries in Sports," Office of Disease Prevention and Health Promotion (ODPHP), U.S. Department of Health and Human Services (HHS), October 1, 2014; Text beginning with the heading "Sports That May Put You at Risk for Eye Injuries" is excerpted from "Sports and Your Eyes," National Eye Institute (NEI), June 16, 2016; Text under the heading "Protect Your Eyes When You Exercise" is excerpted from "Protect Your Eyes When You Exercise," Go4Life, National Institutes of Health (NIH), January 25, 2017; Text under the heading "Protective Eyewear" is excerpted from "Protective Eyewear," National Eye Institute (NEI), June 16, 2016.

baseball is the leading cause. Basketball is a common culprit in athletes aged 15 and older. And boxing and martial arts present a high risk for serious eye injuries.

These eye injuries can be mild ones, but serious injuries like orbital fractures, corneal abrasions, and detached retina can occur. Approximately 13,500 people become legally blind from sports-related eye injuries every year.

Fortunately, the AAO estimates that 90 percent of eye injuries are preventable. Athletes should remember these simple tips to avoid serious eye damage in sports:

- Wear appropriate eye protection, especially in basketball, racket sports, field hockey and soccer. In baseball, ice hockey and men's lacrosse, an athlete should wear a helmet with a polycarbonate shield. Polycarbonate lenses are believed to be 10 times more resistant to impact than other materials. All protective eyewear should comply with American Society for Testing and Materials (ASTM) standards.

- Wear additional protective eyewear, if you wear contact lenses or glasses. Contacts offer no protection against impacts to the eye. Glasses and sunglasses do not provide adequate protection and could shatter upon impact, increasing the danger to the eye.

- Wear eye protection for all sports if you are functionally one-eyed, meaning one eye has normal vision and the other is less than 20/40 vision

- Inspect protective eyewear regularly and replace when it appears worn or damaged.

Last, if an eye injury does occur, every athlete should consider going to an emergency department or consulting an ophthalmologist. Even a seemingly minor injury can actually be potentially serious and lead to loss of vision.

Remember, 90 percent of sports-related eye injuries can be prevented. Let's start taking steps to eliminate these injuries.

Sports That May Put You at Risk for Eye Injuries

If you play sports, you know they can be a lot of fun. The last thing you want to do is miss a game, especially if it's because you're hurt. That's why you should always follow the rules and wear the right safety gear.

Think about your favorite sport. Do you wear anything to protect your eyes, like goggles or a face mask? You might think you don't need protective eyewear, but sports-related eye injuries are serious. Eye injuries are a leading cause of blindness among children in the United States. The good news is that most eye injuries can be prevented with the right protective eyewear.

Check out Table 31.1 below to see examples of some sports that may put you at high risk for eye injuries.

Table 31.1. Sports Prone to Eye Injuries

High-Risk Sports	Moderate-Risk Sports	Low-Risk Sports
Baseball	Badminton	Bicycling
Basketball	Fishing	Diving
Boxing	Football	Gymnastics
Fencing	Golf	Skiing
Hockey	Soccer	Swimming
Lacrosse	Tennis	Track and Field
Paintball		
Racquetball		
Softball		
Squash		
Water Sports		
Wrestling		

Protect Your Eyes When You Exercise

Sports at moderate to high risk for eye injuries include: basketball, baseball, softball, ice hockey, tennis, soccer, volleyball, football, fishing, and golf. Studies show that protective eyewear does not hinder the player's sight while participating in athletics. In fact, some athletes can even play better because they're less afraid of getting hit in the eye.

Play it safe! Protect your eyes:

- Protective eyewear includes safety glasses and goggles, safety shields, and eye guards that are specially designed to provide the right protection for a certain activity.

- You still need protective eyewear that's approved for your sport even if you don't wear glasses or contacts.

- Ordinary prescription glasses, contact lenses, and sunglasses do not protect you from sports-related eye injury. You need to wear safety goggles over them.

- Experts recommend ultra-strong polycarbonate lenses for eye protection. Make sure they are in sport-appropriate frames or goggles.

- Many eye care providers sell protective eyewear, as do some sporting goods stores. Protective eyewear is sport-specific with the proper ASTM standards written on the packaging. This makes it easy to decide which pair is best for each activity.

Quick Tip

Protective eyewear should sit comfortably on your face and not slide off. Try on several pairs before making a final decision.

Protective Eyewear

Whether you're on the basketball court, in chemistry class, or sitting by the pool, wearing protective eyewear is the best way to keep your eyes healthy and injury-free. In fact, the majority of eye injuries can be prevented by wearing the right protective eyewear. Check out the list of activities below to see what you need to protect your eyes.

- **Play basketball or soccer?** Wear sports goggles with polycarbonate lenses.

- **Play baseball?** If you're up to bat, wear a helmet with an attached faceguard. If you're fielding, wear sports goggles.

- **Swimming or playing water sports?** Wear swim goggles to protect your eyes from dirt, germs and bacteria, and pool chemicals.

- **Play ice hockey?** You need a face mask or polycarbonate guard that's attached to a helmet.

- **Are you a football player?** Always wear your helmet with an attached face shield.

- **Play lacrosse?** Girls need protective goggles but have the option to wear headgear with full face protection. Boys are required to wear a helmet with a full face mask. So are goalies, regardless of whether you're a boy or a girl.

- **Into field hockey?** Goalies need helmets with a full face mask. All other players should wear sports goggles. Girls' lacrosse goggles also work for field hockey.

- **Into a racquet sport like squash or racquetball?** Wear sports goggles with polycarbonate lenses.

- **Do you fence?** You need to wear a wire mesh mask so your whole face is protected.

- **Are you a paintball pro?** Always wear your paintball goggles or mask.

- **Going for a bike ride?** Always wear a helmet. You'll also want sunglasses or glasses with clear lenses to protect your eyes from the wind and any bugs.

- **Spending time in the sun?** Wear your sunglasses. They protect your eyes from the sun's ultraviolet (UV) rays, which can damage your eyes. Pick sunglasses that block 99 percent or 100 percent of both UVA and UVB radiation.

Chapter 32

Eye Injuries

Chapter Contents

Section 32.1

Black Eye

"Black Eye," © 2017 Omnigraphics.
Reviewed March 2017.

What Is a Black Eye?

A black eye (periorbital hematoma) is an impact injury that causes broken blood vessels in the tissue around the eye. This results in a bruise and swelling caused by the accumulation of blood and fluids beneath the skin. The skin around the eye is very loose, allowing this area to swell quickly as fluids build up. Despite the common name "black eye," there is usually no injury to the eye itself.

What Causes a Black Eye?

Black eyes are usually caused by an object forcefully hitting the eye or nose. Depending on the location of the blow, one or two black eyes may develop. A strike to the nose typically results in two black eyes. Black eyes can also be caused by surgeries performed on the face, nose, jaw, and some types of dental work.

What Are the Symptoms of a Black Eye?

The term "black eye" is a good indication of the most visible symptoms of this type of injury. Because the area around the eye can bruise easily and turns a dark color quickly, a black eye is easily recognizable. However, dark bruising around the eye is not the only symptom of a black eye. Symptoms of a typical black eye can include:

- Bruising around the eye or nose that appears red, purple, yellow, green, or black
- Swelling around the eye that sometimes causes the eye to close completely
- Pain around the eye or nose
- Blurry vision

A more serious injury to the eye, face, or head can result in additional symptoms, such as:

- Loss of vision

- Seeing double or double vision

- Persistent, severe headache

- Blood collecting on the surface of the eyeball

- Blood or fluid flowing from the eye, ear, or nose

- Inability to move the eye or to look in different directions without turning the head

- Signs of injury to the head or face, including cuts or bruises elsewhere on the face

- Broken teeth

- Broken bones in the face

- Nausea or vomiting

- Dizziness

- Inability to walk

- Unexplained or sudden behavior changes

- Loss of consciousness or fainting

How Is a Black Eye Diagnosed?

One of the most important factors in diagnosing a black eye is to determine whether the injury is limited to the soft tissue around the eye, or if a more critical head injury has occurred. A doctor or other health care provider will typically perform a physical examination to make this determination. Vision is checked by moving an object in front of the patient's face and asking them to follow the movement with their eyes. A light shined in the eye will test for proper dilation of the eye pupil. Special devices may be used to see inside the eye, in order to examine the retina or cornea for any injuries. An examination of the face and head will help determine if there have been any injuries to the skull or facial bones. Further testing may be performed by X-ray or other types of medical imaging.

The occurrence of two black eyes, especially after a forceful blow to the back of the head, may indicate a severe skull fracture. This is a very serious injury that can be life-threatening. Immediate medical attention should be sought if two black eyes appear at the same time.

How Is a Black Eye Treated?

Most black eyes heal on their own within a few days. A black eye can be treated at home with ice packs used for 20 minutes at a time, once every hour. If no improvement is seen after a few days, or if pain, swelling, or bruising persists, medical treatment should be sought. If any of the more serious symptoms described above occur, medical treatment should be sought immediately.

How to Prevent a Black Eye

Black eyes are most commonly caused by sports injuries or accidents. The best method of protection is to always make use of proper safety equipment such as helmets, goggles, or other protective equipment.

What Are the Complications of a Black Eye?

Although most black eyes are surface injuries that heal on their own, there are several serious complications that can develop from this type of injury.

- **Hyphema**—bleeding inside the eye, between the back of the cornea and the front of the iris. This is a medical emergency that can lead to vision loss if left untreated.

- **Subconjunctival hemorrhage**—the white of the eye appears bright red due to bleeding in the eye.

- **Skull fracture**—broken bones in the skull.

- **Damage to the eyeball**—cuts or scratches on the surface of the eye, or object imbedded in the eyeball.

- **Persistent swelling, severe pain, changes in vision**—these symptoms can indicate a more serious problem and medical attention should be sought.

- **Infection**—signs of infection include fever, warmth around the eye, persistent redness, and/or drainage.

- **Retinal detachment**—changes in vision, dizziness, nausea, migraine headaches, seeing flashing lights in the field of vision.

- **Traumatic uveitis and iritis**—pain during exposure to bright light, spots appearing to float in the field of vision, blurred vision, irregularly shaped pupil, redness in the iris.

- **Glaucoma**—a forceful blow to the eye can cause undetected bleeding inside the eye that produces increased pressure on the optic nerve.

- **Orbital floor fracture**—a forceful blow to the eye can push the eyeball back into the eye socket, resulting in pinching of the optic nerve and the muscles that help the eye move. This is a medical emergency that can result in loss of vision if left untreated.

References

1. Cunha, John P. "Black Eye,"MedicineNet.com, June 1, 2015.

2. Hellem, Amy. "Is a Black Eye Serious?" AllAboutVision.com, January 2017.

3. Moss, Dr. Hart. "A Black Eye—How Long Does it Take to Heal?" EyeHealthWeb, n.d.

4. Porter, Daniel. "Black Eye Diagnosis," American Academy of Ophthalmology, March 1, 2017.

Section 32.2

Blowout Fracture

Text in this section is excerpted from "Blowout Fracture,"
© 2017 American Association for Pediatric Ophthalmology
and Strabismus (AAPOS). Reprinted with permission.

What Is a "Blowout" Fracture?

A blowout fracture is a fracture of one or more of the bones surrounding the eye and is commonly referred to as an orbital floor fracture.

What Is the Orbit?

The orbit consists of the bones surrounding the eye. When looking at a skull, the orbit is the hole in the skull encompassing the eye.

What Is the "Floor" of the Orbit?

The bones on the bottom of the orbit are the floor. The bones on the top are the roof and the bones on the side are the walls.

What Is the Function of the Orbit?

The orbit holds the eye in the correct position. The orbit also protects the eye. Because the bones surrounding the eye "stick out" further than the eye, objects tend to hit the orbit and not the eye.

What Causes a Blowout Fracture?

Blowout fractures result from trauma to the orbital bones. When an object hits the orbital bones (usually the eye brow and upper cheek bone) the force is transmitted to the bones. If the force is great enough, the bones buckle and break.

What Are Common Causes of Blowout Fractures?

Any large object with force or speed can cause a blowout fracture. Typical causes include motor vehicle accidents, balls used in sports, fists, and elbows.

What Are the Symptoms of an Orbital Blowout Fracture?

The most common symptoms are bruising, tenderness and swelling around the eye; redness of the eye; double vision, or diplopia (seeing two images at the same time); numbness of the cheek, nose or teeth; nose bleeds (epistaxis).

Symptoms that typically indicate a more serious injury are pain on eye movement, double vision, air under the skin around the eye, and numbness of the cheek/mouth/nose on the side of the injury. Severe trauma may cause facial bone fractures, injury to the eye itself, and injuries to the skull/brain.

How Do You Know If There Is a Fracture?

X-rays and CT scans of the orbit and face are used to make the diagnosis.

Are There Different Types of Blowout Fractures?

Blowout fractures are classified on several features including:

- size (big or small)
- location (front or back)
- bone in place or displaced
- tissue/muscle entrapped in fracture
- accompanying symptoms (double vision, pain, eye position)

A "simple" fracture is one with minimal or no double vision, minimal or no interference with eye movements, and minimal fracture size.

What Can Be Done for a Simple Blowout Fracture?

Most simple blowout fractures usually heal without lasting problems. Treatment consists of:

- ice to decrease swelling
- decongestants to aid in the drainage of blood and fluid accumulating in the sinuses
- avoidance of nose blowing to prevent pressure from propelling the sinus contents into the orbit
- oral steroids in some cases to decrease swelling and scarring
- sometimes oral antibiotics

When Should Surgical Repair of Blowout Fractures Be Considered?

Fractures with persistent symptoms (typically double vision or pain) are usually candidates for surgical repair. Timing of the repair varies, but most often is within two weeks of the injury. Initial repair may consist of any of the following:

- exploration of fracture site and repositioning of bone

- release of trapped tissue from fracture site
- covering of fracture site with synthetic material

What Long-Term Problems May Develop Following Blowout Fractures?

Most fractures heal without long-term effects. However, strabismus surgery (eye muscle surgery) is sometimes necessary for persistent double vision. Occasionally, persistent double vision can be treated with non-surgical methods (prism glasses or botulinum toxin injections).

Section 32.3

Chemical Eye Burns

Text in this section is excerpted from "Chemical Eye Burns,"
© 2017 WebMD LLC. Reprinted with permission.

Chemical exposure to any part of the eye or eyelid may result in a chemical eye burn. Chemical burns represent a small percentage of eye injuries. Some burns to the face involve at least one eye. Although many burns result in only minor discomfort, every chemical exposure or burn should be taken seriously. Permanent damage is possible and can be blinding and life-altering.

The severity of a burn depends on what substance caused it, how long the substance had contact with the eye, and how the injury is treated. Damage is usually limited to the front segment of the eye, including the cornea, (the clear front surface of the eye responsible for good vision, which is most frequently affected), the conjunctiva (the layer covering the white part of the eye), and occasionally the internal eye structures of the eye, including the lens. Burns that penetrate deeper than the cornea are the most severe, often causing cataracts and glaucoma.

Chemical Eye Burn Causes

Most chemical eye injuries occur at work. Industries use a variety of chemicals daily. However, chemical injuries also frequently occur at home from cleaning products or other regular household products; these injuries can be just as dangerous and must be treated seriously and immediately.

Chemical burns to the eye can be divided into three categories: alkali burns, acid burns, and irritants.

The acidity or alkalinity, called the pH, of a substance is measured on a scale from 1–14, with 7 indicating a neutral substance. Substances with pH values less than 7 are acids, while numbers higher than 7 are alkaline; the higher or lower the number, the more acidic or basic a substance is and the more damage it can cause.

- **Alkali burns** are the most dangerous. Alkalis-chemicals that have a high pH-penetrate the surface of the eye and can cause severe injury to both the external structures like the cornea and the internal structures like the lens. In general, more damage occurs with higher pH chemicals.

  - Common alkali substances contain the hydroxides of ammonia, lye, potassium hydroxide, magnesium, and lime.

  - Substances you may have at home that contain these chemicals include fertilizers, cleaning products (ammonia), drain cleaners (lye), oven cleaners, and plaster or cement (lime).

- **Acid burns** result from chemicals with a low pH and are usually less severe than alkali burns because they do not penetrate into the eye as readily as alkaline substances. The exception is a hydrofluoric acid burn, which is as dangerous as an alkali burn. Acids usually damage only the very front of the eye; however, they can cause serious damage to the cornea and also may result in blindness.

  - Common acids causing eye burns include sulfuric acid, sulfurous acid, hydrochloric acid, nitric acid, acetic acid, chromic acid, and hydrofluoric acid.

  - Substances you have at home that may contain these chemicals include glass polish (hydrofluoric acid), vinegar. An automobile battery can explode and cause a sulfuric acid burn. This is one of the most common acidic burns of the eye.

- **Irritants** are substances that have a neutral pH and tend to cause more discomfort to the eye than actual damage.

  - Most household detergents fall into this category.

- Pepper spray is also an irritant. It can cause significant pain but usually does not affect vision and rarely causes any damage to the eye.

Chemical Eye Burn Symptoms

A true loss of vision signifies a very serious burn. Glaucoma, or an increase of the pressure inside the eye, can occur, but may be delayed by hours to days.

Early signs and symptoms of a chemical eye burn are

- Pain

- Redness

- Irritation

- Tearing

- Inability to keep the eye open

- Sensation of something in the eye

- Swelling of the eyelids

- Blurred vision

Self-Care at Home

For all chemical injuries, the first thing you should do is immediately irrigate the eye copiously. Ideally, specific eye irrigating solutions should be used for this, but if none are available regular tap water will do just fine.

- Begin washing your eye before taking any other action and continue for at least 10 minutes. The longer a chemical is in your eye, the more damage will occur. Diluting the substance and washing away any particles that may have been in the chemical are extremely important.

- Ideally, in a work setting, you would be placed in an emergency eyewash or shower station and your eye washed with sterile isotonic saline solution. If sterile saline is not available, use cold tap water.

- If you are at home and do not have special eye wash, step into the shower with your clothes on to wash out your eye.

- Even though it may be uncomfortable, open your eyelids as wide as possible as you rinse them out.

- If an alkali or hydrofluoric acid burn has occurred, continue washing until a doctor arrives or you have been taken to a hospital's emergency department.

When to Seek Medical Care

The next best step if possible is to find out what type of chemical you have been exposed to. You can look on the product label or call your regional Poison Control Center at 800-222-1222 to find out more information about a specific chemical.

If the chemical is an irritant (with a neutral pH) and symptoms are only minor or nonexistent, then you may monitor your condition at home with a call to your ophthalmologist (a medical doctor who specializes in eye care and surgery). Make sure the burn does not worsen. If it does, call your ophthalmologist to arrange an appointment for that day or go to the Emergency Room if an Ophthalmologist is not available.

If you have any question about the danger of a chemical, if you do not know what it is, or if you have significant symptoms, go immediately to the nearest hospital's emergency department.

Any time you experience pain, tearing, redness, irritation, or vision loss, go to a hospital's emergency department for immediate evaluation, even if you believe the chemical is only a mild irritant.

All acid or alkali eye burns require immediate treatment and evaluation by a doctor. You should be taken immediately to the closest emergency department. If you suspect a serious injury may have occurred or are otherwise not able to make the trip to the emergency room quickly, then you should call an ambulance to shorten transport time. All industries are required to keep a Materials Safety Data Sheet (MSDS) on any chemicals being used.

Medical Treatment in the Emergency Room

- **Immediate therapy:** Doctors likely will continue washing your eye. No standard exists for the amount of washing required. Usually, doctors use at least one liter of fluid.

  - Depending on the type of chemical involved, the doctor may test the pH of your eye and continue washing until the pH returns to normal.

377

- You may receive topical anesthetic eyedrops to numb your eye to make washing less painful.

- Doctors will wipe or irrigate away any solid foreign material in your eye.

- **Exams and Tests:** The doctor determines what chemical caused the burn and completes a thorough eye examination.

  - You are given an eye examination using an eye chart to determine how well you can see.

  - Structures surrounding the eye are checked.

  - Eyelids, in particular, require careful assessment. The doctor turns them inside out to look for foreign material.

  - The doctor may stain your eye with a dye called fluorescein to help determine the extent of damage.

- If the burns are minor, you are usually sent home with antibiotic eyedrops and oral pain medications. Occasionally, you may be given dilating eyedrops to help with comfort, and your injured eye may be covered with an eye patch.

- Any significant burn, especially an alkali or hydrofluoric acid burn, may require admission to the hospital.

- For any minor injuries, an ophthalmologist should evaluate you within 24–48 hours of your injury. For any moderate to significant injury, an ophthalmologist should evaluate you before you leave the Emergency Room.

- Your tetanus immunization status may be determined and updated.

Medications after You Go Home

- For very minor injuries, you may need nothing more than artificial tears or lubricants for dry eyes.

- For more significant injuries, you will need prolonged therapy with potentially many medications to heal your eye.

  - Until the surface of the eye heals, it is at a higher risk for an infection; therefore, topical antibiotics may be used in the form of eyedrops or ointments.

  - Topical steroids are used to reduce inflammation and to facilitate healing early in the recovery period after a chemical injury. These medications should be used judiciously under the guidance of an ophthalmologist, because they can cause long-term complications, such as infections and glaucoma.

- Other medications used to support corneal repair include topical citrate and ascorbate drops, oral antibiotics (for example, tetracycline, doxycycline), and oral vitamin C.

- If your eye pressure is too high, glaucoma medications may be used temporarily to control the pressure.

- Pain medications by mouth may be necessary, and dilating eyedrops are often also used to control pain and to aid recovery.

- If your eye has been seriously damaged, you may need a surgery to control glaucoma, remove a cataract, or other procedures to restore a healthy ocular surface and eyelids.

Surgery

- Surgical measures may be necessary after severe chemical injuries when the initial injury has healed.

  - Chemical injuries may necessitate surgery to the eyelids to restore good eyelid closure to protect the eye.

  - If the surface of the eye is severely damaged, a specialized set of cells called Limbal stem cells may be damaged and require replacement to prevent surface scarring.

  - If the cornea becomes opaque (or cloudy) following a chemical injury, a corneal transplant may be required.

  - Chemical injuries, especially from alkaline substances, can also cause cataracts and glaucoma, which may also require later surgical intervention.

Follow-Up

If you are treated for a chemical burn to the eye in a hospital's emergency department, you should see an ophthalmologist within 24 hours. The ophthalmologist determines your continuing care.

Prevention

Safety officials estimate that most chemical eye injuries can be avoided.

- Always wear safety glasses when working with hazardous materials, both at work and at home.

- Children sustain chemical burns most often when they are unsupervised. Keep all hazardous home products away from children.

Outlook

Recovery depends on the type and extent of injury. Every exposure to foreign substances or "chemicals" does not necessarily result in injury.

- Chemical irritants seldom cause permanent damage.

- Recovery from acid and alkali burns depends on the depth of the injury.

The 4 grades of burns are

- Grade 1: You should recover fully.

- Grade 2: You may have some scarring, but your vision should recover.

- Grade 3: Your vision will usually be impaired to some degree.

- Grade 4: Damage to your vision likely will be severe.

Questions to Ask the Doctor

- Is there any sign of significant damage to the eye?

- What medications am I to take, and for how long?

- When am I supposed to visit the doctor for follow up again?

- Is there any chance of permanent vision loss?

Section 32.4

Foreign Objects in the Eye

From the occasional eyelash that wanders uninvited into the eye to the high-speed missile impact from an ejected metal shard, one may find oneself with something in the eye (medically referred to as a foreign body). Depending on what it is and how the injury happened, the foreign body may pierce the eye and cause serious injury or it may simply go away with no long-term problem.

Most people realize that an eyelash in the eye does not require an evaluation by a doctor but that a metal shard in the eye would warrant a visit to your ophthalmologist (a medical doctor who specializes in eye care and surgery), particularly if it has penetrated beyond the superficial layers of the surface of the eye.

Eye Foreign Body Causes

Many eye injuries can be prevented. Something in the eye (a foreign body) is most often the result of improper or no eye protection while working in an environment that exposes one to small flying debris.

Eye Foreign Body Symptoms

- Sharp pain in the eye followed by burning, irritation, tearing, and redness

- Feeling that something is in the eye when moving the eye around while it is closed

- Scratching sensation over the eye when blinking

- Blurred vision or vision loss in the affected eye

- Bleeding into the white part of the eye, which can be either a conjunctival hemorrhage or a subconjunctival hemorrhage. (Sometimes, this is associated with a penetrating injury.)

- Blood layering in front of your iris, the colored area of the eye, and behind the cornea, the clear dome on the front of the eye (This is called hyphema and is often a sign of significant injury.)

When to Seek Medical Care

Because of the specialized nature of eye examination equipment, a foreign body in the eye is usually handled best in an ophthalmologist's office. If an emergency department has the necessary equipment, an ophthalmologist may also see the patient in the emergency department. In some cases, a foreign body in the eye may be handled in an emergency department that has both a properly trained emergency physician and the appropriate equipment.

The most important aspect in deciding to seek medical attention has to do with one's own evaluation of the severity of the injury. A few guidelines should be followed in deciding to have the eyes evaluated. If one does not meet these guidelines, but is concerned that there may be significant damage, then it is always safer to be evaluated by an ophthalmologist or in a hospital's emergency department.

- All children with eye injuries should be evaluated, especially if they complain of any visual problems, scratching sensation, or pain or if the eye is red and has a discharge.

- Adults should seek medical attention for the following:

  - The patient feels something going into the eye after hitting metal on metal, such as hammering a nail.

  - The patient has removed the foreign body from the eye and continues to have a sensation that something is in the eye, or the patient continues to have pain and tearing after removal of the object.

  - The patient is unable to remove the foreign body from the eye.

  - The patient's vision is blurry or otherwise compromised (blind spots, seeing "stars").

  - The patient is bleeding from the eye or the area around the eye (including cuts to the eyelid or eyebrow).

  - Clear or bloody fluid is coming from the eyeball.

Eye Foreign Body Diagnosis

- The first part of an eye examination is to evaluate the vision for acuity (how well one sees).

- The next portion of the examination, usually only performed by an ophthalmologist or a doctor in the emergency department, is the slit lamp examination. While one sits in a chair with their chin on a support, the doctor shines a small slit of light into the eye and looks through a microscope. This helps the doctor to see the cornea, the iris, and the lens, and the fluid in the eye.

  - The doctor starts with a general examination of the visible portions of your eye. The eyelids, eyeball, and iris are examined.

  - During this part of the examination, the doctor looks to make sure that the pupil is symmetric and reacts properly to light, that there is no obvious injury to the eyeball, and that no visible foreign bodies are still in the eye.

  - The eye may be numbed with pain medicine, and a fluorescent dye may be applied to the eye. A blue light may be used to help look for scratches on the cornea or evidence of leaking aqueous fluid, which is the clear fluid that fills the front of the eyeball.

  - While the eye is numbed, a tonometer may be used to check the pressure in the eye.

  - The eyelid may be everted (turned inside out) with a cotton swab to get a better view of the underside of the eyelid.

- Depending on the severity of injury to the eye, the final portion of the examination involves dilating (enlarging) the pupil with eyedrops. Then, the inside of the eye and the retina can be evaluated to ensure that there are no foreign bodies inside the eyeball itself and that there is no damage to the retina.

Eye Foreign Body Self-Care at Home

One should be able to care for minor debris in the eye at home. If one has trouble removing something in the eye or if a larger or sharper object is involved, seek medical attention. If one is wearing a contact lens, it should be removed prior to trying to remove the foreign body.

One should not put the contact lens back into the eye until the eye is completely healed.

- For minor foreign bodies, such as an eyelash, home care is usually adequate.
    - Begin by rinsing the eye with a saline solution (the same solution used to rinse contact lenses). Tap water or distilled water may be used if no saline solution is available. Water will effectively flush out the eye, but the chlorine in most tap water can cause varying levels of irritation. How one washes out the eye is less important than getting it washed out with great amounts of water.
    - A water fountain makes a great eye wash. Just lean over the fountain, turn on the water, and keep the eye open.
    - At a sink, stand over the sink, cup the hands, and put the face into the running water.
    - Hold a glass of water to the eye and tip the head back. Do this multiple times.
    - If one is near a shower, get in and put the eye under the running water.
    - If one is working outside, a garden hose running at a very modest flow will work.
    - If washing the eye is not successful, the object can usually be removed with the tip of a tissue or a cotton swab.
    - Pull back the eyelid by pulling down on the bottom edge of the lower lid or by pulling up on the upper edge of the upper lid.
    - Look up when evaluating for a foreign body under the lower lid.
    - Look down when evaluating for a foreign body under the upper lid. One will often need someone to help in this case.
    - Be very careful not to scrape the tissue or the cotton swab across the cornea, the clear dome over the iris.
- For larger foreign bodies or metal pieces, one should seek medical care, even if they are able to safely remove them at home.
    - If the foreign body is easily accessible and has not penetrated the eyeball, one may be able to remove it carefully with a cotton swab or a tissue.

- If one has any question about penetration of the eye, **do not** remove the object without medical assistance.

- If one cannot remove the object or if one continues to have the sensation that something is in the eye even after the debris is removed, they should seek medical care.

- After the foreign body is removed, the eye may be red and tearing.

- It is very important not to rub the eye or to apply **any** pressure to the eye. If one has punched a hole in the eye (called a ruptured globe or eyeball), one can do **significant** damage by pressing or rubbing your eye. This is especially true with small children who will rub their eyes to try to remove the debris.

- **Do not** put any pressure on the injured eye, because it could cause additional injury to the eye. Do not tape over or patch the eye with any pressure on the injured eye.

Eye Foreign Body Treatment

- For scratches on the cornea (called corneal abrasions), the usual treatment is an antibiotic ointment and/or antibiotic eye-drops and pain medicine. If the abrasion is large (greater than 50 percent of the corneal surface), then it may also be treated with a patch.

- Any noted damage to the iris, the lens, or the retina requires immediate evaluation by an ophthalmologist and may or may not require surgery.

- A ruptured eyeball requires surgery by an ophthalmologist.

- If no other injury is noted, hyphema (blood in between the cornea and the iris) requires close follow-up care with an ophthalmologist.

Eye Foreign Body Follow-Up

- Keeping follow-up appointments is important. Follow-up care is necessary to ensure that the treatment prescribed is effective.

- Depending on the severity of the injury, follow-up care for re-evaluation should be in 1 to 2 days with an ophthalmologist.

Eye Foreign Body Prevention

- Eye protection is the best prevention. Many eye injuries, especially high-speed impacts that may rupture the globe (eyeball), are usually devastating to the eye and could result in vision loss.

- **Always** wear eye protection when working in an environment where flying debris is likely.

- Eye protection should cover not only the front but also the side of the eyes. Regular sunglasses or corrective glasses are **not** sufficient eye protection when working in a high-risk environment. One should wear goggles or safety glasses with side shields.

Eye Foreign Body Prognosis

- The prognosis for corneal abrasions, even large ones, is very good. Most corneal abrasions heal within 48 hours.

- The prognosis for other eye abnormalities is often much less favorable.

  - A ruptured globe (eyeball) often leads to total loss of vision, even with early intervention.

  - Retinal damage usually leads to permanent vision loss. Depending on the extent of the retinal damage, this vision loss could be partial or complete.

  - Depending on the nature of the injury and other associated injuries, damage to the iris may be repairable.

  - Lacerations to the tissues around the eye are often repairable but can lead to varying levels of facial disfigurement.

Chapter 33

Eyelid Disorders

Chapter Contents

Section 33.1

Blepharitis

Text in this section is excerpted from "Facts about Blepharitis,"
National Eye Institute (NEI), August 2009. Reviewed March 2017.

What Is Blepharitis?

Blepharitis is a common condition that causes inflammation of the
eyelids. The condition can be difficult to manage because it tends to
recur.

What Other Conditions Are Associated with Blepharitis?

Complications from blepharitis include:

- **Stye:** A red tender bump on the eyelid that is caused by an
  acute infection of the oil glands of the eyelid.

- **Chalazion:** This condition can follow the development of a stye.
  It is a usually painless firm lump caused by inflammation of the
  oil glands of the eyelid. Chalazion can be painful and red if there
  is also an infection.

- **Problems with the tear film:** Abnormal or decreased oil secre-
  tions that are part of the tear film can result in excess tearing or
  dry eye. Because tears are necessary to keep the cornea healthy,
  tear film problems can make people more at risk for corneal
  infections.

What Causes Blepharitis?

Blepharitis occurs in two forms:

- **Anterior blepharitis** affects the outside front of the eyelid,
  where the eyelashes are attached. The two most common causes
  of anterior blepharitis are bacteria (*Staphylococcus*) and scalp
  dandruff.

- **Posterior blepharitis** affects the inner eyelid (the moist part that makes contact with the eye) and is caused by problems with the oil (meibomian) glands in this part of the eyelid. Two skin disorders can cause this form of blepharitis:

  - acne rosacea, which leads to red and inflamed skin, and

  - scalp dandruff (seborrheic dermatitis).

What Are the Symptoms of Blepharitis?

Symptoms of either form of blepharitis include a foreign body or burning sensation, excessive tearing, itching, sensitivity to light (photophobia), red and swollen eyelids, redness of the eye, blurred vision, frothy tears, dry eye, or crusting of the eyelashes on awakening.

How Is Blepharitis Treated?

Treatment for both forms of blepharitis involves keeping the lids clean and free of crusts. Warm compresses should be applied to the lid to loosen the crusts, followed by a light scrubbing of the eyelid with a cotton swab and a mixture of water and baby shampoo. Because blepharitis rarely goes away completely, most patients must maintain an eyelid hygiene routine for life. If the blepharitis is severe, an eye care professional may also prescribe antibiotics or steroid eye drops.

When scalp dandruff is present, a dandruff shampoo for the hair is recommended as well. In addition to the warm compresses, patients with posterior blepharitis will need to massage their eyelids to clean the oil accumulated in the glands. Patients who also have acne rosacea should have that condition treated at the same time.

Section 33.2

Benign Essential Blepharospasm

Text in this section is excerpted from "Benign Essential
Blepharospasm," Genetics Home Reference (GHR), National
Institutes of Health (NIH), May 2010. Reviewed March 2017.

Benign essential blepharospasm is a condition characterized by
abnormal blinking or spasms of the eyelids. This condition is a type
of dystonia, which is a group of movement disorders involving uncontrolled tensing of the muscles (muscle contractions), rhythmic shaking
(tremors), and other involuntary movements. Benign essential blepharospasm is different from the common, temporary eyelid twitching
that can be caused by fatigue, stress, or caffeine.

The signs and symptoms of benign essential blepharospasm usually appear in mid- to late adulthood and gradually worsen. The
first symptoms of the condition include an increased frequency of
blinking, dry eyes, and eye irritation that is aggravated by wind, air
pollution, sunlight, and other irritants. These symptoms may begin
in one eye, but they ultimately affect both eyes. As the condition
progresses, spasms of the muscles surrounding the eyes cause involuntary winking or squinting. Affected individuals have increasing
difficulty keeping their eyes open, which can lead to severe vision
impairment.

In more than half of all people with benign essential blepharospasm, the symptoms of dystonia spread beyond the eyes to affect
other facial muscles and muscles in other areas of the body. When
people with benign essential blepharospasm also experience involuntary muscle spasms affecting the tongue and jaw (oromandibular
dystonia), the combination of signs and symptoms is known as Meige
syndrome.

Frequency

Benign essential blepharospasm affects an estimated 20,000 to
50,000 people in the United States. For unknown reasons, it occurs in
women more than twice as often as it occurs in men.

Genetic Changes

The causes of benign essential blepharospasm are unknown, although the disorder likely results from a combination of genetic and environmental factors. Certain genetic changes probably increase the likelihood of developing this condition, and environmental factors may trigger the signs and symptoms in people who are at risk.

Studies suggest that this condition may be related to other forms of adult-onset dystonia, including uncontrolled twisting of the neck muscles (spasmodic torticollis) and spasms of the hand and finger muscles (writer's cramp). Researchers suspect that benign essential blepharospasm and similar forms of dystonia are associated with malfunction of the basal ganglia, which are structures deep within the brain that help start and control movement.

Although genetic factors are almost certainly involved in benign essential blepharospasm, no genes have been clearly associated with the condition. Several studies have looked at the relationship between common variations (polymorphisms) in the *DRD5* and *TOR1A* genes and the risk of developing benign essential blepharospasm. These studies have had conflicting results, with some showing an association and others finding no connection. Researchers are working to determine which genetic factors are related to this disorder.

Inheritance Pattern

Most cases of benign essential blepharospasm are sporadic, which means that the condition occurs in people with no history of this disorder or other forms of dystonia in their family.

Less commonly, benign essential blepharospasm has been found to run in families. In some of these families, the condition appears to have an autosomal dominant pattern of inheritance, which means that one copy of an altered gene in each cell is sufficient to cause the disorder. However, no causative genes have been identified.

Other Names for This Condition

- Essential blepharospasm
- Eyelid twitching
- Primary blepharospasm
- Spasm of eyelids

Section 33.3

Blepharophimosis, Ptosis, and Epicanthus Inversus Syndrome (BPES)

Text in this section is excerpted from "Blepharophimosis,
Ptosis, and Epicanthus Inversus Syndrome," Genetics Home
Reference (GHR), National Institutes of Health (NIH), October 2013.
Reviewed March 2017.

Blepharophimosis, ptosis, and epicanthus inversus syndrome (BPES) is a condition that mainly affects development of the eyelids. People with this condition have a narrowing of the eye opening (blepharophimosis), droopy eyelids (ptosis), and an upward fold of the skin of the lower eyelid near the inner corner of the eye (epicanthus inversus). In addition, there is an increased distance between the inner corners of the eyes (telecanthus). Because of these eyelid abnormalities, the eyelids cannot open fully, and vision may be limited.

Other structures in the eyes and face may be mildly affected by BPES. Affected individuals are at an increased risk of developing vision problems such as nearsightedness (myopia) or farsightedness (hyperopia) beginning in childhood. They may also have eyes that do not point in the same direction (strabismus) or "lazy eye" (amblyopia) affecting one or both eyes. People with BPES may also have distinctive facial features including a broad nasal bridge, low-set ears, or a shortened distance between the nose and upper lip (a short philtrum).

There are two types of BPES, which are distinguished by their signs and symptoms. Both types I and II include the eyelid malformations and other facial features. Type I is also associated with an early loss of ovarian function (primary ovarian insufficiency) in women, which causes their menstrual periods to become less frequent and eventually stop before age 40. Primary ovarian insufficiency can lead to difficulty conceiving a child (subfertility) or a complete inability to conceive (infertility).

Genetic Changes

Mutations in the *FOXL2* gene cause BPES types I and II. The *FOXL2* gene provides instructions for making a protein that is active in the eyelids and ovaries. The FOXL2 protein is likely involved in the development of muscles in the eyelids. Before birth and in adulthood, the protein regulates the growth and development of certain ovarian cells and the breakdown of specific molecules.

It is difficult to predict the type of BPES that will result from the many *FOXL2* gene mutations. However, mutations that result in a partial loss of FOXL2 protein function generally cause BPES type II. These mutations probably impair regulation of normal development of muscles in the eyelids, resulting in malformed eyelids that cannot open fully. Mutations that lead to a complete loss of FOXL2 protein function often cause BPES type I. These mutations impair the regulation of eyelid development as well as various activities in the ovaries, resulting in eyelid malformation and abnormally accelerated maturation of certain ovarian cells and the premature death of egg cells.

Inheritance Pattern

This condition is typically inherited in an autosomal dominant pattern, which means one copy of the altered gene in each cell is sufficient to cause the disorder.

In some cases, an affected person inherits the mutation from one affected parent. Other cases result from new mutations in the gene and occur in people with no history of the disorder in their family.

Other Names for This Condition

- Blepharophimosis syndrome

- Blepharophimosis, ptosis, and epicanthus inversus

Chapter 34

Disorders of the Tear Duct

Chapter Contents

Section 34.1

Blocked Tear Duct (Dacryostenosis)

Text in this section is excerpted from "Blocked Tear Duct
(Dacryostenosis) in Children," © 2005-2017 Boston Children's
Hospital. Reprinted with permission.

What Is a Blocked Tear Duct?

As many as 6 percent of newborns have a blocked tear duct in the
eye. This condition is called dacryostenosis or congenital lacrimal duct
obstruction, meaning it's present at birth.

- Tears help clean and lubricate the eye and are produced in the
  lacrimal gland, located under the bone of the eyebrow.

- Tears from the lacrimal gland flow over the eye through tiny
  ducts along the eyelid and drain away from the eye through two
  small openings at the inner corner of the eyelids.

- They then drain into a larger passage from the eye to the inside
  of the nose, called the nasolacrimal duct, or tear duct.

In some babies, the openings into the tear duct haven't formed
properly. This causes a blockage, and the tears have no place to drain.
A blocked tear duct can occur in one or both eyes.

What Are the Symptoms of a Blocked Tear Duct?

Each child may experience symptoms differently, but the most
common symptoms of a blocked tear duct include:

- tears pooling in the corner of your baby's eye

- tears draining down your baby's eyelid and cheek

- mucus or yellowish discharge in the eye

- reddening of the skin from rubbing

Because infants don't produce tears until they are several weeks
old, a blocked tear duct may not be noticeable at birth. A blocked tear

duct may also be noticeable only when a baby cries, or in cold or windy weather when tears are stimulated.

Testing and Diagnosis

A blocked tear duct is usually diagnosed based on a complete medical history and a physical examination of your child. Additional tests are not usually required to confirm the diagnosis.

Treatments

The most common treatment for a blocked tear duct is gently "milking" or massaging the tear duct two to three times a day. Your child's physician will show you how to do this.

If there are symptoms of infection, antibiotics developed specifically for use in the eye may be used.

Fortunately, nearly all blocked tear ducts open on their own, usually by the time the child is 1 year old. If the duct still remains blocked, the duct opening can be enlarged with a small probe. The procedure may need to be repeated, but it's effective in most cases.

Section 34.2

Dacryocystitis

"Dacryocystitis," © 2017 Omnigraphics.
Reviewed March 2017.

Dacryocystitis is a condition that affects the lacrimal sac, a small chamber located near the inner corner of the eye that collects excess tears from the eye's surface and drains them into the nose through the nasolacrimal duct. When this drainage system is obstructed, bacteria may become trapped and cause an infection. Dacryocystitis is characterized by pain, swelling, irritation, redness, and infection of the lacrimal sac.

Types and Causes of Dacryocystitis

There are two main types of dacryocystitis: acute and chronic. Acute dacryocystitis appears suddenly due to the blockage of a tear duct. Some of the possible causes include sinus problems, physical injury, health conditions like tuberculosis, or a cyst or tumor. The blockage causes tears and mucus to accumulate in the lacrimal sac, which creates a breeding ground for bacteria. Chronic dacryocystitis is a persistent, long-lasting condition characterized primarily by excessive watering of the eyes. It may result from an acute case that is not managed properly or from a congenital (present from birth) narrowing or obstruction of the nasolacrimal duct.

Symptoms of Dacryocystitis

The symptoms of chronic dacryocystitis are often limited to excessive tear production in one eye. They may also include one or more of the following common symptoms of acute dacryocystitis:

- pain, redness, and swelling in the inner corner of the eye;
- crusting around the eyelids and eyelashes;
- a painful lump or abscess between the eye and nose;
- oozing of pus from the corner of the eye;
- discharge of pus upon applying pressure to the lacrimal sac;
- swelling that makes it difficult to open the eye;
- fever.

Diagnosis of Dacryocystitis

To diagnose dacryocystitis, an ophthalmologist will evaluate the patient's symptoms and examine the eye to determine whether the drainage system is obstructed. The examination is likely to include looking at the eye and eyelid with a microscope, flushing fluid through the nasolacrimal duct, and taking a sample of fluid discharge from the lacrimal sac to check for bacteria.

Treatment of Dacryocystitis

For acute dacryocystitis caused by a bacterial infection, an eye doctor will typically prescribe an oral antibiotic or a topical antibiotic in the form of ointment or eye drops. Other recommended forms of treatment include applying a warm compress to the lacrimal sac several times a day and gently massaging the nasolacrimal duct to clear out pus and debris. If the symptoms are severe and include feelings of illness along with a fever, the patient should seek emergency treatment at a hospital. Intravenous antibiotics may be needed to prevent the development of potentially fatal complications, such as orbital cellulitis.

For chronic dacryocystitis—or acute dacryocystitis that is caused by a blockage—the eye doctor may recommend a surgical procedure called dacryocystorhinostomy (DCR). DCR is intended to bypass the obstruction in the nasolacrimal duct and restore the flow of tears from the lacrimal sac into the nose. The procedure uses a minimally invasive technique called endonasal approach, which involves inserting an endoscope through the nose into the nasal cavity. The surgeon uses a laser attached to the endoscope to create a hole between the lacrimal sac and the nose, and then inserts a tube to facilitate the drainage of tears.

In another type of surgical treatment, known as balloon dacryoplasty, the surgeon inserts a tiny balloon into the nasolacrimal duct and inflates it to widen a congenital narrowing or blockage. It does not have as high a success rate as DCR, however, and is not recommended for treating acute dacryocystitis.

References

1. Garrity, James. "Dacryocystitis," MSD Manuals, 2017.

2. Kerkar, Pramod. "Dacryocystitis: Types, Causes, Symptoms, Treatment, Surgery," EPainAssist, September 24, 2015.

3. Roth, Ashley. "Everything You Need to Know about Dacryocystitis," EyeHealthWeb, September 2016.

Chapter 35

Computer Vision Syndrome (CVS)

Humans normally blink about 18 times a minute. While staring at a computer—or video game, or handheld device—we blink only half as much, a situation that is resulting in computer vision syndrome (CVS), according to the American Academy of Ophthalmology (AAO).

Experts agree that choosing to stare for long periods at a smartphone or video game will not cause permanent eye damage, but CVS can cause headaches, blurred vision, dry eyes and neck and shoulder pain. Those at greatest risk for developing CVS, also known as digital eyestrain, are those who spend two or more continuous hours in front of a digital device, says the American Optometric Association (AOA). Taking regular breaks from the computer screen and improving the conditions in which we work and play on the computer can help.

"CVS is similar to a repetitive stress issue," said Jo Ann Egan, a registered nurse and vision care services coordinator at the Defense Department's Vision Center of Excellence (VCE). "Really, any break from the computer will help, especially if you just get up from your desk, or look away."

This chapter contains text excerpted from the following sources: Text in this chapter begins with excerpts from "For Digital Eyestrain, Doctors Advise Blink, Look Away," Military Health System (MHS), May 15, 2015; Text beginning with the heading "Symptoms" is excerpted from "Lighting: Computer Use and Visual Displays," Federal Aviation Administration (FAA), U.S. Department of Transportation (DOT), January 24, 2017.

The level of eye discomfort appears to increase with the amount of digital screen use, says the AOA, which recommends some fairly simple measures to prevent or reduce vision problems associated with CVS. Taking steps to control lighting and glare on the device screen, establishing proper working distances and posture for screen viewing, and assuring that minor vision problems are properly corrected can help, according to the AOA.

"As a nurse, I am looking at the whole person, and I would say look at how you are using your electronic devices," said Egan, who is based at VCE's west coast office at Madigan Army Medical Center on Joint Base Lewis-McChord in Tacoma, Washington.

Egan recommends taking regular breaks from the computer and thorough annual eye exams. During the exam, the patient should tell the eye doctor how often he or she uses a computer or other electronic device at work.

For school-age children, ever-increasing use of devices is resulting in similar increases in CVS and eyestrain. Egan suggests children receive a thorough eye exam particularly if a child has complaints or if vision problems are noted during routine pediatric vision screening. Although more studies on CVS and its impact on children need to be done, said Egan, basic common sense works in the meantime.

"Often children do not notice they are having discomfort and they will just keep doing what they are doing. So, having children learn good habits will help," she said.

An even easier rule of thumb for reducing eyestrain is the "20-20-20" rule suggested by eye doctors at the AAO, in which computer users shift their eyes every 20 minutes to look at an object at least 20-feet away for 20 seconds or more. The AAO also adds getting enough sleep to the list of remedies, since the eyes are rested and replenished with nutrients through the act of sleeping.

Lastly, to minimize the development of dry eye when using a computer, the simplest remedy, says the AAO, might also be the easiest to remember. On a note placed near the computer screen, write the following word to fend off symptoms of CVS: "Blink."

Symptoms of Computer Vision Syndrome

- Eyestrain, eye fatigue

- Blurred vision

- Focusing difficulty

- Burning, sore, tearing, or dry eyes

Causes of Computer Vision Syndrome

- Inappropriate lighting
- Glare
- Veiling reflections
- Direct glare
- Inappropriate viewing distance
- Inappropriate viewing angle
- Vision correction inadequate or inappropriate for viewing distance

Part Six

Congenital and Other Disorders That Affect Vision

Chapter 36

Hereditary Disorders Affecting Vision

Chapter Contents

Section 36.1

Achromatopsia

This section includes text excerpted from "Achromatopsia,"
Genetics Home Reference (GHR), National Institutes of
Health (NIH), January 2015.

Achromatopsia is a condition characterized by a partial or total
absence of color vision. People with complete achromatopsia cannot
perceive any colors; they see only black, white, and shades of gray.
Incomplete achromatopsia is a milder form of the condition that allows
some color discrimination.

Achromatopsia also involves other problems with vision, including
an increased sensitivity to light and glare (photophobia), involuntary
back-and-forth eye movements (nystagmus), and significantly reduced
sharpness of vision (low visual acuity). Affected individuals can also
have farsightedness (hyperopia) or, less commonly, nearsightedness
(myopia). These vision problems develop in the first few months of life.

Achromatopsia is different from the more common forms of color
vision deficiency (also called color blindness), in which people can perceive color but have difficulty distinguishing between certain colors,
such as red and green.

Frequency

Achromatopsia affects an estimated 1 in 30,000 people worldwide. Complete achromatopsia is more common than incomplete
achromatopsia.

Complete achromatopsia occurs frequently among Pingelapese
islanders, who live on one of the Eastern Caroline Islands of Micro-
nesia. Between 4 and 10 percent of people in this population have a
total absence of color vision.

Genetic Changes

Achromatopsia results from changes in one of several genes:
CNGA3, *CNGB3*, *GNAT2*, *PDE6C*, or *PDE6H*. A particular *CNGB3*
gene mutation underlies the condition in Pingelapese islanders.

Achromatopsia is a disorder of the retina, which is the light-sensitive tissue at the back of the eye. The retina contains two types of light receptor cells, called rods and cones. These cells transmit visual signals from the eye to the brain through a process called phototransduction. Rods provide vision in low light (night vision). Cones provide vision in bright light (daylight vision), including color vision.

Mutations in any of the genes listed above prevent cones from reacting appropriately to light, which interferes with phototransduction. In people with complete achromatopsia, cones are nonfunctional, and vision depends entirely on the activity of rods. The loss of cone function leads to a total lack of color vision and causes the other vision problems. People with incomplete achromatopsia retain some cone function. These individuals have limited color vision, and their other vision problems tend to be less severe.

Some people with achromatopsia do not have identified mutations in any of the known genes. In these individuals, the cause of the disorder is unknown. Other genetic factors that have not been identified likely contribute to this condition.

Inheritance Pattern

This condition is inherited in an autosomal recessive pattern, which means both copies of the gene in each cell have mutations. The parents of an individual with an autosomal recessive condition each carry one copy of the mutated gene, but they typically do not show signs and symptoms of the condition.

Other Names for This Condition

- Achromatism

- Rod monochromatism

- Total color blindness

Section 36.2

Alström Syndrome

This section contains text excerpted from the following sources:
Text in this section begins with excerpts from "Alström Syndrome,"
Genetics Home Reference (GHR), National Institutes of Health
(NIH), September 2014; Text beginning with the heading
"Symptoms" is excerpted from "Alström Syndrome," Genetic and
Rare Diseases Information Center (GARD), National Center for
Advancing Translational Sciences (NCATS), June 2016.

Alström syndrome is a rare condition that affects many body systems. Many of the signs and symptoms of this condition begin in infancy or early childhood, although some appear later in life.

Alström syndrome is characterized by a progressive loss of vision and hearing, a form of heart disease that enlarges and weakens the heart muscle (dilated cardiomyopathy), obesity, type 2 diabetes mellitus (the most common form of diabetes), and short stature. This disorder can also cause serious or life-threatening medical problems involving the liver, kidneys, bladder, and lungs. Some individuals with Alström syndrome have a skin condition called acanthosis nigricans, which causes the skin in body folds and creases to become thick, dark, and velvety. The signs and symptoms of Alström syndrome vary in severity, and not all affected individuals have all of the characteristic features of the disorder.

Frequency

More than 900 people with Alström syndrome have been reported worldwide.

Genetic Changes

Mutations in the *ALMS1* gene cause Alström syndrome. The *ALMS1* gene provides instructions for making a protein whose function is unknown. Mutations in this gene probably lead to the production of an abnormally short, nonfunctional version of the ALMS1 protein. This protein is normally present at low levels in most tissues, so a loss of the protein's normal function may help explain why the signs and symptoms of Alström syndrome affect many parts of the body.

Inheritance Pattern

This condition is inherited in an autosomal recessive pattern, which means both copies of the gene in each cell have mutations. The parents of an individual with an autosomal recessive condition each carry one copy of the mutated gene, but they typically do not show signs and symptoms of the condition.

Symptoms of Alström Syndrome

The signs and symptoms of Alström syndrome vary among affected individuals. The age that symptoms begin also varies. Symptoms may first appear anywhere from infancy to early adulthood.

Signs and symptoms may include:

- vision abnormalities, specifically cone-rod dystrophy and cataracts

- progressive sensorineural hearing loss in both ears and chronic infection or inflammation of the middle ear

- heart disease that enlarges and weakens the heart muscle (dilated cardiomyopathy)

- excessive eating (hyperphagia) and rapid weight gain leading to obesity

- insulin resistance leading to high levels of insulin in the blood (hyperinsulinemia) and type 2 diabetes mellitus

- elevated levels of fats (lipids) in the blood (hyperlipidemia)

- fatty liver that may progress to significant liver disease

- short stature

- skin findings including abnormally increased coloration and "velvety" thickening of the skin in certain areas of the body (acanthosis nigricans)

- lower hormone levels produced by the male testes or the female ovaries (hypogonadism)

Alström syndrome can also cause serious or life-threatening medical problems involving the liver, kidneys, bladder, and lungs.

Diagnosis of Alström Syndrome

Genetic testing of the *ALMS1* gene is available for Alström syndrome. Although genetic testing is not necessary to make a diagnosis of Alström syndrome, it can be helpful to confirm a diagnosis. If a mutation is not identified in both copies of the *ALMS1* gene of an individual suspected to have Alström syndrome, it does not rule out the diagnosis.

Alström syndrome is diagnosed based on clinical findings (signs and symptoms), medical history, and family history. Making a diagnosis can be complicated by the variation in age of symptom onset from one individual to another.

Alström Syndrome Treatment

There is no specific treatment for Alström syndrome. Treatment is focused on managing the symptoms present in each individual. This may involve a team of specialists including but not limited to: pediatricians, cardiologists, audiologists (hearing specialists), ophthalmologists, endocrinologists, and orthopaedists.

Treatment may include:

- specially-tinted, prescription glasses and vision aids to assist with vision loss

- hearing aids and cochlear implants for hearing loss

- dietary measures, exercise programs, and oral medications and/or insulin to control diabetes

- ACE inhibitors and other medications to manage heart and kidney problems with some individuals requiring a kidney or heart transplant

- hormone therapy if the male testes or female ovaries produce lower than average levels

Prognosis of Alström Syndrome

The prognosis for Alström syndrome varies depending on the progression of symptoms, specifically heart and kidney disease. The lifespan and overall quality of life for individuals with Alström syndrome can be improved by early diagnosis, treatment, surveillance, and proper management of symptoms.

Other Names for Alström Syndrome

- ALMS

- ALSS

- Alstrom syndrome

Section 36.3

Axenfeld-Rieger Syndrome

This section includes text excerpted from "Axenfeld-Rieger Syndrome," Genetic and Rare Diseases Information Center (GARD), National Center for Advancing Translational Sciences (NCATS), December 2016.

Axenfeld-Rieger syndrome is a group of disorders that mainly affects the development of the eye. Common eye symptoms include cornea defects and iris defects. People with this syndrome may have an off-center pupil (corectopia) or extra holes in the eyes that can look like multiple pupils (polycoria). About 50 percent of people with this syndrome develop glaucoma, a condition that increases pressure inside of the eye, and may cause vision loss or blindness.

Even though Axenfeld-Rieger syndrome is primarily an eye disorder, this syndrome can affect other parts of the body. Most people with this syndrome have distinctive facial features and many have issues with their teeth, including unusually small teeth (microdontia) or fewer than normal teeth (oligodontia). Some people have extra folds of skin around their belly button, heart defects, or other more rare birth defects.

There are three types of Axenfeld-Rieger syndrome and each has a different genetic cause. Axenfeld-Rieger syndrome type 1 is caused by mutations in the *PITX2* gene. Axenfeld-Rieger syndrome type 3 is caused by mutations in the *FOXC1* gene. The gene that causes Axenfeld-Rieger syndrome type 2 is not known, but it is located on chromosome 13. Axenfeld-Rieger syndrome has an autosomal dominant pattern of inheritance. Treatment depend on the symptoms.

Symptoms

Axenfeld-Rieger syndrome is an eye disorder. People with this disorder typically have cornea defects, which is the clear cover on the front of the eye. They may have a cloudy cornea or posterior embryotoxin, which is when you can see an opaque ring around the outer edge of the cornea. People with this disorder can also have issues with their iris, which is the colored part of the eye. They typically have iris stands, which is connective tissue that connects the iris with the lens. There may be issues with the pupils as well, which is the black opening in the eye. One of the pupils may be in the wrong location (corectopia), the pupils may be abnormally large or small, or there may be extra pupils (polycoria).

About 50 percent of people with this syndrome develop glaucoma, which is a condition that increases pressure inside of the eye. This may cause vision loss or blindness. People with this syndrome can also have strabismus (cross-eye), cataracts (cloudy lens), macular degeneration (eye disorder that causes vision loss), or coloboma (a hole in a structure in the eye).

Even though Axenfeld-Rieger syndrome is primarily an eye disorder, people with this syndrome can also have symptoms that affect other parts of the body. These symptoms mostly involve the teeth and facial bones. Symptoms affecting the teeth include cone-shaped teeth (peg-like incisors), missing teeth (oligodontia), small teeth (microdontia), and abnormal spacing of the teeth. Symptoms affecting the facial bones may include an underdeveloped jaw, a protruding lower lip, and widely-spaced eyes. Other symptoms include extra folds of skin around the belly button, heart defects, or other more rare birth defects.

Inheritance

Axenfeld-Rieger syndrome is inherited in an autosomal dominant manner.

We have two copies of every gene in our body. In autosomal dominant conditions, if there is a mutation in just one copy of that gene, then that person will develop the condition. This mutation can be inherited from a parent, or it can happen by chance for the first time in that one person, which is called a *de novo* mutation.

Each child of an individual with Axenfeld-Rieger syndrome has a 50 percent chance of inheriting the mutation. Children who inherit the mutation will have Axenfeld-Rieger syndrome, although their symptoms could be more or less severe than their parent's.

Treatment

If glaucoma is present, the goal of treatment is to decrease intraocular pressure (IOP). An annual ophthalmologic exam should be done using several specific exams to detect the presence of glaucoma. Should glaucoma develop, eye drops are usually recommended before surgery. Medications that might be prescribed include those that decrease aqueous output (beta blockers, alpha-agonists and carbonic anhydrase inhibitors). However, alpha-agonists should be used with caution in young children because of possible neurologic effects. Surgery is performed if eye drops are not sufficient in lowering IOP. If surgery is necessary, the procedure of choice is trabeculectomy. Laser surgery may also be indicated. Patients with corectopia (pupil is off center and not located where it should be) and polycoria (more than one pupil is present in the eye) may experience too much sensitivity to light (photophobia), and contact lenses may be helpful.

If the person has additional findings, treatment will depend on the symptoms present, and may include surgery to correct facial or dental problems, heart surgery, or corrective surgery for the cases of hypospadia. Short stature due to a growth hormone deficiency may be treated with growth hormone.

Section 36.4

Bardet-Biedl Syndrome

This section contains text excerpted from the following sources:
Text in this section begins with excerpts from "Bardet-Biedl Syndrome," Genetics Home Reference (GHR), National Institutes of Health (NIH), September 2013. Reviewed March 2017; Text under the heading "Treatment" is excerpted from "Bardet-Biedl Syndrome," Genetic and Rare Diseases Information Center (GARD), National Center for Advancing Translational Sciences (NCATS), July 18, 2016.

Bardet-Biedl syndrome (BBS) is a disorder that affects many parts of the body. The signs and symptoms of this condition vary among affected individuals, even among members of the same family.

Vision loss is one of the major features of BBS. Loss of vision occurs as the light-sensing tissue at the back of the eye (the retina) gradually deteriorates. Problems with night vision become apparent by mid-childhood, followed by blind spots that develop in the side (peripheral) vision. Over time, these blind spots enlarge and merge to produce tunnel vision. Most people with BBS also develop blurred central vision (poor visual acuity) and become legally blind by adolescence or early adulthood.

Obesity is another characteristic feature of BBS. Abnormal weight gain typically begins in early childhood and continues to be an issue throughout life. Complications of obesity can include type 2 diabetes, high blood pressure (hypertension), and abnormally high cholesterol levels (hypercholesterolemia).

Other major signs and symptoms of BBS include the presence of extra fingers or toes (polydactyly), intellectual disability or learning problems, and abnormalities of the genitalia. Most affected males produce reduced amounts of sex hormones (hypogonadism), and they are usually unable to father biological children (infertile). Many people with BBS also have kidney abnormalities, which can be serious or life-threatening.

Additional features of BBS can include impaired speech, delayed development of motor skills such as standing and walking, behavioral problems such as emotional immaturity and inappropriate outbursts, and clumsiness or poor coordination. Distinctive facial features, dental abnormalities, unusually short or fused fingers or toes, and a partial or complete loss of the sense of smell (anosmia) have also been reported in some people with BBS. Additionally, this condition can affect the heart, liver, and digestive system.

Frequency

In most of North America and Europe, BBS has a prevalence of 1 in 140,000 to 1 in 160,000 newborns. The condition is more common on the island of Newfoundland (off the east coast of Canada), where it affects an estimated 1 in 17,000 newborns. It also occurs more frequently in the Bedouin population of Kuwait, affecting about 1 in 13,500 newborns.

Genetic Changes

BBS can result from mutations in at least 14 different genes (often called BBS genes). These genes are known or suspected to play critical roles in cell structures called cilia. Cilia are microscopic, finger-like projections that stick out from the surface of many types of cells. They are involved in cell movement and many different chemical signaling pathways. Cilia are also necessary for the perception of sensory input (such as sight, hearing, and smell). The proteins produced from BBS genes are involved in the maintenance and function of cilia.

Mutations in BBS genes lead to problems with the structure and function of cilia. Defects in these cell structures probably disrupt important chemical signaling pathways during development and lead to abnormalities of sensory perception. Researchers believe that defective cilia are responsible for most of the features of BBS.

About one-quarter of all cases of BBS result from mutations in the *BBS1* gene. Another 20 percent of cases are caused by mutations in the *BBS10* gene. The other BBS genes each account for only a small percentage of all cases of this condition. In about 25 percent of people with BBS, the cause of the disorder is unknown.

In affected individuals who have mutations in one of the BBS genes, mutations in additional genes may be involved in causing or modifying the course of the disorder. Studies suggest that these modifying genes may be known BBS genes or other genes. The additional genetic changes could help explain the variability in the signs and symptoms of BBS. However, this phenomenon appears to be uncommon, and it has not been found consistently in scientific studies.

Inheritance Pattern

BBS is typically inherited in an autosomal recessive pattern, which means both copies of a BBS gene in each cell have mutations. The parents of an individual with an autosomal recessive condition each carry one copy of the mutated gene, but they typically do not show signs and symptoms of the condition.

Treatment

There is no cure for BBS. Treatment generally focuses on the specific signs and symptoms in each individual:

- While there is no therapy for the progressive vision loss, early evaluation by a specialist can help to provide vision aids and mobility training. Additionally, education of affected children should include planning for future blindness.

- Management of obesity may include education, diet, exercise, and behavioral therapies beginning at an early age. Complications of obesity such as abnormally high cholesterol and diabetes mellitus are usually treated as they are in the general population.

- Management of intellectual disability includes early intervention, special education and speech therapy as needed. Many affected adults are able to develop independent living skills.

- Although kidney transplants have been successful, the immunosuppressants used after a transplant may contribute to obesity. Affected individuals may also need surgery for polydactyly (extra fingers and/or toes) or genital abnormalities.

- As children approach puberty, hormone levels should be monitored to determine if hormone replacement therapy is necessary. Additionally, it should not be assumed that affected individuals are infertile—so contraception advice should be offered.

Section 36.5

Coloboma

This section includes text excerpted from "Coloboma," Genetics Home Reference (GHR), National Institutes of Health (NIH), November 2011. Reviewed March 2017.

Coloboma is an eye abnormality that occurs before birth. Colobomas are missing pieces of tissue in structures that form the eye. They may appear as notches or gaps in one of several parts of the eye, including the colored part of the eye called the iris; the retina, which is the specialized light-sensitive tissue that lines the back of the eye; the blood vessel layer under the retina called the choroid; or the optic nerves, which carry information from the eyes to the brain.

Colobomas may be present in one or both eyes and, depending on their size and location, can affect a person's vision. Colobomas affecting the iris, which result in a "keyhole" appearance of the pupil, generally do not lead to vision loss. Colobomas involving the retina result in vision loss in specific parts of the visual field, generally the upper part. Large retinal colobomas or those affecting the optic nerve can cause low vision, which means vision loss that cannot be completely corrected with glasses or contact lenses.

Some people with coloboma also have a condition called **microphthalmia**. In this condition, one or both eyeballs are abnormally small. In some affected individuals, the eyeball may appear to be completely missing; however, even in these cases some remaining eye tissue is generally present. Such severe microphthalmia should be distinguished from another condition called anophthalmia, in which no eyeball forms at all. However, the terms anophthalmia and severe microphthalmia are often used interchangeably. Microphthalmia may or may not result in significant vision loss.

People with coloboma may also have other eye abnormalities, including clouding of the lens of the eye (cataract), increased pressure inside the eye (glaucoma) that can damage the optic nerve, vision problems such as nearsightedness (myopia), involuntary back-and-forth eye movements (nystagmus), or separation of the retina from the back of the eye (retinal detachment).

Some individuals have coloboma as part of a syndrome that affects other organs and tissues in the body. These forms of the condition are described as syndromic. When coloboma occurs by itself, it is described as nonsyndromic or isolated.

Colobomas involving the eyeball should be distinguished from gaps that occur in the eyelids. While these eyelid gaps are also called colobomas, they arise from abnormalities in different structures during early development.

Frequency

Coloboma occurs in approximately 1 in 10,000 people. Because coloboma does not always affect vision or the outward appearance of the eye, some people with this condition are likely undiagnosed.

Genetic Changes

Coloboma arises from abnormal development of the eye. During the second month of development before birth, a seam called the optic fissure (also known as the choroidal fissure or embryonic fissure) closes to form the structures of the eye. When the optic fissure does not close completely, the result is a coloboma. The location of the coloboma depends on the part of the optic fissure that failed to close.

Coloboma may be caused by changes in many genes involved in the early development of the eye, most of which have not been identified. The condition may also result from a chromosomal abnormality affecting one or more genes. Most genetic changes associated with coloboma have been identified only in very small numbers of affected individuals.

The risk of coloboma may also be increased by environmental factors that affect early development, such as exposure to alcohol during pregnancy. In these cases, affected individuals usually have other health problems in addition to coloboma.

Inheritance Pattern

Most often, isolated coloboma is not inherited, and there is only one affected individual in a family. However, the affected individual is still at risk of passing the coloboma on to his or her own children.

In cases when it is passed down in families, coloboma can have different inheritance patterns. Isolated coloboma is sometimes inherited in an autosomal dominant pattern, which means one copy of an altered gene in each cell is sufficient to cause the disorder. Isolated coloboma can also be inherited in an autosomal recessive pattern, which means both copies of a gene in each cell have mutations. The parents of an individual with an autosomal recessive condition each carry one copy of a mutated gene, but they typically do not show signs and symptoms of the condition.

Less commonly, isolated coloboma may have X-linked dominant or X-linked recessive patterns of inheritance. X-linked means that a gene associated with this condition is located on the X chromosome, which is one of the two sex chromosomes. A characteristic of X-linked inheritance is that fathers cannot pass X-linked traits to their sons.

X-linked dominant means that in females (who have two X chromosomes), a mutation in one of the two copies of a gene in each cell is sufficient to cause the disorder. In males (who have only one X chromosome), a mutation in the only copy of a gene in each cell causes the disorder. In most cases, males experience more severe symptoms of the disorder than females.

X-linked recessive means that in females, a mutation would have to occur in both copies of a gene to cause the disorder. In males, one altered copy of a gene in each cell is sufficient to cause the condition. Because it is unlikely that females will have two altered copies of a particular gene, males are affected by X-linked recessive disorders much more frequently than females.

When coloboma occurs as a feature of a genetic syndrome or chromosomal abnormality, it may cluster in families according to the inheritance pattern for that condition, which may be autosomal dominant, autosomal recessive, or X-linked.

Other Names for This Condition

- Congenital ocular coloboma

- Microphthalmia, isolated, with coloboma

- Ocular coloboma

- Uveoretinal coloboma

Section 36.6

Fuchs Endothelial Dystrophy

This section includes text excerpted from "Fuchs Endothelial Dystrophy," Genetics Home Reference (GHR), National Institutes of Health (NIH), June 2011. Reviewed March 2017.

Fuchs endothelial dystrophy is a condition that causes vision problems. The first symptom of this condition is typically blurred vision in the morning that usually clears during the day. Over time, affected individuals lose the ability to see details (visual acuity). People with Fuchs endothelial dystrophy also become sensitive to bright lights.

Fuchs endothelial dystrophy specifically affects the front surface of the eye called the cornea. Deposits called guttae, which are detectable during an eye exam, form in the middle of the cornea and eventually spread. These guttae contribute to the loss of cells in the cornea, leading to vision problems. Tiny blisters may develop on the cornea, which can burst and cause eye pain.

The signs and symptoms of Fuchs endothelial dystrophy usually begin in a person's forties or fifties. A very rare early-onset variant of this condition starts to affect vision in a person's twenties.

Frequency

The late-onset form of Fuchs endothelial dystrophy is a common condition, affecting approximately 4 percent of people over the age of 40. The early-onset variant of Fuchs endothelial dystrophy is rare, although the exact prevalence is unknown.

For reasons that are unclear, women are affected with Fuchs endothelial dystrophy somewhat more frequently than men.

Genetic Changes

The genetics of Fuchs endothelial dystrophy are unclear. Researchers have identified regions of a few chromosomes and several genes that they think may play a role in the development of Fuchs endothelial dystrophy, but many of these associations need to be further tested.

Fuchs endothelial dystrophy affects a thin layer of cells that line the back of the cornea, called corneal endothelial cells. These cells regulate the amount of fluid inside the cornea. An appropriate fluid balance in the cornea is necessary for clear vision. Fuchs endothelial dystrophy occurs when the endothelial cells die, and the cornea becomes swollen with too much fluid. Corneal endothelial cells continue to die over time, resulting in further vision problems. It is thought that mutations in genes that are active (expressed) primarily in corneal endothelial cells or surrounding tissue may lead to the death of corneal endothelial cells, resulting in Fuchs endothelial dystrophy.

Some cases of the early-onset variant of Fuchs endothelial dystrophy are caused by mutations in the *COL8A2* gene. This gene provides instructions for making a protein that is part of type VIII collagen. Type VIII collagen is largely found within the cornea, surrounding the endothelial cells. Specifically, type VIII collagen is a major component of a tissue at the back of the cornea, called Descemet membrane. This membrane is a thin, sheet-like structure that separates and supports corneal endothelial cells. *COL8A2* gene mutations that cause the early-onset variant of Fuchs endothelial dystrophy lead to an abnormal Descemet membrane, which causes the cells to die and leads to the vision problems in people with this condition.

Mutations in unidentified genes are also likely to cause the early-onset variant of Fuchs endothelial dystrophy. The genetic causes of the late-onset form of the disorder are unknown.

Inheritance Pattern

In some cases, Fuchs endothelial dystrophy appears to be inherited in an autosomal dominant pattern, which means one copy of the altered gene in each cell is sufficient to cause the disorder. When this condition is caused by a mutation in the *COL8A2* gene, it is inherited in an autosomal dominant pattern. In addition, an autosomal dominant inheritance pattern is apparent in some situations in which the condition is caused by alterations in an unknown gene.

In many families, the inheritance pattern is unknown.

Some cases result from new mutations in a gene and occur in people with no history of the disorder in their family.

Other Names for This Condition

- Fuchs atrophy

- Fuchs corneal dystrophy

- Fuchs dystrophy

- Fuchs endothelial corneal dystrophy (FECD)

- Fuchs' endothelial dystrophy

Section 36.7

Ocular Albinism

This section includes text excerpted from "Ocular Albinism," Genetic and Rare Diseases Information Center (GARD), National Center for Advancing Translational Sciences (NCATS), August 6, 2015.

Ocular albinism type 1 (OA1) is a genetic eye condition that primarily affects males. Signs and symptoms may include reduced coloring of the iris and retina (ocular hypopigmentation); foveal hypoplasia (underdevelopment); rapid, involuntary eye movements (nystagmus); poor vision; poor depth perception; eyes that do not look in the same direction (strabismus); and increased sensitivity to light. It is caused by mutations in the *GPR143* gene and is inherited in an X-linked recessive manner. Females have been affected in rare instances. Treatment consists of visual correction with eyeglasses or contact lenses; use of sunglasses or special filter glasses for light sensitivity; and in some cases, extraocular muscle surgery to restore alignment and/or improve head posture that is associated with nystagmus.

Signs and Symptoms of Ocular Albinism

- Abnormality of the pupil
- Astigmatism
- Nystagmus
- Ocular albinism
- Photophobia
- Freckling
- Hypoplasia of the fovea
- Strabismus
- Giant melanosomes in melanocytes
- Myopia

Cause of Ocular Albinism

OA1 is caused by mutations in the *GPR143* gene. This gene gives the body instructions for making a protein that plays a role in pigmentation (coloring) of the eyes and skin. It helps control the growth of melanosomes, which are structures inside cells that make and store a pigment called melanin. Melanin also plays a role in vision in the retina. Mutations in the *GPR143* gene can affect the protein's ability to do its job. As a result, melanosomes in skin and retinal cells can grow abnormally large, contributing to the signs and symptoms of the condition. In rare cases, the genetic cause of this condition is unknown.

Ocular Albinism Inheritance

OA1 is usually caused by mutations in the *GPR143* gene. In these cases, the condition is inherited in an X-linked recessive manner. Males are more commonly affected than females. This is because males have only one X chromosome and therefore one copy of the

GPR143 gene. Females have two X chromosomes and therefore two copies of the *GPR143* gene. If females have a mutation in one of their *GPR143* genes, they still have a second normal *GPR143* gene to compensate. Women with one mutated copy of the gene usually do not have vision loss or other significant eye abnormalities. They may have mild changes in retinal pigmentation that can be detected during an eye examination.

Occasionally, females will have more significant signs and symptoms of OA1. This may be due to:

- a phenomenon called skewed X-chromosome inactivation

- inheriting two mutated copies of the *GPR143* gene

- having a partial deletion of the X chromosome

Diagnosis of Ocular Albinism

Making a diagnosis for a genetic or rare disease can often be challenging. Healthcare professionals typically look at a person's medical history, symptoms, physical exam, and laboratory test results in order to make a diagnosis. If you have questions about getting a diagnosis, you should contact a healthcare professional.

Ocular Albinism Treatment

Hypersensitivity to light, often called "photoaversion," "photophobia," or "photodysphoria," is the most incapacitating symptom in some people with OA1. This symptom may be relieved by sunglasses, transition lenses, or special filter glasses, although many prefer not to wear them because of the reduction in vision from the dark lenses when indoors.

Refractive errors should be detected and treated as early as possible with appropriate spectacle correction. Abnormal head posture may be treated with prismatic spectacle correction.

Strabismus surgery is usually not necessary but may be performed for cosmetic purposes, particularly if the strabismus or the face turn is marked or fixed.

Appropriate education for sun-protective lotions and clothing (preferably by an informed dermatologic consultant) is recommended to moderate the lifelong effects of sun exposure.

Children with ocular albinism who are younger than 16 years of age should have an annual ophthalmologic exam (including assessment of refractive error and the need for filter glasses), as well as psychosocial and educational support. Affected adults should have ophthalmologic exams when needed, typically every two to three years.

Ocular Albinism Prognosis

OA1 is a non-progressive disorder. Visual acuity typically remains stable throughout life, even often slowly improving into the mid-teens. Although nystagmus usually develops within the first 3 months of life, it can diminish with time. However, it rarely completely disappears. Because the specific ocular signs and symptoms in affected people can vary, the condition may cause some people to be more visually impaired than others. People with OA1 have a normal life expectancy.

Other Names for Ocular Albinism

- Nettleship-Falls type ocular albinism

- X-linked recessive ocular albinism

- X-linked ocular albinism (XLOA)

Section 36.8

Stargardt Macular Degeneration

This section contains text excerpted from the following sources:
Text in this section begins with excerpts from "Stargardt Macular Degeneration," Genetics Home Reference (GHR), National Institutes of Health (NIH), November 2010. Reviewed March 2017; Text beginning with the heading "Treatment" is excerpted from "Stargardt Disease," Genetic and Rare Diseases Information Center (GARD), National Center for Advancing Translational Sciences (NCATS), June 4, 2014.

Stargardt macular degeneration is a genetic eye disorder that causes progressive vision loss. This disorder affects the retina, the specialized light-sensitive tissue that lines the back of the eye. Specifically, Stargardt macular degeneration affects a small area near the center of the retina called the macula. The macula is responsible for sharp central vision, which is needed for detailed tasks such as reading, driving, and recognizing faces. In most people with Stargardt macular degeneration, a fatty yellow pigment (lipofuscin) builds up in cells underlying the macula. Over time, the abnormal accumulation of this substance can damage cells that are critical for clear central vision. In addition to central vision loss, people with Stargardt macular degeneration have problems with night vision that can make it difficult to navigate in low light. Some affected individuals also have impaired color vision. The signs and symptoms of Stargardt macular degeneration typically appear in late childhood to early adulthood and worsen over time.

Frequency

Stargardt macular degeneration is the most common form of juvenile macular degeneration, the signs and symptoms of which begin in childhood. The estimated prevalence of Stargardt macular degeneration is 1 in 8,000 to 10,000 individuals.

Genetic Changes

In most cases, Stargardt macular degeneration is caused by mutations in the *ABCA4* gene. Less often, mutations in the *ELOVL4* gene cause this condition. The *ABCA4* and *ELOVL4* genes provide instructions for making proteins that are found in light-sensing (photoreceptor) cells in the retina.

The ABCA4 protein transports potentially toxic substances out of photoreceptor cells. These substances form after phototransduction, the process by which light entering the eye is converted into electrical signals that are transmitted to the brain. Mutations in the *ABCA4* gene prevent the ABCA4 protein from removing toxic byproducts from photoreceptor cells. These toxic substances build up and form lipofuscin in the photoreceptor cells and the surrounding cells of the retina, eventually causing cell death. Loss of cells in the retina causes the progressive vision loss characteristic of Stargardt macular degeneration.

The ELOVL4 protein plays a role in making a group of fats called very long-chain fatty acids. The ELOVL4 protein is primarily active (expressed) in the retina, but is also expressed in the brain and skin. The function of very long-chain fatty acids within the retina is unknown. Mutations in the *ELOVL4* gene lead to the formation of ELOVL4 protein clumps (aggregates) that build up and may interfere with retinal cell functions, ultimately leading to cell death.

Inheritance Pattern

Stargardt macular degeneration can have different inheritance patterns.

When mutations in the *ABCA4* gene cause this condition, it is inherited in an autosomal recessive pattern, which means both copies of the gene in each cell have mutations. The parents of an individual with an autosomal recessive condition each carry one copy of the mutated gene, but they typically do not show signs and symptoms of the condition.

When this condition is caused by mutations in the *ELOVL4* gene, it is inherited in an autosomal dominant pattern, which means one copy of the altered gene in each cell is sufficient to cause the disorder.

Treatment

At present there is no cure for Stargardt disease, and there is very little that can be done to slow its progression. Wearing sunglasses to protect the eyes from UVa, UVb and bright light may be of some benefit. Animal studies have shown that taking excessive amounts of vitamin A and beta-carotene could promote the additional accumulation of lipofuscin, as well as a toxic vitamin A derivative called A2E; it is typically recommended that these be avoided by individuals with Stargardt disease. There are possible treatments for Stargardt disease that are being tested, including a gene therapy treatment, which has been given orphan drug status by the European Medicines Agency (EMEA, similar to the U.S. Food and Drug Administration (FDA)). There are also clinical trials involving embryonic stem cell treatments.

Other Names for This Condition

- Juvenile onset macular degeneration
- Stargardt disease
- Stargardt macular dystrophy

Section 36.9

Usher Syndrome

This section includes text excerpted from "Usher Syndrome," Genetics Home Reference (GHR), National Institutes of Health (NIH), June 2016.

Usher syndrome is a condition characterized by partial or total hearing loss and vision loss that worsens over time. The hearing loss is classified as sensorineural, which means that it is caused by abnormalities of the inner ear. The loss of vision is caused by an eye disease called retinitis pigmentosa (RP), which affects the layer of light-sensitive tissue at the back of the eye (the retina). Vision loss occurs as the light-sensing cells of the retina gradually deteriorate. Night vision loss begins first, followed by blind spots that develop in the side (peripheral) vision. Over time, these blind spots enlarge and merge to produce tunnel vision. In some cases, vision is further impaired by clouding of the lens of the eye (cataracts). However, many people with retinitis pigmentosa retain some central vision throughout their lives.

Researchers have identified three major types of Usher syndrome, designated as types I, II, and III. These types are distinguished by their severity and the age when signs and symptoms appear. The types are further divided into subtypes based on their genetic cause.

Most individuals with Usher syndrome type I are born with severe to profound hearing loss. Progressive vision loss caused by retinitis pigmentosa becomes apparent in childhood. This type of Usher syndrome also causes abnormalities of the vestibular system, which is the part of the inner ear that helps maintain the body's balance and orientation in space. As a result of the vestibular abnormalities, children with the condition have trouble with balance. They begin sitting independently and walking later than usual, and they may have difficulty riding a bicycle and playing certain sports.

Usher syndrome type II is characterized by hearing loss from birth and progressive vision loss that begins in adolescence or adulthood. The hearing loss associated with this form of Usher syndrome ranges from mild to severe and mainly affects the ability to hear high-frequency sounds. For example, it is difficult for affected individuals to hear high, soft speech sounds, such as those of the letters d and t. The degree of hearing loss varies within and among families with this condition, and it may become more severe over time. Unlike the other forms of Usher syndrome, type II is not associated with vestibular abnormalities that cause difficulties with balance.

People with Usher syndrome type III experience hearing loss and vision loss beginning somewhat later in life. Unlike the other forms of Usher syndrome, type III is usually associated with normal hearing at birth. Hearing loss typically begins during late childhood or adolescence, after the development of speech, and becomes more severe over time. By middle age, most affected individuals have profound hearing loss. Vision loss caused by retinitis pigmentosa also develops in late childhood or adolescence. Some people with Usher syndrome type III have vestibular abnormalities that cause problems with balance.

Frequency

Usher syndrome is estimated to affect 4 to 5 per 100,000 people, although some studies suggest that the prevalence of the condition may be as high as 1 in 6,000 people. The condition is thought to account for 3 to 6 percent of all childhood deafness and about 50 percent of deaf-blindness in adults.

Types I and II are the most common forms of Usher syndrome in most countries. Type III represents only about 2 percent of all Usher syndrome cases overall. However, type III occurs more frequently in the Finnish population, where it accounts for about 40 percent of cases.

Genetic Changes

Usher syndrome can be caused by mutations in several different genes. Mutations in at least six genes can cause Usher syndrome type I. The most common of these are *MYO7A* gene mutations, followed by mutations in the *CDH23* gene. Usher syndrome type II can result from mutations in three genes; *USH2A* gene mutations account for most cases of type II. Usher syndrome type III is most often caused by mutations in the *CLRN1* gene.

The genes associated with Usher syndrome provide instructions for making proteins involved in normal hearing, balance, and vision. In the inner ear, these proteins are involved in the development and function of specialized cells called hair cells, which help to transmit sound and signals from the inner ear to the brain. In the retina, the proteins contribute to the maintenance of light-sensing cells called rod photoreceptors (which provide vision in low light) and cone photoreceptors (which provide color vision and vision in bright light). For some of the proteins related to Usher syndrome, their exact role in hearing, balance, and vision is unknown.

Most of the gene mutations responsible for Usher syndrome lead to a loss of hair cells in the inner ear and a gradual loss of rods and cones in the retina. Degeneration of these sensory cells causes the hearing loss, balance problems, and vision loss that occur with Usher syndrome.

In some people with Usher syndrome, the genetic cause of the condition has not been identified. Researchers suspect that several additional genes are probably associated with this disorder.

Inheritance Pattern

All of the types of Usher syndrome are inherited in an autosomal recessive pattern, which means both copies of a gene in each cell have a mutation. The parents of an individual with Usher syndrome each carry one copy of the mutated gene, but they do not have any signs and symptoms of the condition.

Other Names for This Condition

- Deafness-retinitis pigmentosa syndrome
- Graefe-Usher syndrome
- Hallgren syndrome
- Retinitis pigmentosa-deafness syndrome
- Usher's syndrome

Section 36.10

Wagener Syndrome

This section contains text excerpted from the following sources:
Text in this section begins with excerpts from "Wagner Syndrome,"
Genetics Home Reference (GHR), National Institutes of Health
(NIH), July 2014; Text beginning with the heading "Treatment" is
excerpted from "Wagner Syndrome," Genetic and Rare Diseases
Information Center (GARD), National Center for Advancing
Translational Sciences (NCATS), January 23, 2017.

Wagner syndrome is a hereditary disorder that causes progressive vision loss. The eye problems that lead to vision loss typically begin in childhood, although the vision impairment might not be immediately apparent.

In people with Wagner syndrome, the light-sensitive tissue that lines the back of the eye (the retina) becomes thin and may separate from the back of the eye (retinal detachment). The blood vessels within the retina (known as the choroid) may also be abnormal. The retina and the choroid progressively break down (degenerate). Some people with Wagner syndrome have blurred vision because of ectopic fovea, an abnormality in which the part of the retina responsible for sharp central vision is out of place. Additionally, the thick, clear gel that fills the eyeball (the vitreous) becomes watery and thin. People with Wagner syndrome develop a clouding of the lens of the eye (cataract). Affected individuals may also experience nearsightedness (myopia), progressive night blindness, or a narrowing of their field of vision.

Vision impairment in people with Wagner syndrome can vary from near normal vision to complete loss of vision in both eyes.

Frequency

Wagner syndrome is a rare disorder, although its exact prevalence is unknown. Approximately 300 affected individuals have been described worldwide; about half of these individuals are from the Netherlands.

Genetic Changes

Mutations in the *VCAN* gene cause Wagner syndrome. The *VCAN* gene provides instructions for making a protein called versican. Versican is found in the extracellular matrix, which is the intricate lattice of proteins and other molecules that forms in the spaces between cells. Versican interacts with many of these proteins and molecules to facilitate the assembly of the extracellular matrix and ensure its stability. Within the eye, versican interacts with other proteins to maintain the structure and gel-like consistency of the vitreous.

VCAN gene mutations that cause Wagner syndrome lead to insufficient levels of versican in the vitreous. Without enough versican to interact with the many proteins of the vitreous, the structure becomes unstable. This lack of stability in the vitreous affects other areas of the eye and contributes to the vision problems that occur in people with Wagner syndrome. It is unknown why *VCAN* gene mutations seem solely to affect vision.

Inheritance Pattern

This condition is inherited in an autosomal dominant pattern, which means one copy of the altered gene in each cell is sufficient to cause the disorder.

Treatment

There is no cure for Wagner syndrome, but there may be ways to manage the symptoms. Refractive errors (such as myopia) can be corrected by glasses or contact lenses. Cataracts should be removed via standard protocols by an experienced eye care professional. Retinal breaks can be treated with laser retinopexy (gas bubble placement) or cryotherapy (use of subzero temperatures to treat tissue damage). All individuals with Wagner syndrome should be seen yearly a vitreoretinal specialist for an ophthalmologic evaluation.

Other Names for This Condition

- Erosive vitreoretinopathy
- ERVR

- Hyaloideoretinal degeneration of Wagner
- Wagner syndrome type 1
- Wagner vitreoretinal degeneration
- WGN1

Chapter 37

Other Congenital Disorders Affecting Vision

Chapter Contents

Section 37.1

Anophthalmia and Microphthalmia

This section includes text excerpted from "Facts about Anophthalmia/
Microphthalmia," Division of Birth Defects and Developmental
Disabilities (NCBDDD), Centers for Disease Control and
Prevention (CDC), December 10, 2015.

Anophthalmia and microphthalmia are birth defects of a baby's
eye(s). Anophthalmia is a birth defect where a baby is born without
one or both eyes. Microphthalmia is a birth defect in which one or both
eyes did not develop fully, so they are small.

What Is Anophthalmia and Microphthalmia?

Anophthalmia and microphthalmia develop during pregnancy and
can occur alone, with other birth defects, or as part of a syndrome.
Anophthalmia and microphthalmia often result in blindness or limited
vision.

Occurrence

Anophthalmia and microphthalmia are rare. Researchers estimate
that about 1 in every 5,300 babies born in the United States will have
anophthalmia or microphthalmia. This means about 780 U.S. babies
are born with these conditions each year.

Causes and Risk Factors

The causes of anophthalmia and microphthalmia among most
infants are unknown. Some babies have anophthalmia or microphthalmia because of a change in their genes or chromosomes. Anophthalmia
and microphthalmia can also be caused by taking certain medicines,
like isotretinoin (Accutane®) or thalidomide, during pregnancy. These
medicines can lead to a pattern of birth defects, which can include
anophthalmia or microphthalmia. These defects might also be caused
by a combination of genes and other factors, such as the things the

mother comes in contact with in the environment or what the mother eats or drinks, or certain medicines she uses during pregnancy.

Like many families of children with a birth defect, Centers for Disease Control and Prevention (CDC) wants to find out what causes them. Understanding the factors that are more common among babies with a birth defect will help us learn more about the causes.

CDC continues to study birth defects, such as anophthalmia and microphthalmia, and how to prevent them. If you are pregnant or thinking about becoming pregnant, talk with your doctor about ways to increase your chances of having a healthy baby.

Diagnosis

Anophthalmia and microphthalmia can either be diagnosed during pregnancy or after birth. During pregnancy, doctors can often identify anophthalmia and microphthalmia through an ultrasound or a Computerized tomography (CT) scan (special X-ray test) and sometimes with certain genetic testing. After birth, a doctor can identify anophthalmia and microphthalmia by examining the baby. A doctor will also perform a thorough physical exam to look for any other birth defects that may be present.

Treatment

There is no treatment available that will create a new eye or that will restore complete vision for those affected by anophthalmia or microphthalmia. A baby born with one of these conditions should be seen by a team of special eye doctors:

- an ophthalmologist, a doctor specially trained to care for eyes

- an ocularist, a healthcare provider who is specially trained in making and fitting prosthetic eyes

- an oculoplastic surgeon, a doctor who specializes in surgery for the eye and eye socket

The eye sockets are critical for a baby's face to grow and develop properly. If a baby has one of these conditions, the bones that shape the eye socket may not grow properly. Babies can be fitted with a plastic structure called a conformer that can help the eye socket and bones to grow properly. As babies get older, these devices will need to be enlarged to help expand the eye socket. Also, as children age, they can be fitted for an artificial eye.

A team of eye specialists should frequently monitor children with these conditions early in life. If other conditions arise, like a cataract or detached retina, children might need surgery to repair these other conditions. If anophthalmia or microphthalmia affects only one eye, the ophthalmologist can suggest ways to protect and preserve sight in the healthy eye. Depending on the severity of anophthalmia and microphthalmia, children might need surgery. It is important to talk to their team of eye specialists to determine the best plan of action.

Babies born with these conditions can often benefit from early intervention and therapy to help their development and mobility.

Section 37.2

Bietti Crystalline Dystrophy

This section includes text excerpted from "Bietti Crystalline Dystrophy," Genetics Home Reference (GHR), National Institutes of Health (NIH), November 2012. Reviewed March 2017.

Bietti crystalline dystrophy is a disorder in which numerous small, yellow or white crystal-like deposits of fatty (lipid) compounds accumulate in the light-sensitive tissue that lines the back of the eye (the retina). The deposits damage the retina, resulting in progressive vision loss.

People with Bietti crystalline dystrophy typically begin noticing vision problems in their teens or twenties. They experience a loss of sharp vision (reduction in visual acuity) and difficulty seeing in dim light (night blindness). They usually lose areas of vision (visual field loss), most often side (peripheral) vision. Color vision may also be impaired.

The vision problems may worsen at different rates in each eye, and the severity and progression of symptoms varies widely among affected individuals, even within the same family. However, most people with this condition become legally blind by their forties or fifties. Most affected individuals retain some degree of vision, usually in the center of the visual field, although it is typically blurry and cannot be corrected by glasses or contact lenses. Vision impairment that cannot be improved with corrective lenses is called low vision.

Frequency

Bietti crystalline dystrophy has been estimated to occur in 1 in 67,000 people. It is more common in people of East Asian descent, especially those of Chinese and Japanese background. Researchers suggest that Bietti crystalline dystrophy may be underdiagnosed because its symptoms are similar to those of other eye disorders that progressively damage the retina.

Genetic Changes

Bietti crystalline dystrophy is caused by mutations in the *CYP4V2* gene. This gene provides instructions for making a member of the cytochrome P450 family of enzymes. These enzymes are involved in the formation and breakdown of various molecules and chemicals within cells. The CYP4V2 enzyme is involved in a multi-step process called fatty acid oxidation in which lipids are broken down and converted into energy, but the enzyme's specific function is not well understood. *CYP4V2* gene mutations that cause Bietti crystalline dystrophy impair or eliminate the function of this enzyme and are believed to affect lipid breakdown. However, it is unknown how they lead to the specific signs and symptoms of Bietti crystalline dystrophy. For unknown reasons, the severity of the signs and symptoms differs significantly among individuals with the same *CYP4V2* gene mutation.

Inheritance Pattern

This condition is inherited in an autosomal recessive pattern, which means both copies of the gene in each cell have mutations. The parents of an individual with an autosomal recessive condition each carry one copy of the mutated gene, but they typically do not show signs and symptoms of the condition.

Other Names for This Condition

- BCD
- Bietti crystalline corneoretinal dystrophy
- Bietti crystalline retinopathy
- Bietti tapetoretinal degeneration with marginal corneal dystrophy

Section 37.3

Congenital Stationary Night Blindness

This section includes text excerpted from "Autosomal
Recessive Congenital Stationary Night Blindness," Genetics Home
Reference (GHR), National Institutes of Health (NIH), January 2014.

Autosomal Recessive Congenital Stationary Night Blindness

Autosomal recessive congenital stationary night blindness is a disorder of the retina, which is the specialized tissue at the back of the eye that detects light and color. People with this condition typically have difficulty seeing and distinguishing objects in low light (night blindness). For example, they may not be able to identify road signs at night or see stars in the night sky. They also often have other vision problems, including loss of sharpness (reduced acuity), nearsightedness (myopia), involuntary movements of the eyes (nystagmus), and eyes that do not look in the same direction (strabismus).

The vision problems associated with this condition are congenital, which means they are present from birth. They tend to remain stable (stationary) over time.

Frequency

Autosomal recessive congenital stationary night blindness is likely a rare disease; however, its prevalence is unknown.

Genetic Changes

Mutations in several genes can cause autosomal recessive congenital stationary night blindness. Each of these genes provide instructions for making proteins that are found in the retina. These proteins are involved in sending (transmitting) visual signals from cells called rods, which are specialized for vision in low light, to cells called bipolar cells, which relay the signals to other retinal cells. This signaling is an essential step in the transmission of visual information from the eyes to the brain.

Mutations in two genes, *GRM6* and *TRPM1*, cause most cases of this condition. These genes provide instructions for making proteins that are necessary for bipolar cells to receive and relay signals. Mutations in other genes involved in the same bipolar cell signaling pathway are likely responsible for a small percentage of cases of autosomal recessive congenital stationary night blindness.

Gene mutations that cause autosomal recessive congenital stationary night blindness disrupt the transmission of visual signals between rod cells and bipolar cells or interfere with the bipolar cells' ability to pass on these signals. As a result, visual information received by rod cells cannot be effectively transmitted to the brain, leading to difficulty seeing in low light. The cause of the other vision problems associated with this condition is unclear. It has been suggested that the mechanisms that underlie night blindness can interfere with other visual systems, causing myopia, reduced visual acuity, and other impairments.

Some people with autosomal recessive congenital stationary night blindness have no identified mutation in any of the known genes. The cause of the disorder in these individuals is unknown.

Inheritance Pattern

This condition is inherited in an autosomal recessive pattern, which means both copies of the gene in each cell have mutations. The parents of an individual with an autosomal recessive condition each carry one copy of the mutated gene, but they typically do not show signs and symptoms of the condition.

Other Names for This Condition

- Autosomal recessive complete congenital stationary night blindness

- Autosomal recessive incomplete congenital stationary night blindness

Section 37.4

Color Blindness

This section includes text excerpted from "Facts about Color
Blindness," National Eye Institute (NEI), February 2015.

What Is Color Blindness?

Most of us share a common color vision sensory experience. Some
people, however, have a color vision deficiency, which means their perception of colors is different from what most of us see. The most severe
forms of these deficiencies are referred to as color blindness. People
with color blindness aren't aware of differences among colors that are
obvious to the rest of us. People who don't have the more severe types
of color blindness may not even be aware of their condition unless
they're tested in a clinic or laboratory.

Inherited color blindness is caused by abnormal photopigments.
These color-detecting molecules are located in cone-shaped cells within
the retina, called cone cells. In humans, several genes are needed for
the body to make photopigments, and defects in these genes can lead
to color blindness.

There are three main kinds of color blindness, based on photopigment defects in the three different kinds of cones that respond to blue,
green, and red light. Red-green color blindness is the most common,
followed by blue-yellow color blindness. A complete absence of color
vision – total color blindness – is rare.

Sometimes color blindness can be caused by physical or chemical
damage to the eye, the optic nerve, or parts of the brain that process
color information. Color vision can also decline with age, most often
because of cataract—a clouding and yellowing of the eye's lens.

Who Gets Color Blindness?

As many as 8 percent of men and 0.5 percent of women with Northern
European ancestry have the common form of red-green color blindness.

Men are much more likely to be color blind than women because
the genes responsible for the most common, inherited color blindness

are on the X chromosome. Males only have one X chromosome, while females have two X chromosomes. In females, a functional gene on only one of the X chromosomes is enough to compensate for the loss on the other. This kind of inheritance pattern is called X-linked, and primarily affects males. Inherited color blindness can be present at birth, begin in childhood, or not appear until the adult years.

How Genes Are Inherited

Genes are bundled together on structures called chromosomes. One copy of each chromosome is passed by a parent at conception through egg and sperm cells. The X and Y chromosomes, known as sex chromosomes, determine whether a person is born female (XX) or male (XY) and also carry other traits not related to gender.

In X-linked inheritance, the mother carries the mutated gene on one of her X chromosomes and will pass on the mutated gene to 50 percent of her children. Because females have two X chromosomes, the effect of a mutation on one X chromosome is offset by the normal gene on the other X chromosome. In this case the mother will not have the disease, but she can pass on the mutated gene and so is called a carrier. If a mother is a carrier of an X-linked disease (and the father is not affected), there is a:

- 1 in 2 chance that a son will have the disease,

- 1 in 2 chance that a daughter will be a carrier of the disease,

- No chance that a daughter will have the disease.

In autosomal recessive inheritance, it takes two copies of the mutant gene to give rise to the disease. An individual who has one copy of a recessive gene mutation is known as a carrier. When two carriers have a child, there is a:

- 1 in 4 chance of having a child with the disease,

- 1 in 2 chance of having a child who is a carrier,

- 1 in 4 chance of having a child who neither has the disease nor is a carrier.

In autosomal dominant inheritance, it takes just one copy of the mutant gene to bring about the disease. When an affected parent with one dominant gene mutation has a child, there is a 1 in 2 chance that a child will inherit the disease.

How Do We See Color?

What color is a strawberry? Most of us would say red, but do we all see the same red? Color vision depends on our eyes and brain working together to perceive different properties of light.

We see the natural and artificial light that illuminates our world as white, although it is actually a mixture of colors that, perceived on their own, would span the visual spectrum from deep blue to deep red. You can see this when rain separates sunlight into a rainbow or a glass prism separates white light into a multi-color band. The color of light is determined by its wavelength. Longer wavelength corresponds to red light and shorter wavelength corresponds to blue light.

Strawberries and other objects reflect some wavelengths of light and absorb others. The reflected light we perceive as color. So, a strawberry is red because its surface is only reflecting the long wavelengths we see as red and absorbing the others. An object appears white when it reflects all wavelengths and black when it absorbs all wavelengths.

Vision begins when light enters the eye and the cornea and lens focus it onto the retina, a thin layer of tissue at the back of the eye that contains millions of light-sensitive cells called photoreceptors. Some photoreceptors are shaped like rods and some are shaped like cones. In each eye there are many more rods than cones—approximately 120 million rods compared to only 6 million cones. Rods and cones both contain photopigment molecules that undergo a chemical change when they absorb light. This chemical change acts like an on-switch, triggering electrical signals that are then passed from the retina to the visual parts of the brain.

Rods and cones are different in how they respond to light. Rods are more responsive to dim light, which makes them useful for night vision. Cones are more responsive to bright light, such as in the daytime when light is plentiful.

Another important difference is that all rods contain only one photopigment, while cones contain one of three different photopigments. This makes cones sensitive to long (red), medium (green), or short (blue) wavelengths of light. The presence of three types of photopigments, each sensitive to a different part of the visual spectrum, is what gives us our rich color vision.

Humans are unusual among mammals for our trichromatic vision—named for the three different types of photopigments we have. Most mammals, including dogs, have just two photopigment types. Other creatures, such as butterflies, have more than three. They may be able to see colors we can only imagine.

Most of us have a full set of the three different cone photopigments and so we share a very similar color vision experience, but because the human eye and brain together translate light into color, each of us sees colors differently. The differences may be slight. Your blue may be more blue than someone else's, or in the case of color blindness, your red and green may be someone else's brown.

What Are the Different Types of Color Blindness?

The most common types of color blindness are inherited. They are the result of defects in the genes that contain the instructions for making the photopigments found in cones. Some defects alter the photopigment's sensitivity to color, for example, it might be slightly more sensitive to deeper red and less sensitive to green. Other defects can result in the total loss of a photopigment. Depending on the type of defect and the cone that is affected problems can arise with red, green, or blue color vision.

Red-Green Color Blindness

The most common types of hereditary color blindness are due to the loss or limited function of red cone (known as protan) or green cone (deutran) photopigments. This kind of color blindness is commonly referred to as red-green color blindness.

Protanomaly: In males with protanomaly, the red cone photopigment is abnormal. Red, orange, and yellow appear greener and colors are not as bright. This condition is mild and doesn't usually interfere with daily living. Protanomaly is an X-linked disorder estimated to affect 1 percent of males.

Protanopia: In males with protanopia, there are no working red cone cells. Red appears as black. Certain shades of orange, yellow, and green all appear as yellow. Protanopia is an X-linked disorder that is estimated to affect 1 percent of males.

Deuteranomaly: In males with deuteranomaly, the green cone photopigment is abnormal. Yellow and green appear redder and it is difficult to tell violet from blue. This condition is mild and doesn't interfere with daily living. Deuteranomaly is the most common form of color blindness and is an X-linked disorder affecting 5 percent of males.

Deuteranopia: In males with deuteranopia, there are no working green cone cells. They tend to see reds as brownish-yellow and greens as beige. Deuteranopia is an X-linked disorder that affects about 1 percent of males.

Blue-Yellow Color Blindness

Blue-yellow color blindness is rarer than red-green color blindness. Blue-cone (tritan) photopigments are either missing or have limited function.

Tritanomaly: People with tritanomaly have functionally limited blue cone cells. Blue appears greener and it can be difficult to tell yellow and red from pink. Tritanomaly is extremely rare. It is an autosomal dominant disorder affecting males and females equally.

Tritanopia: People with tritanopia, also known as blue-yellow color blindness, lack blue cone cells. Blue appears green and yellow appears violet or light grey. Tritanopia is an extremely rare autosomal recessive disorder affecting males and females equally.

Complete Color Blindness

People with complete color blindness (monochromacy) don't experience color at all and the clearness of their vision (visual acuity) may also be affected.

There are two types of monochromacy:

Cone monochromacy: This rare form of color blindness results from a failure of two of the three cone cell photopigments to work. There is red cone monochromacy, green cone monochromacy, and blue cone monochromacy. People with cone monochromacy have trouble distinguishing colors because the brain needs to compare the signals from different types of cones in order to see color. When only one type of cone works, this comparison isn't possible. People with blue cone monochromacy, may also have reduced visual acuity, near-sightedness, and uncontrollable eye movements, a condition known as nystagmus. Cone monochromacy is an autosomal recessive disorder.

Rod monochromacy or achromatopsia: This type of monochromacy is rare and is the most severe form of color blindness. It is present at birth. None of the cone cells have functional photopigments. Lacking all cone vision, people with rod monochromacy see the world in black, white, and gray. And since rods respond to dim light, people with rod monochromacy tend to be photophobic—very uncomfortable in bright environments. They also experience nystagmus. Rod monochromacy is an autosomal recessive disorder.

How Is Color Blindness Diagnosed?

Eye care professionals use a variety of tests to diagnose color blindness. These tests can quickly diagnose specific types of color blindness.

- The **Ishihara Color Test** is the most common test for red-green color blindness. The test consists of a series of colored circles, called Ishihara plates, each of which contains a collection of dots in different colors and sizes. Within the circle are dots that form a shape clearly visible to those with normal color vision, but invisible or difficult to see for those with red-green color blindness.

- The **Cambridge Color Test** uses a visual array similar to the Ishihara plates, except displayed on a computer monitor. The goal is to identify a C shape that is different in color from the background. The "C" is presented randomly in one of four orientations. When test-takers see the "C," they are asked to press one of four keys that correspond to the orientation.

- The **anomaloscope** uses a test in which two different light sources have to be matched in color. Looking through the eyepiece, the viewer sees a circle. The upper half is a yellow light that can be adjusted in brightness. The lower half is a combination of red and green lights that can be mixed in variable proportions. The viewer uses one knob to adjust the brightness of the top half, and another to adjust the color of the lower half. The goal is to make the upper and lower halves the same brightness and color.

- The **HRR Pseudoisochromatic Color Test** is another red-green color blindness test that uses color plates to test for color blindness.

- The **Farnsworth-Munsell 100 Hue Test** uses a set of blocks or pegs that are roughly the same color but in different hues (shades of the color). The goal is to arrange them in a line in order of hue. This test measures the ability to discriminate subtle color changes. It is used by industries that depend on the accurate color perception of its employees, such as graphic design, photography, and food quality inspection.

- The **Farnsworth Lantern Test** is used by the U.S. military to determine the severity of color blindness. Those with mild forms pass the test and are allowed to serve in the armed forces.

Are There Treatments for Color Blindness?

There is no cure for color blindness. However, people with red-green color blindness may be able to use a special set of lenses to help them perceive colors more accurately. These lenses can only be used outdoors under bright lighting conditions. Visual aids have also been developed to help people cope with color blindness. There are iPhone and iPad apps, for example, that help people with color blindness discriminate among colors. Some of these apps allow users to snap a photo and tap it anywhere on the image to see the color of that area. More sophisticated apps allow users to find out both color and shades of color. These kinds of apps can be helpful in selecting ripe fruits such as bananas, or finding complementary colors when picking out clothing.

How Does Color Blindness Affect Daily Life?

Color blindness can make it difficult to read color-coded information such as bar graphs and pie charts. This can be particularly troubling for children who aren't yet diagnosed with color blindness, since educational materials are often color-coded. Children with red-green color blindness may also have difficulty reading a green chalkboard when yellow chalk is used. Art classes, which require selecting appropriate colors of paint or crayons, may be challenging.

Color blindness can go undetected for some time since children will often try to hide their disorder. It's important to have children tested, particularly boys, if there is a family history of color blindness. Many school systems offer vision screening tests that include color blindness testing. Once a child is diagnosed, he or she can learn to ask for help with tasks that require color recognition.

Simple everyday tasks like cooking meat to the desired color or selecting ripe produce can be a challenge for adults. Children might find food without bright color as less appetizing. Traffic lights pose challenges, since they have to be read by the position of the light. Since most lights are vertical, with green on bottom and red on top, if a light is positioned horizontally, a color blind person has to do a quick mental rotation to read it. Reading maps or buying clothes that match colors can also be difficult. However, these are relatively minor inconveniences and most people with color blindness learn to adapt.

Section 37.5

Down Syndrome

This section includes text excerpted from documents published
by two public domain sources. Text under headings marked 1
are excerpted from "Birth Defects: Facts about Down Syndrome,"
Division of Birth Defects and Developmental Disabilities (NCBDDD),
Centers for Disease Control and Prevention (CDC), March 3, 2016;
text under heading marked 2 are excerpted from "Down Syndrome,"
Eunice Kennedy Shriver National Institute of Child Health and
Human Development (NICHD), February 16, 2017.

What Is Down Syndrome?[1]

Down syndrome is a condition in which a person has an extra chromosome. Chromosomes are small "packages" of genes in the body. They determine how a baby's body forms during pregnancy and how the baby's body functions as it grows in the womb and after birth. Typically, a baby is born with 46 chromosomes. Babies with Down syndrome have an extra copy of one of these chromosomes, chromosome 21. A medical term for having an extra copy of a chromosome is 'trisomy.' Down syndrome is also referred to as Trisomy 21. This extra copy changes how the baby's body and brain develop, which can cause both mental and physical challenges for the baby.

Even though people with Down syndrome might act and look similar, each person has different abilities. People with Down syndrome usually have an IQ (a measure of intelligence) in the mildly-to-moderately low range and are slower to speak than other children.

Some common physical features of Down syndrome include:

- a flattened face, especially the bridge of the nose

- almond-shaped eyes that slant up

- a short neck

- small ears

- a tongue that tends to stick out of the mouth

- tiny white spots on the iris (colored part) of the eye

- small hands and feet
- a single line across the palm of the hand (palmar crease)
- small pinky fingers that sometimes curve toward the thumb
- poor muscle tone or loose joints
- shorter in height as children and adults

Types of Down Syndrome[1]

There are three types of Down syndrome. People often can't tell the difference between each type without looking at the chromosomes because the physical features and behaviors are similar.

- **Trisomy 21:** About 95 percent of people with Down syndrome have Trisomy 21. With this type of Down syndrome, each cell in the body has 3 separate copies of chromosome 21 instead of the usual 2 copies.

- **Translocation Down syndrome:** This type accounts for a small percentage of people with Down syndrome (about 3%). This occurs when an extra part or a whole extra chromosome 21 is present, but it is attached or "translocated" to a different chromosome rather than being a separate chromosome 21.

- **Mosaic Down syndrome:** This type affects about 2 percent of the people with Down syndrome. Mosaic means mixture or combination. For children with mosaic Down syndrome, some of their cells have 3 copies of chromosome 21, but other cells have the typical two copies of chromosome 21. Children with mosaic Down syndrome may have the same features as other children with Down syndrome. However, they may have fewer features of the condition due to the presence of some (or many) cells with a typical number of chromosomes.

Vision Problems[2]

More than 60 percent of children with Down syndrome have vision problems, including cataracts (clouding of the eye lens) that may be present at birth. The risk of cataract increases with age. Other eye problems that are more likely in children with Down syndrome are near-sightedness, "crossed" eyes, and rapid, involuntary eye movements. Glasses, surgery, or other treatments usually improve vision. The American Academy of Pediatrics (AAP) recommends that infants with Down syndrome be examined by a pediatric eye specialist during the newborn period, and then have vision exams regularly as recommended.

Occurrence[1]

Down syndrome remains the most common chromosomal condition diagnosed in the United States. Each year, about 6,000 babies born in the United States have Down syndrome. This means that Down syndrome occurs in about 1 out of every 700 babies.

Causes and Risk Factors[1]

The extra chromosome 21 leads to the physical features and developmental challenges that can occur among people with Down syndrome. Researchers know that Down syndrome is caused by an extra chromosome, but no one knows for sure why Down syndrome occurs or how many different factors play a role.

One factor that increases the risk for having a baby with Down syndrome is the mother's age. Women who are 35 years or older when they become pregnant are more likely to have a pregnancy affected by Down syndrome than women who become pregnant at a younger age. However, the majority of babies with Down syndrome are born to mothers less than 35 years old, because there are many more births among younger women.

Diagnosis[1]

There are two basic types of tests available to detect Down syndrome during pregnancy. Screening tests are one type and diagnostic tests are another type. A screening test can tell a woman and her healthcare provider whether her pregnancy has a lower or higher chance of having Down syndrome. So screening tests help decide whether a diagnostic test might be needed. Screening tests do not provide an absolute diagnosis, but they are safer for the mother and the baby. Diagnostic tests can typically detect whether or not a baby will have Down syndrome, but they can be more risky for the mother and baby. Neither screening nor diagnostic tests can predict the full impact of Down syndrome on a baby; no one can predict this.

Screening tests

Screening tests often include a combination of a blood test, which measures the amount of various substances in the mother's blood (e.g., Maternal Serum Alpha-Fetoprotein Screening (MS-AFP), Triple Screen, Quad-screen), and an ultrasound, which creates a picture of the baby. During an ultrasound, one of the things the technician looks at is the fluid behind the baby's neck. Extra fluid in this region could indicate a genetic problem. These screening tests can help determine the baby's risk of Down syndrome. Rarely, screening tests can give an abnormal result even when there is nothing wrong with the baby. Sometimes, the test results are normal and yet they miss a problem that does exist.

A test available since 2010 for certain chromosome problems, including Down syndrome, screens the mother's blood to detect small pieces of the developing baby's deoxyribonucleic acid (DNA) that are circulating in the mother's blood. This test is recommended for women who are more likely to have a pregnancy affected by Down syndrome. The test is typically completed during the first trimester (first 3 months of pregnancy) and it is becoming more widely available.

Diagnostic Tests

Diagnostic tests are usually performed after a positive screening test in order to confirm a Down syndrome diagnosis. Types of diagnostic tests include:

- Chorionic villus sampling (CVS)—examines material from the placenta

- Amniocentesis—examines the amniotic fluid (the fluid from the sac surrounding the baby)

- Percutaneous umbilical blood sampling (PUBS)—examines blood from the umbilical cord

These tests look for changes in the chromosomes that would indicate a Down syndrome diagnosis.

Treatments[1]

Down syndrome is a lifelong condition. Services early in life will often help babies and children with Down syndrome to improve their physical and intellectual abilities. Most of these services focus on helping children with Down syndrome develop to their full potential. These services include speech, occupational, and physical therapy, and they are typically offered through early intervention programs in each state. Children with Down syndrome may also need extra help or attention in school, although many children are included in regular classes.

Section 37.6

Duane Syndrome

This section includes text excerpted from "Learning about Duane Syndrome," National Human Genome Research Institute (NHGRI), December 26, 2013. Reviewed March 2017.

What Is Duane Syndrome?

Duane syndrome (DS) is a rare, congenital (present from birth) eye movement disorder. Most patients are diagnosed by the age of 10 years and DS is more common in girls (60 percent of the cases) than boys (40 percent of the cases).

DS is a miswiring of the eye muscles, causing some eye muscles to contract when they shouldn't and other eye muscles not to contract when they should. People with DS have a limited (and sometimes absent) ability to move the eye outward toward the ear (abduction) and, in most cases, a limited ability to move the eye inward toward the nose (adduction).

Often, when the eye moves toward the nose, the eyeball also pulls into the socket (retraction), the eye opening narrows and, in some cases, the eye will move upward or downward. Many patients with DS develop a face turn to maintain binocular vision and compensate for improper turning of the eyes.

In about 80 percent of cases of DS, only one eye is affected, most often the left. However, in some cases, both eyes are affected, with one eye usually more affected than the other.

Other names for this condition include: Duane Retraction Syndrome (or DR syndrome), Eye Retraction Syndrome, Retraction Syndrome, Congenital retraction syndrome and Stilling-Turk-Duane Syndrome.

In 70 percent of DS cases, this is the only disorder the individual has. However, other conditions and syndromes have been found in association with DS. These include malformation of the skeleton, ears, eyes, kidneys and nervous system, as well as:

- Okihiro syndrome, an association of DS with forearm malformation and hearing loss,

453

- Wildervanck syndrome, fusion of neck vertebrae and hearing loss,

- Holt-Oram syndrome, abnormalities of the upper limbs and heart,

- Morning Glory syndrome, abnormalities of the optic disc or "blind spot," and

- Goldenhar syndrome, malformation of the jaw, cheek and ear, usually on one side of the face.

What Are the Symptoms of Duane Syndrome?

Clinically, Duane syndrome is often subdivided into three types, each with associated symptoms.

- **Type 1:** The affected eye, or eyes, has limited ability to move outward toward the ear, but the ability to move inward toward the nose is normal or nearly so. The eye opening narrows and the eyeball pulls in when looking inward toward the nose, however the reverse occurs when looking outward toward the ear. About 78 percent of all DS cases are Type 1.

- **Type 2:** The affected eye, or eyes, has limited ability to move inward toward the nose, but the ability to move outward toward the ear is normal or nearly so. The eye opening narrows and the eyeball pulls in when looking inward toward the nose. About 7 percent of all DS cases are Type 2.

- **Type 3:** The affected eye, or eyes, has limited ability to move both inward toward the nose and outward toward the ears. The eye opening narrows and the eyeball pulls in when looking inward toward the nose. About 15 percent of all DS cases are Type 3.

Each of these three types can be further classified into three subgroups, depending on where the eyes are when the individual looks straight (the primary gaze):

- **Subgroup A:** The affected eye is turned inward toward the nose (esotropia).

- **Subgroup B:** The affected eye is turned outward toward the ear (exotropia).

- **Subgroup C:** The eyes are in a straight, primary position.

What Causes Duane Syndrome?

Common thought is that DS is a miswiring of the medial and the lateral rectus muscles, the muscles that move the eyes. Also, patients with DS lack the abducens nerve, the sixth cranial nerve, which is involved in eye movement. However, the etiology or origin of these malfunctions is, at present, a mystery.

Many researchers believe that DS results from a disturbance—either by genetic or environmental factors—during embryonic development. Since the cranial nerves and ocular muscles are developing between the third and eighth week of pregnancy, this is most likely when the disturbance happens.

Presently, it appears that several factors may be involved in causing DS. Therefore it is doubtful that a single mechanism is responsible for this condition.

How Is Duane Syndrome Diagnosed?

The diagnosis of DS is based on clinical findings. Mutations in the *CHN1* gene are associated with familial isolated Duane syndrome. Direct sequencing of the *CHN1* gene is available as a clinical test, and has to date detected missense mutations in seven patients and affected family members. The CHN1 mutations have not been found to be a common cause of simplex Duane retraction syndrome.

What Do We Know about Heredity and Duane Syndrome?

Most likely, both genetic and environmental factors play a role in the development of DS. For those cases that show evidence of having a genetic cause, both dominant and recessive forms of DS have been found. (When a gene is dominant, only one gene from one parent is needed for the individual to express it physically. However, when a gene is recessive, a copy of the gene from both parents is needed for expression.)

The chromosomal location of the proposed gene for this syndrome is currently unknown. Some research shows that more than one gene may be involved. There is evidence that a gene involved in the development of DS is located on chromosome 2. Also, deletions of chromosomal material from chromosomes 4 and 8, as well as the presence of an extra marker chromosome thought to be derived from chromosome 22, have been linked to DS.

Section 37.7

Gillespie Syndrome

This section includes text excerpted from "Gillespie Syndrome,"
Genetics Home Reference (GHR), National Institutes of
Health (NIH), July 2014.

Gillespie syndrome is a disorder that involves eye abnormalities, problems with balance and coordinating movements (ataxia), and mild to moderate intellectual disability.

Gillespie syndrome is characterized by **aniridia**, which is the absence of the colored part of the eye (the iris). In most affected individuals, only part of the iris is missing (partial aniridia) in both eyes, but in some affected individuals, partial aniridia affects only one eye, or the entire iris is missing (complete aniridia) in one or both eyes. The absence of all or part of the iris can cause blurry vision (reduced visual acuity) and increased sensitivity to light (photophobia). Rapid, involuntary eye movements (nystagmus) can also occur in Gillespie syndrome.

The balance and movement problems in Gillespie syndrome result from underdevelopment (hypoplasia) of a part of the brain called the cerebellum. This abnormality can cause delayed development of motor skills such as walking. In addition, difficulty controlling the muscles in the mouth can lead to delayed speech development. The difficulties with coordination generally become noticeable in early childhood when the individual is learning these skills. People with Gillespie syndrome usually continue to have an unsteady gait and speech problems. However, the problems do not get worse over time, and in some cases they improve slightly.

Other features of Gillespie syndrome can include abnormalities in the bones of the spine (vertebrae) and malformations of the heart.

Frequency

The prevalence of Gillespie syndrome is unknown. Only a few dozen affected individuals have been described in the medical literature. It has been estimated that Gillespie syndrome accounts for about 2 percent of cases of aniridia.

Genetic Changes

Gillespie syndrome can be caused by mutations in the *PAX6* gene. The *PAX6* gene provides instructions for making a protein that is involved in early development, including the development of the eyes and brain. The PAX6 protein attaches (binds) to specific regions of deoxyribonucleic acid (DNA) and regulates the activity of other genes. On the basis of this role, the PAX6 protein is called a transcription factor.

Mutations in the *PAX6* gene result in the absence of the PAX6 protein or production of a nonfunctional PAX6 protein that is unable to bind to DNA and regulate the activity of other genes. This lack of functional protein disrupts embryonic development, especially the development of the eyes and brain, leading to the signs and symptoms of Gillespie syndrome.

Most people with Gillespie syndrome do not have mutations in the *PAX6* gene. In these affected individuals, the cause of the disorder is unknown.

Inheritance Pattern

In some cases, including those in which Gillespie syndrome is caused by *PAX6* gene mutations, the condition occurs in an autosomal dominant pattern, which means one copy of the altered gene in each cell is sufficient to cause the disorder. Some affected individuals inherit the mutation from one affected parent. Other cases result from new mutations in the gene and occur in people with no history of the disorder in their family.

Gillespie syndrome can also be inherited in an autosomal recessive pattern, which means both copies of a gene in each cell have mutations. The gene or genes involved in these cases are unknown. The parents of an individual with an autosomal recessive condition each carry one copy of the mutated gene, but they typically do not show signs and symptoms of the condition.

Other Names for This Condition

- Aniridia-cerebellar ataxia-intellectual disability
- Aniridia-cerebellar ataxia-mental deficiency
- Aniridia, cerebellar ataxia, and mental retardation
- Partial aniridia-cerebellar ataxia-oligophrenia

Section 37.8

Horner Syndrome

This section includes text excerpted from "Horner Syndrome,"
Genetics Home Reference (GHR), National Institutes of
Health (NIH), April 2013. Reviewed March 2017.

Horner syndrome is a disorder that affects the eye and surrounding tissues on one side of the face and results from paralysis of certain nerves. Horner syndrome can appear at any time of life; in about 5 percent of affected individuals, the disorder is present from birth (congenital).

Horner syndrome is characterized by drooping of the upper eyelid (ptosis) on the affected side, a constricted pupil in the affected eye (miosis) resulting in unequal pupil size (anisocoria), and absent sweating (anhidrosis) on the affected side of the face. Sinking of the eye into its cavity (enophthalmos) and a bloodshot eye often occur in this disorder. In people with Horner syndrome that occurs before the age of 2, the colored part (iris) of the eyes may differ in color (iris heterochromia), with the iris of the affected eye being lighter in color than that of the unaffected eye. Individuals who develop Horner syndrome after age 2 do not generally have iris heterochromia.

The abnormalities in the eye area related to Horner syndrome do not generally affect vision or health. However, the nerve damage that causes Horner syndrome may result from other health problems, some of which can be life-threatening.

Frequency

About 1 in 6,250 babies are born with Horner syndrome. The incidence of Horner syndrome that appears later is unknown, but it is considered an uncommon disorder.

Genetic Changes

Although congenital Horner syndrome can be passed down in families, no associated genes have been identified. Horner syndrome that appears after the newborn period (acquired Horner syndrome) and most cases of congenital Horner syndrome result from damage to nerves called the cervical sympathetics. These nerves belong to the part of the nervous system that controls involuntary functions (the autonomic nervous system). Within the autonomic nervous system, the nerves are part of a subdivision called the sympathetic nervous system. The cervical sympathetic nerves control several functions in the eye and face such as dilation of the pupil and sweating. Problems with the function of these nerves cause the signs and symptoms of Horner syndrome. Horner syndrome that occurs very early in life can lead to iris heterochromia because the development of the pigmentation (coloring) of the iris is under the control of the cervical sympathetic nerves.

Damage to the cervical sympathetic nerves can be caused by a direct injury to the nerves themselves, which can result from trauma that might occur during a difficult birth, surgery, or accidental injury. The nerves related to Horner syndrome can also be damaged by a benign or cancerous tumor, for example a childhood cancer of the nerve tissues called a neuroblastoma.

Horner syndrome can also be caused by problems with the artery that supplies blood to the head and neck (the carotid artery) on the affected side, resulting in loss of blood flow to the nerves. Some individuals with congenital Horner syndrome have a lack of development (agenesis) of the carotid artery. Tearing of the layers of the carotid artery wall (carotid artery dissection) can also lead to Horner syndrome.

The signs and symptoms of Horner syndrome can also occur during a migraine headache. When the headache is gone, the signs and symptoms of Horner syndrome usually also go away.

Some people with Horner syndrome have neither a known problem that would lead to nerve damage nor any history of the disorder in their family. These cases are referred to as idiopathic Horner syndrome.

Inheritance Pattern

Horner syndrome is usually not inherited and occurs in individuals with no history of the disorder in their family. Acquired Horner syndrome and most cases of congenital Horner syndrome have nongenetic causes. Rarely, congenital Horner syndrome is passed down within a family in a pattern that appears to be autosomal dominant, which means one copy of an altered gene in each cell is sufficient to cause the disorder. However, no genes associated with Horner syndrome have been identified.

Other Names for This Condition

- Bernard-Horner syndrome

- Horner's syndrome

- Oculosympathetic palsy

- von Passow syndrome

Section 37.9

WAGR Syndrome

This section includes text excerpted from "WAGR syndrome,"
Genetics Home Reference (GHR), National Institutes of
Health (NIH), January 2014.

WAGR syndrome is a disorder that affects many body systems and
is named for its main features: Wilms tumor, anirida, genitourinary
anomalies, and intellectual disability (formerly referred to as mental
retardation).

People with WAGR syndrome have a 45 to 60 percent chance of
developing Wilms tumor, a rare form of kidney cancer. This type of
cancer is most often diagnosed in children but is sometimes seen in
adults.

Most people with WAGR syndrome have aniridia, an absence of
the colored part of the eye (the iris). This can cause reduction in the
sharpness of vision (visual acuity) and increased sensitivity to light
(photophobia). Aniridia is typically the first noticeable sign of WAGR
syndrome. Other eye problems may also develop, such as clouding of
the lens of the eyes (cataracts), increased pressure in the eyes (glaucoma), and involuntary eye movements (nystagmus).

Abnormalities of the genitalia and urinary tract (genitourinary
anomalies) are seen more frequently in males with WAGR syndrome
than in affected females. The most common genitourinary anomaly in
affected males is undescended testes (cryptorchidism). Females may
not have functional ovaries and instead have undeveloped clumps of
tissue called streak gonads. Females may also have a heart-shaped

(bicornate) uterus, which makes it difficult to carry a pregnancy to term.

Another common feature of WAGR syndrome is intellectual disability. Affected individuals often have difficulty processing, learning, and properly responding to information. Some individuals with WAGR syndrome also have psychiatric or behavioral problems including depression, anxiety, attention deficit hyperactivity disorder (ADHD), obsessive-compulsive disorder (OCD), or a developmental disorder called autism that affects communication and social interaction.

Other signs and symptoms of WAGR syndrome can include childhood-onset obesity, inflammation of the pancreas (pancreatitis), and kidney failure. When WAGR syndrome includes childhood-onset obesity, it is often referred to as WAGRO syndrome.

Frequency

The prevalence of WAGR syndrome ranges from 1 in 500,000 to one million individuals. It is estimated that one-third of people with aniridia actually have WAGR syndrome. Approximately 7 in 1,000 cases of Wilms tumor can be attributed to WAGR syndrome.

Genetic Changes

WAGR syndrome is caused by a deletion of genetic material on the short (p) arm of chromosome 11. The size of the deletion varies among affected individuals.

The signs and symptoms of WAGR syndrome are related to the loss of multiple genes on the short arm of chromosome 11. WAGR syndrome is often described as a contiguous gene deletion syndrome because it results from the loss of several neighboring genes. The *PAX6* and *WT1* genes are always deleted in people with the typical signs and symptoms of this disorder. Because changes in the *PAX6* gene can affect eye development, researchers think that the loss of the *PAX6* gene is responsible for the characteristic eye features of WAGR syndrome. The *PAX6* gene may also affect brain development. Wilms tumor and genitourinary abnormalities are often the result of mutations in the *WT1* gene, so deletion of the *WT1* gene is very likely the cause of these features in WAGR syndrome.

In people with WAGRO syndrome, the chromosome 11 deletion includes an additional gene, *BDNF*. This gene is active (expressed) in the brain and plays a role in the survival of nerve cells (neurons). The protein produced from the *BDNF* gene is thought to be involved in the management of eating, drinking, and body weight. Loss of the *BDNF* gene is likely responsible for childhood-onset obesity in people with WAGRO syndrome. People with WAGRO syndrome may be at greater risk of neurological problems such as intellectual disability and autism than those with WAGR syndrome. It is unclear whether this increased risk is due to the loss of the *BDNF* gene or other nearby genes.

Research is ongoing to identify additional genes deleted in people with WAGR syndrome and to determine how their loss leads to the other features of the disorder.

Inheritance Pattern

Most cases of WAGR syndrome are not inherited. They result from a chromosomal deletion that occurs as a random event during the formation of reproductive cells (eggs or sperm) or in early fetal development. Affected people typically have no history of the disorder in their family.

Some affected individuals inherit a chromosome 11 with a deleted segment from an unaffected parent. In these cases, the parent carries a chromosomal rearrangement called a balanced translocation, in which no genetic material is gained or lost. Balanced translocations usually do not cause any health problems; however, they can become unbalanced as they are passed to the next generation. Children who inherit an unbalanced translocation can have a chromosomal rearrangement with extra or missing genetic material. Individuals with WAGR syndrome who inherit an unbalanced translocation are missing genetic material from the short arm of chromosome 11, which results in an increased risk of Wilms tumor, aniridia, genitourinary anomalies, and intellectual disability.

Other Names for This Condition

- 11p deletion syndrome
- 11p partial monosomy syndrome
- WAGR complex
- WAGR contiguous gene syndrome
- Wilms tumor-aniridia-genital anomalies-retardation syndrome
- Wilms tumor-aniridia-genitourinary anomalies-MR syndrome
- Wilms tumor, aniridia, genitourinary anomalies, and mental retardation syndrome

Chapter 38

Infectious Diseases Affecting Vision

Chapter Contents

Section 38.1

Acanthamoeba *Keratitis*

This section includes text excerpted from "Basics of Parasitic/
Amebic Keratitis," Centers for Disease Control and
Prevention (CDC), November 17, 2014.

What Is Acanthamoeba *Keratitis?*

Acanthamoeba keratitis, or AK, is a rare but serious infection of
the eye that can cause permanent vision loss or blindness. This infection is caused by a tiny ameba (single-celled living organism) called
Acanthamoeba. *Acanthamoeba* causes *Acanthamoeba* keratitis when
it infects the cornea, the clear dome that covers the colored part of
the eye.

What Are the Symptoms of Acanthamoeba *Keratitis?*

Symptoms of AK include:

• sensation of something in the eye

• eye pain

• eye redness

• blurred vision

• sensitivity to light

• excessive tearing

If you experience any of these symptoms, remove your contact lenses
(if you wear them) and call your eye doctor right away. AK is a rare
condition, but if left untreated it can result in vision loss or blindness.

Where Is Acanthamoeba *Found?*

Acanthamoeba is very common in nature and can be found in bodies of water (for example, lakes and oceans) and soil. It can also be
found in tap water, heating, ventilating, and air conditioning units,

and whirlpools. Infection of the eye occurs when the *Acanthamoeba* organisms contained in water or contact lens solution enter the eye through small scrapes that can be caused by contact lens wear or other minor eye injuries. The *Acanthamoeba* organism has to make contact directly with the eyes in order to cause AK, so this type of corneal infection cannot occur from drinking or inhaling water that has this ameba in it. AK cannot be spread from person to person.

What Puts People at Risk for Acanthamoeba *Keratitis?*

In the United States, an estimated 85 percent of AK cases occur in contact lens wearers. For people who wear contact lenses, the risk of getting *Acanthamoeba* keratitis is higher if they:

- Do not store or handle contact lenses properly. This can include not washing hands before touching contact lenses, not rubbing and rinsing lenses after taking them out, and not storing them in the recommended contact lens solution.

- Do not disinfect contact lenses properly. This can include using tap water to clean the lenses or lens case, or adding fresh solution to existing used solution in the case instead of using only fresh solution when storing contact lenses.

- Swim, use a hot tub, or shower while wearing lenses.

- Have a history of trauma to the cornea, such as a previous eye injury.

How Is Acanthamoeba *Keratitis Diagnosed?*

Early diagnosis is important because early treatment can prevent AK infections from becoming more severe. The infection is usually diagnosed by an eye doctor based on symptoms, lab results from a scraping of the eye, and/or through a close-up eye exam that allows the eye doctor to see the ameba.

How Is Acanthamoeba *Keratitis Treated?*

AK can be difficult to treat, and the best treatment regimen for each patient should be determined by an eye doctor. AK usually requires aggressive medical and surgical treatment. If you think that your eye may be infected with *Acanthamoeba*, see an eye doctor immediately.

Section 38.2

Bacterial Keratitis

This section includes text excerpted from "Basics of Bacterial Keratitis," Centers for Disease Control and Prevention (CDC), April 7, 2014.

What Is Bacterial Keratitis?

Bacterial keratitis is an infection of the cornea (the clear dome covering the colored part of the eye) that is caused by bacteria. It can affect contact lens wearers, and also sometimes people who do not wear contact lenses. Types of bacteria that commonly cause bacterial keratitis include:

- *Pseudomonas aeruginosa*
- *Staphylococcus aureus*

What Are the Symptoms of Bacterial Keratitis?

Symptoms of bacterial keratitis include:

- eye pain
- eye redness
- blurred vision
- sensitivity to light
- excessive tearing
- eye discharge

If you experience any of these symptoms, remove your contact lenses (if you wear them) and call your eye doctor right away. If left untreated, bacterial keratitis can result in vision loss or blindness.

Where Are These Bacteria Found?

Bacteria are common in nature and found in the environment and on the human body. *Pseudomonas* bacteria can be found in soil and water. *Staphylococcus aureus* bacteria normally live on human skin and on the protective lining inside the body called the mucous membrane. Bacterial keratitis cannot be spread from person to person.

What Puts People at Risk for Bacterial Keratitis?

Risks for developing bacterial keratitis include:

- wearing contact lenses, especially:
  - overnight wear
  - temporary reshaping of the cornea (to correct nearsightedness) by wearing a rigid contact lens overnight, otherwise known as orthokeratology (Ortho-K)
  - not disinfecting contact lenses well
  - not cleaning contact lens cases
  - storing or rinsing contact lenses in water
  - using visibly contaminated lens solution
  - "topping off" lens solution rather than discarding used solution and replacing
  - sharing non-corrective contact lenses used for cosmetic purposes
- recent eye injury
- eye disease
- weakened immune system
- problems with the eyelids or tearing

How Is Bacterial Keratitis Diagnosed?

It is critical that when you first notice unusual eye irritation that you remove your contact lenses and not wear them again until instructed to do so by your eye doctor. Your eye doctor will examine your eye. He or she may take a tiny scraping of your cornea and send a sample to a laboratory to be analyzed.

Section 38.3

Fungal Keratitis

This section includes text excerpted from "Basics of
Fungal Keratitis," Centers for Disease Control and
Prevention (CDC), October 10, 2014.

What Is Fungal Keratitis?

Fungal keratitis is an infection of the cornea (the clear dome covering the colored part of the eye) that is caused by a fungus. Some fungi
that have been known to commonly cause fungal keratitis include:

- *Fusarium* species
- *Aspergillus* species
- *Candida* species

What Are the Symptoms of Fungal Keratitis?

Symptoms of fungal keratitis include:

- eye pain
- eye redness
- blurred vision
- sensitivity to light
- excessive tearing
- eye discharge

If you experience any of these symptoms, remove your contact
lenses (if you wear them) and call your eye doctor right away. Fungal
keratitis is a very rare condition, but if left untreated, it can become
serious and result in vision loss or blindness.

Where Are These Fungi Found?

Fusarium and *Aspergillus* species live in the environment. *Candida* species normally live on human skin and on the protective lining

inside the body called the mucous membrane. Fungal keratitis is most common in tropical and sub-tropical regions of the world, but can also occur in areas of the world with milder temperatures. It cannot be spread from person to person.

What Puts People at Risk for Fungal Keratitis?

The most common way that someone gets fungal keratitis is after experiencing trauma to the eye—especially trauma caused by a stick, thorn, or plant.

Risks for developing fungal keratitis include:

- recent eye trauma, particularly involving plants (for example, thorns or sticks)
- underlying eye disease
- weakened immune system
- contact lens use

How Is Fungal Keratitis Diagnosed?

Your eye doctor will examine your eye and may possibly take a tiny scraping of your cornea. The sample will be sent to a laboratory to be analyzed.

How Is Fungal Keratitis Treated?

Fungal keratitis must be treated with prescription antifungal medicine for several months. Patients who do not get better after skin treatment and oral antifungal medications may require surgery, including corneal transplantation.

How Do You Prevent Fungal Keratitis?

Protective eyewear is recommended for people who are at risk for eye trauma involving plants, such as agricultural workers.

Section 38.4

HSV (Herpes Simplex Virus) Keratitis

This section includes text excerpted from "Basics of HSV
(Herpes Simplex Virus) Keratitis," Centers for Disease
Control and Prevention (CDC), April 7, 2014.

What Is HSV (Herpes Simplex Virus) Keratitis?

HSV (Herpes Simplex Virus) keratitis is an infection of the cornea—
the clear dome that covers the colored part of the eye—that is caused
by HSV. The infection usually heals without damaging the eye, but
more severe infections can lead to scarring of the cornea or blindness.
HSV keratitis is a major cause of blindness worldwide. HSV-1, which
is the type of HSV that also causes cold sores on the mouth, is the most
common cause of corneal infections.

What Are the Symptoms of HSV Keratitis?

Symptoms of HSV keratitis include:

- eye pain
- eye redness
- blurred vision
- sensitivity to light
- watery discharge

If you experience any of these symptoms, remove your contact
lenses (if you wear them) and call your eye doctor right away. If left
untreated, HSV keratitis can result in vision loss or blindness.

Where Is HSV found?

HSV is only found in humans and is spread through direct contact with someone who is infected with the virus. Most HSV keratitis
infections happen after another part of the body—most commonly the
mouth—has already been infected by HSV. HSV keratitis is often the
result of a "flare up" (reactivation) of the earlier infection.

What Puts People at Risk for HSV Keratitis?

People who have had HSV keratitis are at risk for recurrences of the same infection. For these people, wearing contact lenses may further increase the risk.

People most at risk for HSV-1 (but not necessarily HSV keratitis) are:

- female

- non-Hispanic black or Mexican American

- born outside the United States

- sexually active, or have had 3 or more lifetime sex partners

How Is HSV Keratitis Diagnosed?

HSV keratitis is usually diagnosed based on a patient's health history and findings from an eye exam. Lab testing is not usually necessary, but certain lab tests may further help to confirm HSV-1.

How Is HSV Keratitis Treated?

The treatment of HSV keratitis usually involves medicine, including eye drops or antiviral medications taken by mouth. Surgery is rarely necessary but may be considered if scarring on the eye from HSV keratitis causes vision problems. Each case of HSV keratitis is unique, and an eye doctor should determine the best treatment for each patient. While some treatments can greatly lower the severity and recurrence of symptoms, there is no cure for HSV.

Section 38.5

Histoplasmosis

This section contains text excerpted from the following sources: Text beginning with the heading "What Is Histoplasmosis?" is excerpted from "Histoplasmosis: Protecting Workers at Risk," Centers for Disease Control and Prevention (CDC), June 6, 2014; Text beginning with the heading "Diagnosis and Testing for Histoplasmosis" is excerpted from "Histoplasmosis," Centers for Disease Control and Prevention (CDC), November 21, 2015.

What Is Histoplasmosis?

Histoplasmosis is an infectious disease caused by inhaling the spores of a fungus called *Histoplasma capsulatum*. Histoplasmosis is not contagious; it cannot be transmitted from an infected person or animal to someone else.

Histoplasmosis primarily affects a person's lungs, and its symptoms vary greatly. The vast majority of infected people are asymptomatic (have no apparent ill effects), or they experience symptoms so mild they do not seek medical attention and may not even realize that their illness was histoplasmosis. If symptoms do occur, they will usually start within 3 to 17 days after exposure, with an average of 10 days. Histoplasmosis can appear as a mild, flu-like respiratory illness and has a combination of symptoms, including malaise (a general ill feeling), fever, chest pain, dry or nonproductive cough, headache, loss of appetite, shortness of breath, joint and muscle pains, chills, and hoarseness. A chest X-ray can reveal distinct markings on an infected person's lungs.

Chronic lung disease due to histoplasmosis resembles tuberculosis and can worsen over months or years. Special antifungal medications are needed to arrest the disease. The most severe and rarest form of this disease is disseminated histoplasmosis, which involves spreading of the fungus to other organs outside the lungs. Disseminated histoplasmosis is fatal if untreated, but death can also occur in some patients even when medical treatment is received. People with weakened immune systems are at the greatest risk for developing severe and disseminated histoplasmosis. Included in this high-risk group are persons with acquired immunodeficiency syndrome (AIDS) or cancer and persons receiving cancer chemotherapy; high-dose, long-term steroid therapy; or other immunosuppressive drugs.

Presumed Ocular Histoplasmosis

Impaired vision and even blindness develop in some people because of a rare condition called "presumed ocular histoplasmosis." The factors causing this condition are poorly understood. Results of laboratory tests suggest that presumed ocular histoplasmosis is associated with hypersensitivity to *H. capsulatum* and not from direct exposure of the eyes to the microorganism. What delayed events convert the condition from asymptomatic to symptomatic are also unknown.

Who Can Get Histoplasmosis and What Jobs and Activities Put People at Risk for Exposure to H. Capsulatum Spores?

Anyone working at a job or present near activities where material contaminated with *H. capsulatum* becomes airborne can develop histoplasmosis if enough spores are inhaled. After an exposure, how ill a person becomes varies greatly and most likely depends on the number of spores inhaled and a person's age and susceptibility to the disease. The number of inhaled spores needed to cause disease is unknown. Infants, young children, and older persons, in particular those with chronic lung disease, are at increased risk for developing symptomatic histoplasmosis.

The U.S. Public Health Service (USPHS) and the Infectious Diseases Society of America (IDSA) have jointly published guidelines for the prevention of opportunistic infections in persons infected with the human immunodeficiency virus (HIV). The USPHS/IDSA Prevention of Opportunistic Infections Working Group recommended that HIV-infected persons "should avoid activities known to be associated with increased risk (e.g., cleaning chicken coops, disturbing soil beneath bird-roosting sites, and exploring caves)." HIV-infected persons should consult their healthcare provider about appropriate exposure precautions that should be taken for any activity with a risk of exposure to *H. capsulatum*.

Below is a partial list of occupations and hobbies with risks for exposure to *H. capsulatum* spores. Appropriate exposure precautions should be taken by these people and others whenever contaminated soil, bat droppings, or bird manure are disturbed.

- bridge inspector or painter
- chimney cleaner
- construction worker
- demolition worker
- farmer
- gardener
- heating and air-conditioning system installer or service person
- microbiology laboratory worker
- pest control worker
- restorer of historic or abandoned buildings
- roofer
- spelunker (cave explorer)

If someone who engages in these activities develops flu-like symptoms days or even weeks after disturbing material that might be contaminated with *H. capsulatum*, and the illness worsens rather than subsides after a few days, medical care should be sought and the healthcare provider informed about the exposure.

Diagnosis and Testing for Histoplasmosis

How Is Histoplasmosis Diagnosed?

Healthcare providers rely on your medical and travel history, symptoms, physical examinations, and laboratory tests to diagnose histoplasmosis. The most common way that healthcare providers test for histoplasmosis is by taking a blood sample or a urine sample and sending it to a laboratory.

Healthcare providers may do imaging tests such as chest X-rays or CT scans of your lungs. They may also collect a sample of fluid from your respiratory tract or perform a tissue biopsy, in which a small sample of affected tissue is taken from the body and examined under a microscope. Laboratories may also see if *Histoplasma* will grow from body fluids or tissues (this is called a culture).

Where Can I Get Tested for Histoplasmosis?

Most healthcare providers can order a test for histoplasmosis.

How Long Will It Take to Get My Test Results?

It depends on the type of test. Results from a blood test or a urine test will usually be available in a few days. If your healthcare provider sends a sample to a laboratory to be cultured, the results could take a couple of weeks.

Treatment for Histoplasmosis

For some people, the symptoms of histoplasmosis will go away without treatment. However, prescription antifungal medication is needed to treat severe histoplasmosis in the lungs, chronic histoplasmosis, and infections that have spread from the lungs to other parts of the body (disseminated histoplasmosis). Itraconazole is one type of antifungal medication that's commonly used to treat histoplasmosis. Depending on the severity of the infection and the person's immune status, the course of treatment can range from 3 months to 1 year.

Section 38.6

Toxoplasmosis

This section includes text excerpted from "Toxoplasmosis,"
Centers for Disease Control and Prevention (CDC),
January 10, 2013. Reviewed March 2017.

What Is Toxoplasmosis?

A single-celled parasite called *Toxoplasma gondii* causes a disease known as toxoplasmosis. While the parasite is found throughout the world, more than 60 million people in the United States may be infected with the *Toxoplasma* parasite. Of those who are infected, very few have symptoms because a healthy person's immune system usually keeps the parasite from causing illness. However, pregnant women and individuals who have compromised immune systems should be cautious; for them, a *Toxoplasma* infection could cause serious health problems.

How Do People Get Toxoplasmosis?

A *Toxoplasma* infection occurs by:

- Eating undercooked, contaminated meat (especially pork, lamb, and venison)

- Accidental ingestion of undercooked, contaminated meat after handling it and not washing hands thoroughly (*Toxoplasma* cannot be absorbed through intact skin).

- Eating food that was contaminated by knives, utensils, cutting boards and other foods that have had contact with raw, contaminated meat.

- Drinking water contaminated with *Toxoplasma gondii*.

- Accidentally swallowing the parasite through contact with cat feces that contain *Toxoplasma*. This might happen by

  - cleaning a cat's litter box when the cat has shed *Toxoplasma* in its feces

  - touching or ingesting anything that has come into contact with cat feces that contain *Toxoplasma*

  - accidentally ingesting contaminated soil (e.g., not washing hands after gardening or eating unwashed fruits or vegetables from a garden)

- Mother-to-child (congenital) transmission.

- Receiving an infected organ transplant or infected blood via transfusion, though this is rare.

Ocular Toxoplasmosis

Eye disease (most frequently retinochoroiditis) from *Toxoplasma* infection can result from congenital infection or infection after birth by any of the modes of transmission discussed above. Eye lesions from congenital infection are often not identified at birth but occur in 20–80 percent of infected persons by adulthood. However, in the United States <2 percent of persons infected after birth develop eye lesions. Eye infection leads to an acute inflammatory lesion of the retina, which resolves leaving retinochoroidal scarring.

The eye disease can reactivate months or years later, each time causing more damage to the retina. If the central structures of the retina are involved there will be a progressive loss of vision that can lead to blindness.

What Are the Signs and Symptoms of Toxoplasmosis?

Symptoms of the infection vary.

- Most people who become infected with *Toxoplasma gondii* are not aware of it.
- Some people who have toxoplasmosis may feel as if they have the "flu" with swollen lymph glands or muscle aches and pains that last for a month or more.
- Severe toxoplasmosis, causing damage to the brain, eyes, or other organs, can develop from an acute *Toxoplasma* infection or one that had occurred earlier in life and is now reactivated. Severe cases are more likely in individuals who have weak immune systems, though occasionally, even persons with healthy immune systems may experience eye damage from toxoplasmosis.
- Signs and symptoms of **ocular toxoplasmosis** can include reduced vision, blurred vision, pain (often with bright light), redness of the eye, and sometimes tearing. Ophthalmologists sometimes prescribe medicine to treat active disease. Whether or not medication is recommended depends on the size of the eye lesion, the location, and the characteristics of the lesion (acute active, versus chronic not progressing). An ophthalmologist will provide the best care for ocular toxoplasmosis.
- Most infants who are infected while still in the womb have no symptoms at birth, but they may develop symptoms later in life. A small percentage of infected newborns have serious eye or brain damage at birth.

Who Is at Risk for Developing Severe Toxoplasmosis?

People who are most likely to develop severe toxoplasmosis include:

- Infants born to mothers who are newly infected with *Toxoplasma gondii* during or just before pregnancy.
- Persons with severely weakened immune systems, such as individuals with AIDS, those taking certain types of chemotherapy, and those who have recently received an organ transplant.

What Should I Do If I Think I Am at Risk for Severe Toxoplasmosis?

If you are planning to become pregnant, your healthcare provider may test you for *Toxoplasma gondii*. If the test is positive it means you have already been infected sometime in your life. There usually is little need to worry about passing the infection to your baby. If the test is negative, take necessary precautions to avoid infection.

If you are already pregnant, you and your healthcare provider should discuss your risk for toxoplasmosis. Your healthcare provider may order a blood sample for testing.

If you have a weakened immune system, ask your doctor about having your blood tested for *Toxoplasma*. If your test is positive, your doctor can tell you if and when you need to take medicine to prevent the infection from reactivating. If your test is negative, it means you need to take precautions to avoid infection.

What Should I Do If I Think I May Have Toxoplasmosis?

If you suspect that you may have toxoplasmosis, talk to your healthcare provider. Your provider may order one or more varieties of blood tests specific for toxoplasmosis. The results from the different tests can help your provider determine if you have a *Toxoplasma gondii* infection and whether it is a recent (acute) infection.

What Is the Treatment for Toxoplasmosis?

Once a diagnosis of toxoplasmosis is confirmed, you and your healthcare provider can discuss whether treatment is necessary. In an otherwise healthy person who is not pregnant, treatment usually is not needed. If symptoms occur, they typically go away within a few weeks to months. For pregnant women or persons who have weakened immune systems, medications are available to treat toxoplasmosis.

How Can I Prevent Toxoplasmosis?

There are several general sanitation and food safety steps you can take to reduce your chances of becoming infected with *Toxoplasma gondii*.

Cook food to safe temperatures. A food thermometer should be used to measure the internal temperature of cooked meat. Do not sample meat until it is cooked. United States Department of Agriculture (USDA) recommends the following for meat preparation.

For Whole Cuts of Meat (excluding poultry)

Cook to at least 145°F (63°C) as measured with a food thermometer placed in the thickest part of the meat, then allow the meat to rest* for three minutes before carving or consuming.

For Ground Meat (excluding poultry)

Cook to at least 160°F (71°C); ground meats do not require a rest* time.

For All Poultry (whole cuts and ground)

Cook to at least 165°F (74°C), and for whole poultry allow the meat to rest* for three minutes before carving or consuming.

According to USDA, "A 'rest time' is the amount of time the product remains at the final temperature, after it has been removed from a grill, oven, or other heat source. During the three minutes after meat is removed from the heat source, its temperature remains constant or continues to rise, which destroys pathogens."

- Freeze meat for several days at sub-zero (0°F) temperatures before cooking to greatly reduce chance of infection.

- Peel or wash fruits and vegetables thoroughly before eating.

- Do not eat raw or undercooked oysters, mussels, or clams (these may be contaminated with *Toxoplasma* that has washed into sea water).

- Do not drink unpasteurized goat's milk.

- Wash cutting boards, dishes, counters, utensils, and hands with hot soapy water after contact with raw meat, poultry, seafood, or unwashed fruits or vegetables.

- Wear gloves when gardening and during any contact with soil or sand because it might be contaminated with cat feces that contain *Toxoplasma*. Wash hands with soap and warm water after gardening or contact with soil or sand.

- Teach children the importance of washing hands to prevent infection.

If I Am at Risk, Can I Keep My Cat?

Yes, you may keep your cat if you are a person at risk for a severe infection (e.g., you have a weakened immune system or are pregnant); however, there are several safety precautions to avoid being exposed to *Toxoplasma gondii*:

- Ensure the cat litter box is changed daily. The *Toxoplasma* parasite does not become infectious until 1 to 5 days after it is shed in a cat's feces.

- If you are pregnant or immunocompromised:
  - Avoid changing cat litter if possible. If no one else can perform the task, wear disposable gloves and wash your hands with soap and warm water afterwards.
  - Keep cats indoors.
  - Do not adopt or handle stray cats, especially kittens. Do not get a new cat while you are pregnant.
- Feed cats only canned or dried commercial food or well-cooked table food, not raw or undercooked meats.
- Keep your outdoor sandboxes covered.

Your veterinarian can answer any other questions you may have regarding your cat and risk for toxoplasmosis.

Once Infected with Toxoplasma Is My Cat Always Able to Spread the Infection to Me?

No, cats only spread *Toxoplasma* in their feces for a few weeks following infection with the parasite. Like humans, cats rarely have symptoms when infected, so most people do not know if their cat has been infected. The *Toxoplasma* shedding in feces will go away on its own; therefore it does not help to have your cat or your cat's feces tested for *Toxoplasma*.

Section 38.7

Trachoma

This section contains text excerpted from the following sources: Text in this section begins with excerpts from "Hygiene-Related Diseases," Centers for Disease Control and Prevention (CDC), December 28, 2009. Reviewed March 2017; Text under the heading "Impact" is excerpted from "Trachoma," U.S. Agency for International Development (USAID), September 22, 2016.

Trachoma is the world's leading cause of preventable blindness of infectious origin. Caused by the bacterium *Chlamydia trachomatis*, trachoma is easily spread through direct personal contact, shared towels and clothes, and flies that have come in contact with the eyes or nose of an infected person. If left untreated, repeated trachoma infections can cause severe scarring of the inside of the eyelid and can cause the eyelashes to scratch the cornea (trichiasis). In addition to causing pain, trichiasis permanently damages the cornea and can lead to irreversible blindness. Trachoma, which spreads in areas that lack adequate access to water and sanitation, affects the most marginalized communities in the world.

The World Health Organization (WHO) has targeted trachoma for elimination by 2020 through an innovative, multi-faceted public health strategy known as S.A.F.E.:

- **S**urgery to correct the advanced, blinding stage of the disease (trichiasis),

- **A**ntibiotics to treat active infection,

- **F**acial cleanliness, and

- **E**nvironmental improvements in the areas of water and sanitation to reduce disease transmission

The comprehensive SAFE strategy combines measures for the treatment of active infection and trichiasis (S&A) with preventive measures to reduce disease transmission (F&E). Implementation of the full SAFE strategy in endemic areas increases the effectiveness of trachoma programs. The F and E components of SAFE, which reduce disease transmission, are particularly critical to achieving sustainable elimination of trachoma.

The "F" in the SAFE strategy refers to facial cleanliness. Because trachoma is transmitted through close personal contact, it tends to occur in clusters, often infecting entire families and communities. Children, who are more likely to touch their eyes and have unclean faces that attract eye-seeking flies, are especially vulnerable to infection, as are women, the traditional caretakers of the home. Therefore, the promotion of good hygiene practices, such as hand washing and the washing of children's faces at least once a day with water, is a key step in breaking the cycle of trachoma transmission.

The "E" in the SAFE strategy refers to environmental change. Improvements in community and household sanitation, such as the provision of household latrines, help control fly populations and breeding grounds. Increased access to water facilitates good hygiene practices and is vital to achieving sustainable elimination of the disease. Separation of animal quarters from human living space, as well as safe handling of food and drinking water, are also important environmental measures that affected communities can take within a trachoma control program.

Impact

Trachoma is responsible for the visual impairment of an estimated 1.8 million people worldwide, half a million of whom are irreversibly blind. Trachoma is commonly found in areas with limited access to adequate water, sanitation, and basic hygiene. More than 232 million people in 51 countries are at risk.

- Trachoma can result in loss of vision, blindness, loss of social status, stigmatization and can place a tremendous economic burden on individuals, families, and communities.

- Children have high infection rates, and as a result of their frequent contact with their female caretakers, women are almost twice as likely as men to develop trichiasis from trachoma.

- Blindness from trachoma strikes adults in their prime years (30–40 years of age), hindering their ability to care for themselves and their families.

- The disease's long-term effects can have an impact on multiple generations of families.

- Globally, trachoma causes between an estimated U.S. $3–6 billion loss in productivity per year.

Chapter 39

Fungal Infections Affecting Vision

Fungal eye infections are extremely rare, but they can be very serious. The most common way for someone to develop a fungal eye infection is as a result of an eye injury, particularly if the injury was caused by plant material such as a stick or a thorn. Inflammation or infection of the cornea (the clear, front layer of the eye) is known as keratitis, and inflammation or infection in the interior of the eye is called endophthalmitis. Many different types of fungi can cause eye infections.

Definition of Fungal Eye Infections

Eye infections can be caused by many different organisms, including bacteria, viruses, amoeba, and fungi.

Types of Fungal Eye Infections

Fungal infections can affect different parts of the eye.

- **Keratitis** is an infection of the clear, front layer of the eye (the cornea).

This chapter includes text excerpted from "Fungal Eye Infections," Centers for Disease Control and Prevention (CDC), January 27, 2017.

- **Endophthalmitis** is an infection of the inside of the eye (the vitreous and/or aqueous humor). There are two types of endophthalmitis: exogenous and endogenous.

  - Exogenous fungal endophthalmitis occurs after fungal spores enter the eye from an external source.

  - Endogenous endophthalmitis occurs when a bloodstream infection (for example, candidemia) spreads to one or both eyes.

Types of Fungi That Cause Eye Infections

Many of different types of fungi can cause eye infections. Common types include:

- *Fusarium*—a fungus that lives in the environment, especially in soil and on plants

- *Aspergillus*—a common fungus that lives in indoor and outdoor environments

- *Candida*—a type of yeast that normally lives on human skin and on the protective lining inside the body called the mucous membrane

Symptoms of Fungal Eye Infections

In people who have had exposures that put them at risk for fungal eye infections, the symptoms of a fungal eye infection can appear anywhere from several days to several weeks after the fungi enter the eye. The symptoms of a fungal eye infection are similar to the symptoms of other types of eye infections (such as those caused by bacteria) and can include:

- eye pain

- eye redness

- blurred vision

- sensitivity to light

- excessive tearing

- eye discharge

If you have any of these symptoms, call your eye doctor right away. If you wear contact lenses, remove them immediately. Fungal eye infections are very rare, but if they aren't treated, they can become serious and result in permanent vision loss or blindness.

Fungal Eye Infections Risk and Prevention

Who Gets Fungal Eye Infections?

Fungal eye infections usually occur in association with the following:

- eye injury, particularly with plant matter (for example, thorns or sticks)
- eye surgery (most commonly, cataract surgery)
- chronic eye disease involving the surface of the eye
- wearing contact lenses
- exposure to contaminated medical products that come in contact with the eye
- fungal bloodstream infection (like candidemia)

In addition to the risk factors listed above, people who have diabetes, weakened immune system, or use corticosteroids may be more likely to develop fungal eye infections than people without these conditions.

How Can I Prevent a Fungal Eye Infection?

Protective eyewear is recommended for people who are at risk for eye injuries involving plant matter, such as agricultural workers.

People who wear contact lenses should make sure to follow proper contact lens care practices.

Sources of Fungal Eye Infections

Fungal eye infections can't spread from person to person.

The most common way for someone to get a fungal eye infection is as a result of an eye injury, particularly if the injury was caused by plant material such as a stick or a thorn. Some fungi that cause eye infections, such as *Fusarium*, live in the environment, often association with plant material, and fungi can enter the eye and cause infection after an injury.

Less often, infection can occur after eye surgery or another type of invasive eye procedure such as an injection. Some fungal eye infections have been traced to contaminated medical products such as contact lens solution, irrigation solution and dye used during eye surgery, or corticosteroids injected directly into the eye. Rarely, fungal eye infections can happen after a fungal bloodstream infection such as candidemia spreads to the eye.

Fungal Eye Infection Diagnosis and Testing

To diagnose a fungal eye infection, your eye doctor will examine your eye and might take a small sample of tissue or fluid from your eye. The sample will be sent to a laboratory to be examined under a microscope or cultured. Polymerase chain reaction (PCR) and confocal microscopy are also being used as newer, faster forms of diagnosis; however, culture is the standard method for the definitive diagnosis of a fungal eye infection.

Treatment for Fungal Eye Infections

The treatment for a fungal eye infection depends on:

- the type of fungus
- the severity of the infection
- the parts of the eye that are affected

Possible forms of treatment for fungal eye infections include:

- antifungal eye drops
- antifungal medication given as a pill or through a vein
- antifungal medication injected directly into the eye
- eye surgery

All types of fungal eye infections must be treated with prescription antifungal medication, usually for several weeks to months. Natamycin is a topical (meaning it's given in the form of eye drops) antifungal medication that works well for fungal infections involving the outer layer of the eye, particularly those caused by fungi such as *Aspergillus* and *Fusarium*. However, infections that are deeper and more severe may require treatment with antifungal medication such as amphotericin B, fluconazole, or voriconazole. These medications can be given by mouth, through a vein, or injected directly into the eye. Patients whose infections don't get better after using antifungal medications may need surgery, including corneal transplantation, removal of vitreous gel from the interior of the eye (vitrectomy), or, in extreme cases, removal of the eye (enucleation).

Fungal Eye Infection Statistics

- **Fungal keratitis:** The exact incidence of fungal keratitis in the general population is unknown, but it's thought to be more common in warmer climates where the fungi that cause these infections are likely more common in the environment.

- **Exogenous fungal endophthalmitis** (fungi enter the eye from outside the body): Endophthalmitis is a very rare complication of eye injury or eye surgery; in the United States, it occurs as a postsurgical complication in approximately 0.1 percent of all cataract surgeries. Furthermore, only a small percentage of these infections are caused by fungi; bacterial endophthalmitis is more common.

- **Endogenous fungal endophthalmitis** (fungi enter the eye as a result of an existing bloodstream infection): Endogenous endophthalmitis is extremely rare and is less common than exogenous endophthalmitis; studies have estimated that only 2 to 15 percent of all endophthalmitis cases are endogenous. Candida species are the most common cause of endogenous fungal endophthalmitis. An estimated 1 percent of patients with candidemia develop *Candida* endophthalmitis.

Chapter 40

Stroke and Vision Loss

What Is Stroke?

A stroke is a "brain attack" that occurs when the blood, which brings oxygen to your brain, stops flowing and brain cells die. Nearly 795,000 people in the U.S. have a stroke each year.

How Does Vision Loss Relate to Stroke?

Vision loss can be both a symptom and result of a stroke. Temporary vision loss can be a sign of impending stroke and requires immediate medical attention.

Vision complications due to a stroke depend on where the stroke occurs. The majority of visual processing occurs in the occipital lobe, in the back of the brain. Most strokes affect one side of the brain. If the right occipital lobe is injured, the left field of vision in each eye may be affected. A stroke that affects the left occipital lobe may disturb the right field of vision in each eye. Rarely, both sides of the brain are affected, which can result in blindness.

Up to a quarter of stroke survivors may have vision loss. While most stroke patients with vision loss do not fully recover their vision, partial recovery or natural vision improvement is possible, usually in the first months after a stroke. Proper diagnosis and a vision rehabilitation plan can help improve most daily activities, self-esteem and feelings of independence.

What Are the Types of Vision Loss?

The most common type of vision loss with a stroke is loss of half of the visual field in each eye (homonymous hemianopia). Other types include loss of a quarter of the vision field (homonymous quadrantanopia) and an island-like area of blindness (scotoma). An automated visual field test provides proper diagnosis.

What Are Other Possible Vision Problems Following a Stroke?

The brain stem is the starting point for three pairs of nerves that control eye movements. A stroke in this area can result in only one eye moving correctly. This can cause double vision or the inability of both eyes to look in a particular direction.

Also originating in the brain stem is the sensation that objects at which one is looking are moving. A stroke in this area may lead to reading difficulties because the normal sense of stability is affected.

Loss of feeling may occur on the eye's surface, making blinking difficult, not allowing an eyelid to properly close or causing a droopy lid or blurry vision.

A stroke may also interfere with visually comprehending, understanding or recognizing objects. Visual agnosia is the inability to recognize or interpret objects by sight and often causes an inability to recognize familiar faces or objects.

How Can Vision Loss Be Treated?

A neuro-ophthalmologist or neurooptometrist can diagnose and recommend a vision rehabilitation plan. Vision rehabilitation includes different types of therapies.

Compensatory Vision Therapy

Compensatory vision therapy includes prisms, visual field awareness systems and scanning.

Prism and visual field awareness systems typically compensate for vision loss by shifting images from the non-seeing to the seeing visual field.

Scanning training is another compensatory therapy, which helps improve functional use of the remaining visual field by training the eyes to scan more efficiently toward and away from the field loss.

Restorative Vision Therapy

Vision Restoration Therapy (VRT) makes use of the brain's ability to reorganize neural connections to improve vision. It is a noninvasive neurostimulation therapy program customized for each specific type of vision loss. While the patient fixates on a central point, light stimuli are presented in a specific pattern targeting neuronal structures with the highest recovery potential.

Warning Signs of Stroke

Learn the many warning signs of a stroke. Act FAST and call 9-1-1 immediately at any sign of a stroke. Use FAST to remember warning signs:

- **FACE**: Ask the person to smile. Does one side of the face droop?

- **ARMS**: Ask the person to raise both arms. Does one arm drift downward?

- **SPEECH**: Ask the person to repeat a simple phrase. Is their speech slurred or strange?

- **TIME**: If you observe any of these signs, call 9-1-1 immediately.

Chapter 41

Traumatic Brain Injury and Vision Loss

Traumatic brain injury (TBI) occurs when the brain is harmed by an external force, such as a violent blow to the head or an object penetrating the skull. More than 1.4 million Americans receive treatment for TBI every year, while millions more suffer mild brain injuries—such as a concussion—and do not seek medical treatment. TBI can disrupt normal brain functioning and produce sensory, cognitive, or physical impairments that may be temporary or permanent. Many people with a TBI, or even a mild head injury, experience problems with their eyes and vision.

Situations that cause TBI can also cause trauma to the eyes or vision system, resulting in such sight-threatening conditions as retinal detachment, vitreous hemorrhage, or optic nerve damage. In addition to injuring the eyes directly, however, TBI can also cause vision problems by damaging parts of the brain involved in processing visual input from the eyes, such as the occipital lobe. Vision involves not only seeing with the eyes, but also interpreting, making sense of, and developing appropriate responses to visual images. Vision accounts for around 85 percent of the sensory input that is processed by the brain, and it affects perception, cognition, learning, motor skills, and other systems in the body. As a result, vision problems related to TBI can have a significant impact on people's everyday activities and overall quality of life.

"Traumatic Brain Injury and Vision Loss," © 2017 Omnigraphics. Reviewed March 2017.

Common Types of Vision Problems

An accident that injures the brain can also cause physical injury to the eyes and vision system. Some of the potentially serious injuries that create vision problems include the following:

- **Retinal detachment:** The retina is a thin layer of photore-active cells at the back of the eye that turns light images into nerve impulses and sends them to the brain for processing. A violent blow to the head can cause the retina to tear loose from the back of the eye. Without prompt medical treatment, retinal detachment can result in permanent blindness.

- **Optic nerve damage:** When TBI causes swelling of the brain, the increased pressure within the skull can cut off blood circulation to the optic nerve. Damage to the optic nerve can disrupt the flow of visual input from the eyes to the brain, sometimes resulting in permanent vision loss.

- **Vitreous hemorrhage:** The vitreous is a clear, jelly-like substance that fills the rear portion of the eye and allows light to pass through to the retina. A brain injury can break blood vessels in the eye and allow blood to enter the vitreous. Although such hemorrhages can disrupt vision temporarily, most cases clear up over time without causing permanent damage.

Symptoms of Vision Problems

Many other vision problems associated with TBI occur due to damage to parts of the brain involved in processing visual signals from the eyes. The symptoms vary depending on the extent of the injury, the parts of the brain that are affected, and the patient's individual recovery process. Some of the symptoms of vision problems that commonly result from traumatic brain injuries include the following:

- blurry vision

- double vision

- sensitivity to light

- headaches when performing visual tasks

- motion sickness, nausea, or vomiting when performing visual tasks

- difficulty reading

- difficulty with visual attention, concentration, comprehension, or memory

- visual balance disorders

- decreased peripheral vision or reduction of visual field

- inability to maintain visual contact or focus

- difficulty with eye movements, including the ability to: change focus from near to distant objects; track moving objects; shift gaze quickly from one object to another; and achieve the eye teaming or alignment required for binocular vision and depth perception.

Impact of Vision Problems

The vision symptoms experienced by people with TBI can affect many aspects of their daily lives, including the ability to work, go to school, drive a car, participate in recreational activities, and perform self-care tasks. Some of the difficulties caused by dysfunction in the brain's ability to process visual images include the following:

- **Difficulty with reading or close work:** Many people with TBI or concussion experience blurry near vision, which can make it hard to read or look at a computer screen. They may find it difficult to focus on near objects, or text may appear to move or jump around.

- **Struggles with pain or discomfort:** Swelling inside the skull often causes headaches, eye pain, and nausea or motion sickness when performing visual tasks.

- **Issues with movement or balance:** Many people with TBI have trouble tracking moving objects with their eyes or judging the relative location of objects in space. They may feel as if the floor is tilted, or they may become dizzy when they turn around or lean to the side.

- **Difficulty processing and understanding visual information:** Injury to the occipital lobe can make it difficult for the brain to make sense of images seen by the eyes. People with TBI may find it difficult to scan for visual information, focus visual attention on objects, or recall visual information.

- **Anxiety or irritability in certain environments:** Visual problems associated with TBI may cause people to feel uncomfortable or distressed when confronted with certain visual input, such as bright lights, complex patterns, or rapid motion.

- **Struggles with loss of vision or visual field:** People with decreased vision, double vision, or visual field loss face a risk of physical harm from bumping into objects, being struck by objects, or tripping over objects.

Treatment of Vision Problems

It is important to seek medical attention for any type of head injury that results in vision problems. Treatment for TBI-related vision problems depends on the type of problem and underlying cause. An optometrist or ophthalmologist can provide treatment for eye issues that can be corrected with surgery, patching, corrective eyeglasses, magnifying eyeglasses, or special lenses, such as prism lenses. Eye doctors who specialize in visual problems related to TBI, such as neuro-ophthalmologists, may be needed for more complex problems involving the brain's visual processing center. Occupational therapists, vision rehabilitation therapists, and low vision specialists can also provide exercises, training, and adaptive devices aimed at decreasing or eliminating TBI-related vision problems.

Management of Vision Problems

People with TBI can also use a number of strategies to adapt or manage the associated vision problems. Some suggestions include the following:

- Take frequent breaks to give the eyes and brain a rest while reading, using a computer, watching television, or doing other vision-dependent activities.

- Use magnifying lenses or increase print size and contrast on computer screens to make things easier to see.

- Avoid bright, fluorescent, and flashing lights or other visual input that might prove irritating to the eyes or brain.

- Wear tinted sunglasses to reduce glare and use glare-reducing filters on computer screens.

- Reduce visual input and overload by decluttering your home and work environment.

- Use adaptive devices like talking appliances, audio books, screen-reading software and apps, and mobility canes to help with reduced vision or vision loss.

References

1. "About Vision Problems Associated with Brain Injuries," Optometrists Network, 2017.

2. Metcalf, Eric. "Head Injuries Can Lead to Serious Vision Problems," Everyday Health, January 20, 2009.

3. Politzer, Thomas. "Introduction to Vision and Brain Injury," Neuro-Optometric Rehabilitation Association, n.d.

4. Powell, Janet M., Alan Weintraub, Laura Dreer, and Tom Novack. "Vision Problems and Traumatic Brain Injury," Model Systems Knowledge Translation Center, 2014.

Chapter 42

Diabetes and Eye Problems

Chapter Contents

Section 42.1

Diabetic Eye Disease

This section includes text excerpted from "Diabetic Eye Disease,"
National Institute of Diabetes and Digestive and Kidney
Diseases (NIDDK), May 2015.

How Can Diabetes Affect My Eyes?

Too much glucose, also called sugar, in your blood from diabetes can damage four parts of your eye:

- **Retina.** The retina is the tissue that lines the back of your eye. The retina converts light coming into your eye into visual messages through the optic nerve to your brain. The macula is the small, sensitive, center part of the retina that gives sharp, detailed vision.

- **Lens.** The lens of your eye is clear and is located behind the iris, the colored part of your eye. The lens helps to focus light, or an image, on the retina.

- **Vitreous gel.** The vitreous gel is a clear, colorless mass that fills the rear of your eye, between the retina and lens.

- **Optic nerve.** The optic nerve, at the back of your eye, is your eye's largest sensory nerve. The optic nerve connects your eye to your brain, carries visual messages from the retina to your brain, and sends messages between your brain and your eye muscles.

Diabetes damage to your eyes—called diabetic eye disease—can cause permanent vision loss, including low vision and blindness. Low vision means that even with regular glasses, contact lenses, medicine, or surgery, you can't see well enough to easily complete everyday tasks.

How Does Diabetes Affect the Retina?

Over time, having high blood glucose levels from diabetes can damage the tiny blood vessels on the retina. Diabetic retinopathy is the medical term for damage to the retina from diabetes.

500

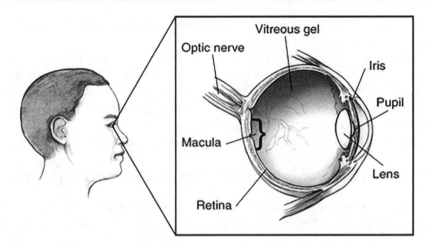

Figure 42.1. *The Human Eye*

Retina damage happens slowly. First, the retina's blood vessels swell. As retina damage worsens, the blood vessels become blocked and cut off the retina's oxygen supply. In response, new, weak blood vessels grow on the retina and the surface of the vitreous gel. These blood vessels break easily and leak blood into the vitreous gel. The leaking blood keeps light from reaching the retina.

When that happens, you may see floating spots or almost total darkness. One of your eyes may be damaged more than the other, or both eyes may have the same amount of damage. Sometimes the blood clears out by itself. However, you might need surgery to remove the blood.

You might not have any problems with your vision until the damage is severe, so you should have an eye exam at least once a year, even if your vision seems fine. Call your eye doctor right away if you notice any changes in your vision.

Over the years, the swollen and weak blood vessels can form scar tissue and pull the retina away from the back of your eye. If the retina pulls away, a condition called detached retina, you may see floating spots or flashing lights. You may feel as if a curtain has been pulled over part of what you are looking at. A detached retina can cause vision loss or blindness if you don't take care of it quickly. See an ophthalmologist—a doctor who diagnoses and treats all eye diseases—right away if you have these symptoms.

Some people with diabetic retinopathy also have a problem called macular edema. Macular edema, or swelling, can happen in any stage of retinopathy. Swelling in the macula is caused by leaking fluid from the retina's damaged blood vessels.

Macular edema is the most common cause of vision loss for people with diabetes. Your vision loss can be mild to severe if the edema is not treated, so it is important to have an eye exam at least once a year. You can have an eye exam with an ophthalmologist or an optometrist—a primary eye care provider who prescribes glasses and contact lenses and diagnoses and treats certain conditions and diseases of the eye.

What Are the Symptoms of Diabetes Retina Problems?

Often, no symptoms appear during the early stages of diabetes retina problems. As retina problems worsen, your symptoms might include

- blurry or double vision

- rings, flashing lights, or blank spots in your vision

- dark or floating spots in your vision

- pain or pressure in one or both of your eyes

- trouble seeing things out of the corners of your eyes

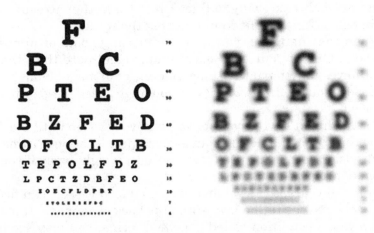

Figure 42.2. *Normal Vision and Blurry Vision*

How Can My Eye Doctor Tell Whether I Have Diabetes Retina Problems?

Your eye doctor can tell whether you have diabetes retina problems during a dilated eye exam. In a dilated eye exam, your eye doctor will use eye drops to enlarge your pupils. Your pupil is the opening at the center of the iris.

Enlarging your pupils allows your eye doctor to see more of the inside of your eyes to check for signs of disease. Your eye doctor will use a special magnifying lens to look at your retina and optic nerve for signs of damage and other eye problems.

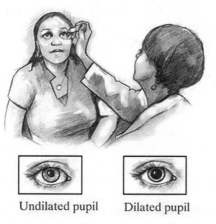

Undilated pupil   Dilated pupil

Figure 42.3. *Dilated Eye Exam*

At the time of your dilated eye exam, your eye doctor also will conduct other tests to measure

- pressure in your eyes

- your side, or peripheral, vision

- how well you see at various distances

Have a dilated eye exam at least once a year, even if your vision seems fine. Regular exams can prevent most instances of severe vision loss or blindness from diabetes eye problems. These exams can also help you protect your vision and make sure you are seeing at your best.

You may need to see an ophthalmologist to have a test called an eye angiogram.

For this test, you will be given eye drops to dilate your pupils. You will be asked to place your chin on a camera's chin rest and your forehead against a support bar to keep your head still during the test. Your ophthalmologist will take pictures of the insides of your eyes. A dye is injected into a vein in your arm. As the dye reaches your eyes and moves through your eyes' blood vessels, the camera takes more pictures.

This test will show whether you have abnormal or leaking blood vessels on your retina and help your ophthalmologist decide the best treatment.

Will I Have Diabetes Retina Problems?

The longer you've had diabetes, the more likely you are to have diabetes retina problems. You are less likely to have diabetes retina problems, or will have milder problems if you have them, if you keep your blood glucose numbers close to your targets. Targets are numbers you aim for.

How Are Diabetes Retina Problems Treated?

You can help your diabetes retina problems by controlling your

- blood glucose
- blood pressure
- cholesterol and triglycerides, or types of blood fat

If your retinopathy still does not improve, then you may need other treatments.

What Other Eye Problems Can Occur in People with Diabetes?

People with diabetes can have the following eye problems more often and at a younger age than people who do not have diabetes:

- **Cataract.** A cataract is a clouding of the normally clear lens that causes blurry vision. You need surgery to remove a cataract. During surgery, the ophthalmologist takes the lens out and puts in a plastic lens that is similar to a contact lens. The plastic lens stays in your eye permanently.

- **Glaucoma.** Glaucoma is a group of diseases that may be caused by an increase in eye pressure. Glaucoma can damage the optic nerve and result in vision loss and blindness. People with diabetes are more likely to get a severe type of glaucoma in which abnormal blood vessels grow in the front part of your eye. Your ophthalmologist will treat glaucoma with eye drops, pills, or surgery to control your eye pressure.

- **Neuropathy.** Neuropathy is nerve damage. Damage to the nerves in the feet or legs is the most common nerve damage from diabetes. However, diabetes can also affect the nerves to the eye. Having high blood glucose from diabetes causes decreased blood supply to the optic nerve. You may suddenly have double vision, drooping of your eyelid, or pain over your eye. Some people have full or partial paralysis of their eye muscles. This type of neuropathy tends to improve by itself over a period of weeks to months. If it doesn't, you may need to wear a patch over one eye or use a special lens to try to align your eyes.

What Can I Do If I Already Have Some Vision Loss from Diabetes Retina Problems?

If you already have some vision loss from diabetes retina problems that cannot be corrected by treatment, ask your eye doctor about low vision services and devices that can help you make the most of your remaining vision. Ask for a referral to a specialist in low vision. Many community organizations and agencies offer information about low vision counseling and training, and other special services for people with vision problems.

Section 42.2

Stay on TRACK to Prevent Blindness from Diabetes

This section contains text excerpted from the following sources: Text beginning with the heading "Diabetes: A Statistical Picture" is excerpted from "Stay on TRACK to Prevent Blindness from Diabetes," National Eye Institute (NEI), November 2, 2015: Text under the heading "How Can I Keep My Eyes Healthy?" is excerpted from "Diabetic Eye Disease," National Institute of Diabetes and Digestive and Kidney Diseases (NIDDK), May 2015.

Diabetes: A Statistical Picture

- Diabetes affects more than 9 percent of the U.S. population.

- More than 1 in 3 people have prediabetes.

- Everyone with diabetes is at risk for diabetic retinopathy—the number one cause of vision loss and blindness in working-age adults.

Eleven Million People to Be at Risk by 2030

You can't feel it. You can't see it—until it's too late. Diabetic retinopathy, the most common form of diabetic eye disease, is the leading cause of blindness in adults age 20–74. It occurs when diabetes damages blood vessels in the retina.

Diabetic retinopathy affects 7.7 million Americans, and that number is projected to increase to more than 11 million people by 2030.

Dr. Paul Sieving, director of the National Eye Institute (NEI), says, "Only about half of all people with diabetes get an annual comprehensive dilated eye exam, which is essential for detecting diabetic eye disease early, when it is most treatable."

With no early symptoms, diabetic eye disease—a group of conditions including cataract, glaucoma, and diabetic retinopathy—can affect anyone with type 1 or type 2 diabetes. African Americans, American Indians / Alaska Natives, and Hispanics/Latinos are at higher risk for losing vision or going blind from diabetes. The longer a person has diabetes, the greater the risk for diabetic eye disease. Once vision is lost, it often cannot be restored.

Keeping diabetes under control is key to slowing the progression of vision complications like diabetic retinopathy. There are important steps people with diabetes can take to keep their health on TRACK:

- **T**ake your medications as prescribed by your doctor.

- **R**each and maintain a healthy weight.

- **A**dd physical activity to your daily routine.

- **C**ontrol your ABC's—A1C, blood pressure, and cholesterol levels.

- **K**ick the smoking habit.

Additionally, people with diabetes should have annual comprehensive dilated eye exams to help protect their sight. Early detection, timely treatment, and appropriate follow-up care can reduce a person's risk for severe vision loss from diabetic eye disease by 95 percent.

"More than ever, it's important for people with diabetes to have a comprehensive dilated eye exam at least once a year. New treatments are being developed all the time, and we are learning that different treatments may work best for different patients. What hasn't changed is that early treatment is always better," says Dr. Suber Huang, chair of the Diabetic Eye Disease Subcommittee for NEI's National Eye Health Education Program (NEHEP) and member of the NEI-funded Diabetic Retinopathy Clinical Research Network (DRCR.net). "There has never been a more hopeful time in the treatment of diabetic retinopathy," he adds.

Remember, if you have diabetes, make annual comprehensive dilated eye exams part of your self-management routine. Living with diabetes can be challenging, but you don't have to lose your vision or go blind because of it.

How Can I Keep My Eyes Healthy?

You can keep your eyes healthy by taking these steps:

- Keep your blood glucose numbers as close to your targets as you can. Improving your blood glucose numbers can greatly lower your risk for retinopathy. Your doctor will work with you to set your target blood glucose numbers and teach you what to do if your numbers are too high or too low.

- Keep your blood pressure as close to your target as you can. High blood pressure can damage the tiny blood vessels on the retina. Have your blood pressure checked at every medical visit. Ask your doctor whether you need medicine or a combination of medicines to control your blood pressure. If your doctor prescribes blood pressure medicine, take it regularly.

- Have a healthy diet and be physically active to reduce your need for medicines to control your blood glucose, blood pressure, cholesterol, and triglycerides.

- If you smoke, stop smoking.

- Call your eye doctor right away if you have any signs of eye problems, especially sudden vision loss.

- Have a dilated eye exam at least once a year, even if your vision seems fine.

Section 42.3

Diabetic Retinopathy and Diabetic Macular Edema (DME)

This section includes text excerpted from "Facts about Diabetic Eye Disease," National Eye Institute (NEI), September 2015.

What Is Diabetic Eye Disease?

Diabetic eye disease is a group of eye conditions that can affect people with diabetes.

- **Diabetic retinopathy** affects blood vessels in the light-sensitive tissue called the retina that lines the back of the eye. It is the most common cause of vision loss among people with diabetes and the leading cause of vision impairment and blindness among working-age adults.

- **Diabetic macular edema (DME).** A consequence of diabetic retinopathy, DME is swelling in an area of the retina called the macula.

Diabetic eye disease also includes cataract and glaucoma:

- **Cataract** is a clouding of the eye's lens. Adults with diabetes are 2–5 times more likely than those without diabetes to develop cataract. Cataract also tends to develop at an earlier age in people with diabetes.

- **Glaucoma** is a group of diseases that damage the eye's optic nerve—the bundle of nerve fibers that connects the eye to the brain. Some types of glaucoma are associated with elevated pressure inside the eye. In adults, diabetes nearly doubles the risk of glaucoma.

All forms of diabetic eye disease have the potential to cause severe vision loss and blindness.

Diabetic Retinopathy

What Causes Diabetic Retinopathy?

Chronically high blood sugar from diabetes is associated with damage to the tiny blood vessels in the retina, leading to diabetic retinopathy. The retina detects light and converts it to signals sent through the optic nerve to the brain. Diabetic retinopathy can cause blood vessels in the retina to leak fluid or hemorrhage (bleed), distorting vision. In its most advanced stage, new abnormal blood vessels proliferate (increase in number) on the surface of the retina, which can lead to scarring and cell loss in the retina.

Diabetic retinopathy may progress through four stages:

1. **Mild nonproliferative retinopathy.** Small areas of balloon-like swelling in the retina's tiny blood vessels, called microaneurysms, occur at this earliest stage of the disease. These microaneurysms may leak fluid into the retina.

2. **Moderate nonproliferative retinopathy.** As the disease progresses, blood vessels that nourish the retina may swell and distort. They may also lose their ability to transport blood. Both conditions cause characteristic changes to the appearance of the retina and may contribute to DME.

3. **Severe nonproliferative retinopathy.** Many more blood vessels are blocked, depriving blood supply to areas of the retina. These areas secrete growth factors that signal the retina to grow new blood vessels.

4. **Proliferative diabetic retinopathy (PDR).** At this advanced stage, growth factors secreted by the retina trigger the proliferation of new blood vessels, which grow along the inside surface of the retina and into the vitreous gel, the fluid that fills the eye. The new blood vessels are fragile, which makes them more likely to leak and bleed. Accompanying scar tissue can contract and cause retinal detachment—the pulling away of the retina from underlying tissue, like wallpaper peeling away from a wall. Retinal detachment can lead to permanent vision loss.

What Is Diabetic Macular Edema (DME)?

DME is the buildup of fluid (edema) in a region of the retina called the macula. The macula is important for the sharp, straight-ahead vision that is used for reading, recognizing faces, and driving. DME is the most common cause of vision loss among people with diabetic retinopathy. About half of all people with diabetic retinopathy will develop DME. Although it is more likely to occur as diabetic retinopathy worsens, DME can happen at any stage of the disease.

Who Is at Risk for Diabetic Retinopathy?

People with all types of diabetes (type 1, type 2, and gestational) are at risk for diabetic retinopathy. Risk increases the longer a person has diabetes. Between 40 and 45 percent of Americans diagnosed with diabetes have some stage of diabetic retinopathy, although only about half are aware of it. Women who develop or have diabetes during pregnancy may have rapid onset or worsening of diabetic retinopathy.

Symptoms and Detection

What Are the Symptoms of Diabetic Retinopathy and DME?

The early stages of diabetic retinopathy usually have no symptoms. The disease often progresses unnoticed until it affects vision. Bleeding from abnormal retinal blood vessels can cause the appearance of "floating" spots. These spots sometimes clear on their own. But without prompt treatment, bleeding often recurs, increasing the risk of permanent vision loss. If DME occurs, it can cause blurred vision.

How Are Diabetic Retinopathy and DME Detected?

Diabetic retinopathy and DME are detected during a comprehensive dilated eye exam that includes:

- **Visual acuity testing.** This eye chart test measures a person's ability to see at various distances.

- **Tonometry.** This test measures pressure inside the eye.

- **Pupil dilation.** Drops placed on the eye's surface dilate (widen) the pupil, allowing a physician to examine the retina and optic nerve.

- **Optical coherence tomography (OCT).** This technique is similar to ultrasound but uses light waves instead of sound waves to capture images of tissues inside the body. OCT provides detailed images of tissues that can be penetrated by light, such as the eye.

A comprehensive dilated eye exam allows the doctor to check the retina for:

- changes to blood vessels

- leaking blood vessels or warning signs of leaky blood vessels, such as fatty deposits

- swelling of the macula (DME)

- changes in the lens

- damage to nerve tissue

If DME or severe diabetic retinopathy is suspected, a fluorescein angiogram may be used to look for damaged or leaky blood vessels. In this test, a fluorescent dye is injected into the bloodstream, often into an arm vein. Pictures of the retinal blood vessels are taken as the dye reaches the eye.

Prevention and Treatment

How Can People with Diabetes Protect Their Vision?

Vision lost to diabetic retinopathy is sometimes irreversible. However, early detection and treatment can reduce the risk of blindness by 95 percent. Because diabetic retinopathy often lacks early symptoms, people with diabetes should get a comprehensive dilated eye exam at least once a year. People with diabetic retinopathy may need eye exams more frequently. Women with diabetes who become pregnant should have a comprehensive dilated eye exam as soon as possible. Additional exams during pregnancy may be needed.

Studies such as the Diabetes Control and Complications Trial (DCCT) have shown that controlling diabetes slows the onset and worsening of diabetic retinopathy. DCCT study participants who kept their blood glucose level as close to normal as possible were significantly less likely than those without optimal glucose control to develop diabetic retinopathy, as well as kidney and nerve diseases. Other trials have shown that controlling elevated blood pressure and cholesterol can reduce the risk of vision loss among people with diabetes.

Treatment for diabetic retinopathy is often delayed until it starts to progress to PDR, or when DME occurs. Comprehensive dilated eye exams are needed more frequently as diabetic retinopathy becomes more severe. People with severe nonproliferative diabetic retinopathy have a high risk of developing PDR and may need a comprehensive dilated eye exam as often as every 2 to 4 months.

How Is DME Treated?

DME can be treated with several therapies that may be used alone or in combination.

Anti-VEGF Injection Therapy. Anti-VEGF drugs are injected into the vitreous gel to block a protein called vascular endothelial growth factor (VEGF), which can stimulate abnormal blood vessels to grow and leak fluid. Blocking VEGF can reverse abnormal blood vessel growth and decrease fluid in the retina. Available anti-VEGF drugs include Avastin (bevacizumab), Lucentis (ranibizumab), and Eylea (aflibercept). Lucentis and Eylea are approved by the U.S. Food and Drug Administration (FDA) for treating DME. Avastin was approved by the FDA to treat cancer, but is commonly used to treat eye conditions, including DME.

The National Eye Institute (NEI)-sponsored Diabetic Retinopathy Clinical Research Network compared Avastin, Lucentis, and Eylea in a clinical trial. The study found all three drugs to be safe and effective for treating most people with DME. Patients who started the trial with 20/40 or better vision experienced similar improvements in vision no matter which of the three drugs they were given. However, patients who started the trial with 20/50 or worse vision had greater improvements in vision with Eylea.

Most people require monthly anti-VEGF injections for the first six months of treatment. Thereafter, injections are needed less often: typically three to four during the second six months of treatment, about four during the second year of treatment, two in the third year, one in the fourth year, and none in the fifth year. Dilated eye exams may be needed less often as the disease stabilizes.

Avastin, Lucentis, and Eylea vary in cost and in how often they need to be injected, so patients may wish to discuss these issues with an eye care professional.

Focal/grid macular laser surgery. In focal/grid macular laser surgery, a few to hundreds of small laser burns are made to leaking blood vessels in areas of edema near the center of the macula. Laser burns for DME slow the leakage of fluid, reducing swelling in the retina. The procedure is usually completed in one session, but some people may need more than one treatment. Focal/grid laser is sometimes applied before anti-VEGF injections, sometimes on the same day or a few days after an anti-VEGF injection, and sometimes only when DME fails to improve adequately after six months of anti-VEGF therapy.

Corticosteroids. Corticosteroids, either injected or implanted into the eye, may be used alone or in combination with other drugs or laser surgery to treat DME. The Ozurdex (dexamethasone) implant is for short-term use, while the Iluvien (fluocinolone acetonide) implant is longer lasting. Both are biodegradable and release a sustained dose of corticosteroids to suppress DME. Corticosteroid use in the eye increases the risk of cataract and glaucoma. DME patients who use corticosteroids should be monitored for increased pressure in the eye and glaucoma.

How Is Proliferative Diabetic Retinopathy (PDR) Treated?

For decades, PDR has been treated with scatter laser surgery, sometimes called panretinal laser surgery or panretinal photocoagulation. Treatment involves making 1,000 to 2,000 tiny laser burns in areas of the retina away from the macula. These laser burns are intended to cause abnormal blood vessels to shrink. Although treatment can be completed in one session, two or more sessions are sometimes required. While it can preserve central vision, scatter laser surgery may cause some loss of side (peripheral), color, and night vision. Scatter laser surgery works best before new, fragile blood vessels have started to bleed. Studies have shown that anti-VEGF treatment not only is effective for treating DME, but is also effective for slowing progression of diabetic retinopathy, including PDR, so anti-VEGF is increasingly used as a first-line treatment for PDR.

What Is a Vitrectomy?

A vitrectomy is the surgical removal of the vitreous gel in the center of the eye. The procedure is used to treat severe bleeding into the vitreous, and is performed under local or general anesthesia. Ports (temporary watertight openings) are placed in the eye to allow the surgeon to insert and remove instruments, such as a tiny light or a small vacuum called a vitrector. A clear salt solution is gently pumped into the eye through one of the ports to maintain eye pressure during surgery and to replace the removed vitreous. The same instruments used during vitrectomy also may be used to remove scar tissue or to repair a detached retina.

Vitrectomy may be performed as an outpatient procedure or as an inpatient procedure, usually requiring a single overnight stay in the hospital. After treatment, the eye may be covered with a patch for days to weeks and may be red and sore. Drops may be applied to the eye to reduce inflammation and the risk of infection. If both eyes require vitrectomy, the second eye usually will be treated after the first eye has recovered.

What If Treatment Doesn't Improve Vision?

An eye care professional can help locate and make referrals to low vision and rehabilitation services and suggest devices that may help make the most of remaining vision. Many community organizations and agencies offer information about low vision counseling, training, and other special services for people with visual impairment. A nearby school of medicine or optometry also may provide low vision and rehabilitation services.

Chapter 43

Other Disorders with Eye-Related Complications

Chapter Contents

Section 43.1

Acquired Immune Deficiency Syndrome (AIDS)

This section contains text excerpted from the following sources: Text under the heading "Ocular Complications of AIDS" is excerpted from "Longitudinal Study of Ocular Complications of AIDS (LSOCA)," ClinicalTrials.gov, U.S. National Institutes of Health (NIH), June 2015; Text under the heading "Cytomegalovirus Retinitis" is excerpted from "Studies of Ocular Complications of AIDS (SOCA)— Ganciclovir-Cidofovir CMV Retinitis Trial (GCCRT)," ClinicalTrials. gov, U.S. National Institutes of Health (NIH), July 2015; Text under the heading "Transmission and Symptoms of Cytomegalovirus" is excerpted from "Cytomegalovirus (CMV)," U.S. Department of Veterans Affairs (VA), August 9, 2016.

Ocular Complications of AIDS

Ocular abnormalities in patients with AIDS were first reported in 1982. The most common finding is a non-infectious "HIV retinopathy," characterized by cotton wool spots, intraretinal hemorrhages, and/or microaneurysms. These changes occur in approximately 50 percent of patients with AIDS. HIV retinopathy alone is not typically associated with clinical loss of vision, but functional deficits in patients with AIDS without other ocular complications may be due to this phenomenon.

Cytomegalovirus (CMV) retinitis has had the most clinical importance of all the associated complications of AIDS. It is commonly seen in late stage AIDS, and even when treated has the potential to cause substantial loss of vision. CMV retinitis is also the most costly AIDS-related opportunistic infection; the mean monthly cost of treatment has been estimated at $7,825. The incidence of CMV retinitis has varied with changes in the therapeutic and prophylactic strategies for AIDS and its complications. It has been on the decline in recent years related to the increased use of highly active anti-retroviral therapy (HAART).

Other ocular complications of AIDS such as ocular toxoplasmosis, herpes zoster retinitis, and pneumocystis choroidopathy occur less frequently than CMV retinitis and HIV retinopathy. Their frequency has also changed over the course of the AIDS epidemic.

Because the epidemiology of AIDS is rapidly evolving, with HIV becoming more like a chronic disease, new information is needed on the incidence and course of ocular complications. There is little information about the effect of HAART therapy over time on changes in immune status and the risk of ocular complications of AIDS. More information is also needed to determine who is at risk for developing ocular complications of AIDS, and how treatment is affecting their visual function, quality of life, and survival.

Cytomegalovirus Retinitis

CMV is among the most frequently encountered opportunistic infections in patients with AIDS. In the era of prophylaxis for pneumocystic pneumonia, CMV disease is estimated to affect 45 percent of patients with AIDS sometime between the diagnosis of AIDS and death. Retinitis has been estimated to account for up to 85 percent of CMV disease in these patients, making CMV retinitis the most common ocular infection encountered. CMV retinitis is a relatively late-stage manifestation, associated with cluster of differentiation 4 (CD4) + T-cell counts < 100 cells/μL and often < 50 cells/μL.

All currently available treatments for CMV suppress viral replication but do not eliminate the virus from the body. Discontinuation of therapy is associated with a prompt relapse of the retinitis. Despite the use of chronic suppressive therapy, relapse of the retinitis generally occurs, at least with systemically administered anti-CMV drugs.

The first two treatments approved for CMV retinitis were intravenous ganciclovir and intravenous foscarnet. Both are given by daily intravenous infusions and therefore require central venous catheters. The development of newer treatments has focused not only on efficacious treatments, but also on treatments that do not require central venous catheters. Available treatments now include oral ganciclovir, the ganciclovir intraocular device, and intravenous cidofovir.

Transmission and Symptoms of Cytomegalovirus

Cytomegalovirus (or CMV) is passed by close contact through sex and through saliva, urine, and other body fluids. It can be passed from mother to child during pregnancy and by breast-feeding. If you are not infected, using condoms during sex may help prevent infection.

Many people are infected with this virus, though they have no symptoms. In HIV-positive people with low CD4 counts, the infection can be extremely serious. Symptoms can include:

- blind spots in vision, loss of peripheral vision

- headache, difficulty concentrating, sleepiness

- mouth ulcers

- pain in the abdomen, bloody diarrhea

- fever, fatigue, weight loss

- shortness of breath

- lower back pain

- confusion, apathy, withdrawal, personality changes

Section 43.2

Adie Syndrome

This section includes text excerpted from "Adie Syndrome," Genetic and Rare Diseases Information Center (GARD), National Center for Advancing Translational Sciences (NCATS), February 16, 2017.

Adie syndrome is a neurological disorder affecting the pupil of the eye and the autonomic nervous system. It is characterized by one eye with a pupil that is larger than normal that constricts slowly in bright light (tonic pupil), along with the absence of deep tendon reflexes, usually in the Achilles tendon. In most cases, the cause of Adie syndrome is unknown. Some cases may result from trauma, surgery, lack of blood flow, or infection. Treatment may not be necessary. Glasses and eye drops may help when treatment is needed.

The term Adie syndrome is used when both the pupil and deep tendon reflexes are affected. When only the pupil is affected, the disorder may be referred to as Adie pupil.

Symptoms of Adie Syndrome

Adie syndrome is characterized by one eye with a pupil that is larger than normal that constricts slowly in bright light (tonic pupil), along with the absence of deep tendon reflexes, usually in the Achilles tendon. It typically begins gradually in one eye, and often progresses to involve the other eye. At first, it may only cause the loss of deep tendon reflexes on one side of the body, but then progress to the other side. The eye and reflex symptoms may not appear at the same time. People with Adie syndrome may also sweat excessively, sometimes only on one side of the body. The combination of these 3 symptoms—abnormal pupil size, loss of deep tendon reflexes, and excessive sweating—is usually called **Ross syndrome**, although some doctors will still diagnosis the condition as a variant of Adie syndrome. Some individuals will also have cardiovascular abnormalities. The symptoms of Adie syndrome can appear on their own, or in association with other diseases of the nervous system, such as Sjogren syndrome or migraine.

Cause of Adie Syndrome

In most cases, the cause of Adie syndrome is unknown (idiopathic). The tonic pupil in Adie syndrome is believed to result from inflammation or damage to the ciliary ganglion (a cluster of nerve cells found behind the eye) or damage to the postganglionic nerves. The ciliary ganglion is part of the parasympathetic nervous system, a component of the autonomic nervous system. It helps control the pupil's response to light and other stimuli. In most cases, damage to the ciliary ganglion or postganglionic nerves is caused by an infection. Damage may also result from autoimmune processes, tumors, trauma, and complications of surgery.

The loss of deep tendon reflexes in Adie syndrome is believed to be caused by damage to the dorsal root ganglion, a cluster of nerve cells in the root of the spinal nerves.

In rare cases, Adie syndrome may be inherited. In these cases, it appears to follow an autosomal dominant pattern of inheritance.

Diagnosis of Adie Syndrome

Making a diagnosis for a genetic or rare disease can often be challenging. Healthcare professionals typically look at a person's medical history, symptoms, physical exam, and laboratory test results in order to make a diagnosis. If you have questions about getting a diagnosis, you should contact a healthcare professional.

Treatment of Adie Syndrome

Doctors may prescribe reading glasses to compensate for impaired vision in the affected eye, and pilocarpine drops to be applied 3 times

daily to constrict the dilated pupil. This may help with depth perception and reduce glare. For many, these strategies improve vision. Tho-
racic sympathectomy, which severs the involved sympathetic nerve,
is the definitive treatment for excessive sweating.

Other Names for Adie Syndrome

- Adie's Pupil

- Holmes-Adie syndrome (HAS)

- Tonic, sluggishly reacting pupil and hypoactive or absent tendon
  reflexes

Section 43.3

Behçet Disease

This section includes text excerpted from "Behçet's Disease,"
National Institute of Arthritis and Musculoskeletal and Skin
Diseases (NIAMS), August 2015.

What Is Behçet Disease?

The disease was first described in 1937 by Dr. Hulusi Behçet, a
dermatologist in Turkey. Behçet disease is now recognized as a chronic
condition that causes canker sores or ulcers in the mouth and on the
genitals, and inflammation in parts of the eye. In some people, the disease also results in arthritis (swollen, painful, stiff joints), skin problems, and inflammation of the digestive tract, brain, and spinal cord.

Who Gets Behçet Disease?

Behçet disease is common in the Middle East, Asia, and Japan; it
is rare in the United States. In Middle Eastern and Asian countries,
the disease affects more men than women. In the United States, the
opposite is true. Behçet disease tends to develop in people in their
twenties or thirties, but people of all ages can develop this disease.

What Causes Behçet Disease?

The exact cause of Behçet disease is unknown. Most symptoms of the disease are caused by inflammation of the blood vessels. Inflammation is a characteristic reaction of the body to injury or disease and is marked by four signs: swelling, redness, heat, and pain. Doctors think that an autoinflammatory reaction may cause the blood vessels to become inflamed, but they do not know what triggers this reaction. Under normal conditions, the immune system protects the body from diseases and infections by killing harmful "foreign" substances, such as germs, that enter the body. In an autoinflammatory reaction, the immune system mistakenly attacks and harms the body's own tissues.

Behçet disease is not contagious; it is not spread from one person to another. Researchers think that two factors are important for a person to get Behçet disease. First, it is believed that abnormalities of the immune system make some people susceptible to the disease. Scientists think that this susceptibility may be inherited; that is, it may be due to one or more specific genes. Second, something in the environment, possibly a bacterium or virus, might trigger or activate the disease in susceptible people.

What Are the Symptoms of Behçet Disease?

Behçet disease affects each person differently. Some people have only mild symptoms, such as canker sores or ulcers in the mouth or on the genitals. Others have more severe signs, such as meningitis, which is an inflammation of the membranes that cover the brain and spinal cord. Meningitis can cause fever, a stiff neck, and headaches. More severe symptoms usually appear months or years after a person notices the first signs of Behçet disease. Symptoms can last for a long time or may come and go in a few weeks. Typically, symptoms appear, disappear, and then reappear. The times when a person is having symptoms are called flares. Different symptoms may occur with each flare; the problems of the disease often do not occur together. To help the doctor diagnose Behçet disease and monitor its course, patients may want to keep a record of which symptoms occur and when. Because many conditions mimic Behçet disease, doctors must observe the lesions (injuries) caused by the disorder to make an accurate diagnosis.

Common symptoms of Behçet disease include mouth sores, genital sores, other skin lesions, inflammation of parts of the eye, and arthritis.

- **Mouth sores** (known as oral aphthosis and aphthous stomatitis) affect almost all people with Behçet disease. Individual sores or ulcers are usually identical to canker sores, which are common in many people. They are often the first symptom that a person notices and may occur long before any other symptoms appear. The sores usually have a red border and several may appear at the same time. They may be painful and can make eating difficult. Mouth sores go away in 10 to 14 days but often come back. Small sores usually heal without scarring, but larger sores may scar.

- **Genital sores** affect more than half of all people with Behçet disease and most commonly appear on the scrotum in men and vulva in women. The sores look similar to the mouth sores and may be painful. After several outbreaks, they may cause scarring.

- **Skin problems** are a common symptom of Behçet disease. Skin sores often look red or resemble pus-filled bumps or a bruise. The sores are red and raised, and typically appear on the legs and on the upper torso. In some people, sores or lesions may appear when the skin is scratched or pricked. When doctors suspect that a person has Behçet disease, they may perform a pathergy test, in which they prick the skin with a small needle; 1 to 2 days after the test, people with Behçet disease may develop a red bump where the doctor pricked the skin. However, only half of the Behçet patients in Middle Eastern countries and Japan have this reaction. It is less commonly observed in patients from the United States, but if this reaction occurs, then Behçet disease is likely.

- **Uveitis** involves inflammation of the middle or back part of the eye (the uvea) including the iris, and occurs in more than half of all people with Behçet disease. This symptom is more common among men than women and typically begins within 2 years of the first symptoms. Eye inflammation can cause blurred vision; rarely, it causes pain and redness. Because partial loss of vision or blindness can result if the eye frequently becomes inflamed, patients should report these symptoms to their doctor immediately.

- **Arthritis**, which is inflammation of the joints, occurs in more than half of all people with Behçet disease. Arthritis causes pain, swelling, and stiffness in the joints, especially in the knees, ankles, wrists, and elbows. Arthritis that results from Behçet disease usually lasts a few weeks and does not cause permanent damage to the joints.

In addition to mouth and genital sores, other skin lesions, eye inflammation, and arthritis, Behçet disease may also cause blood clots and inflammation in the central nervous system and digestive organs.

Vascular System

Some people with Behçet disease have blood clots resulting from inflammation in the veins (thrombophlebitis), usually in the legs. Symptoms include pain and tenderness in the affected area. The area may also be swollen and warm. Because thrombophlebitis can have severe complications, people should report symptoms to their doctor immediately. A few patients may experience artery problems such as aneurysms (balloon-like swelling of the artery wall).

Central Nervous System

In the United States, Behçet disease affects the central nervous system in an estimated one-fifth to one-quarter of people with the disease. The central nervous system includes the brain and spinal cord. Its function is to process information and coordinate thinking, behavior, sensation, and movement. Behçet disease can cause inflammation of the brain and the thin membrane that covers and protects the brain and spinal cord. This condition is called meningoencephalitis. People with meningoencephalitis may have fever, headache, stiff neck, and difficulty coordinating movement, and should report any of these symptoms to their doctor immediately. If this condition is left untreated, a stroke (blockage or rupture of blood vessels in the brain) can result.

Digestive Tract

Rarely, Behçet disease causes inflammation and ulceration (sores) throughout the digestive tract that are identical to the aphthous lesions in the mouth and genital area.

This leads to abdominal pain, diarrhea, and/or bleeding. Because these symptoms are very similar to symptoms of other diseases of the digestive tract, such as ulcerative colitis and Crohn's disease, careful evaluation is essential to rule out these other diseases.

How Is Behçet Disease Diagnosed?

Diagnosing Behçet disease is very difficult because no specific test confirms it. Less than half of people initially thought to have Behçet disease actually have it. When a patient reports symptoms, the doctor must conduct an examination and rule out other conditions with similar symptoms. Because it may take several months or even years for all the common symptoms to appear, the diagnosis may not be made for a long time. A patient may even visit several different kinds of doctors before the diagnosis is made.

These symptoms are key to a diagnosis of Behçet disease:

• Mouth sores at least three times in 12 months.

• Any two of the following symptoms: recurring genital sores, eye inflammation with loss of vision, characteristic skin lesions, or positive pathergy (skin prick test).

Besides finding these signs, the doctor must rule out other conditions with similar symptoms, such as Crohn's disease and reactive arthritis. The doctor also may recommend that the patient see an eye specialist to identify possible complications related to eye inflammation. A dermatologist may perform a biopsy of mouth, genital, or skin lesions to help distinguish Behçet from other disorders.

What Kind of Doctor Treats a Person with Behçet Disease?

Because the disease affects different parts of the body, a patient probably will see several different doctors. It may be helpful to both the doctors and the patient for one doctor to manage the complete treatment plan. This doctor can coordinate the treatments and monitor any side effects from the various medications that the patient takes.

A rheumatologist (a doctor specializing in arthritis and other inflammatory disorders) often manages a patient's treatment and treats joint disease. The following specialists also treat other symptoms that affect the different body systems:

• A gynecologist, who treats genital sores in women.

• An urologist, who treats genital sores in men and women.

• A dermatologist, who treats genital sores in men and women and skin and mucous membrane problems.

• An ophthalmologist, who treats eye inflammation.

- A gastroenterologist, who treats digestive tract symptoms.

- A hematologist, who treats disorders of the blood.

- A neurologist, who treats central nervous system symptoms.

How Is Behçet Disease Treated?

Although there is no cure for Behçet disease, people usually can control symptoms with proper medication, rest, exercise, and a healthy lifestyle. The goal of treatment is to reduce discomfort and prevent serious complications such as disability from arthritis or blindness. The type of medicine and the length of treatment depend on the person's symptoms and their severity. It is likely that a combination of treatments will be needed to relieve specific symptoms. Patients should tell each of their doctors about all of the medicines they are taking so that the doctors can coordinate treatment.

Topical Medicine

Topical medicine is applied directly on the sores to relieve pain and discomfort. For example, doctors prescribe rinses, gels, or ointments. Creams are used to treat skin and genital sores. The medicine usually contains corticosteroids (which reduce inflammation), other anti-inflammatory drugs, or an anesthetic, which relieves pain.

Oral Medicine

Doctors also prescribe medicines taken by mouth to reduce inflammation throughout the body, suppress the overactive immune system, and relieve symptoms. Doctors may prescribe one or more of the medicines described below to treat the various symptoms of Behçet disease.

- **Corticosteroids.** A corticosteroid medication is prescribed to reduce pain and inflammation throughout the body for people with severe joint pain, skin sores, eye disease, or central nervous system symptoms. Patients must carefully follow the doctor's instructions about when to take a corticosteroid and how much to take. It also is important not to stop taking the medicine suddenly, because the medicine alters the body's production of the natural corticosteroid hormones. Long-term use of these medications can have side effects such as osteoporosis (a disease that leads to bone fragility), weight gain, delayed wound healing, persistent heartburn, and elevated blood pressure. However, these side effects are rare when they are taken at low doses for a short time. It is important that people with the disease see their doctor regularly to monitor possible side effects. Corticosteroids are useful in early stages of disease and for acute severe flares. They are of limited use for long-term management of central nervous system and serious eye complications.

- **Immunosuppressive drugs.** These medicines (in addition to corticosteroids) help control an overactive immune system, which occurs in Behçet disease, and reduce inflammation throughout the body and lessen the number of disease flares. Doctors may use immunosuppressive drugs when a person has eye disease or central nervous system involvement. These medicines are very strong and can have serious side effects. Patients must see their doctor regularly for blood tests to detect and monitor side effects.

Doctors may prescribe other medications to reduce inflammation and treat specific manifestations of the disease.

Rest and Exercise

Although rest is important during flares, doctors usually recommend moderate exercise, such as swimming or walking, when the symptoms have improved or disappeared. Exercise can help people with Behçet disease keep their joints strong and flexible.

Section 43.4

Graves Disease

This section includes text excerpted from "Graves' Disease," National Institute of Diabetes and Digestive and Kidney Diseases (NIDDK), August 2012. Reviewed March 2017.

What Is Graves Disease?

Graves disease, also known as toxic diffuse goiter, is the most common cause of hyperthyroidism in the United States. Hyperthyroidism is a disorder that occurs when the thyroid gland makes more thyroid hormone than the body needs.

The Thyroid

The thyroid is a 2-inch-long, butterfly-shaped gland in the front of the neck below the larynx, or voice box. The thyroid makes two thyroid hormones, triiodothyronine (T_3) and thyroxine (T_4). T_3 is made from T_4 and is the more active hormone, directly affecting the tissues. Thyroid hormones circulate throughout the body in the bloodstream and act on virtually every tissue and cell in the body.

Thyroid hormones affect metabolism, brain development, breathing, heart and nervous system functions, body temperature, muscle strength, skin dryness, menstrual cycles, weight, and cholesterol levels. Hyperthyroidism causes many of the body's functions to speed up.

Thyroid hormone production is regulated by another hormone called thyroid-stimulating hormone (TSH), which is made by the pituitary gland in the brain. When thyroid hormone levels in the blood are low, the pituitary releases more TSH. When thyroid hormone levels are high, the pituitary responds by decreasing TSH production.

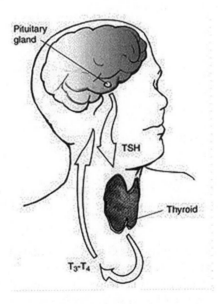

Figure 43.1. *Production of Thyroid Hormones*

The thyroid's production of thyroid hormones – T_3 and T_4 – is regulated by thyroid-stimulating hormone (TSH), which is made by the pituitary gland.

Autoimmune Disorder

Graves disease is an autoimmune disorder. Normally, the immune system protects the body from infection by identifying and destroying bacteria, viruses, and other potentially harmful foreign substances. But in autoimmune diseases, the immune system attacks the body's own cells and organs.

With Graves disease, the immune system makes an antibody called thyroid-stimulating immunoglobulin (TSI)—sometimes called TSH receptor antibody—that attaches to thyroid cells. TSI mimics TSH and stimulates the thyroid to make too much thyroid hormone. Sometimes the TSI antibody instead blocks thyroid hormone production, leading to conflicting symptoms that may make correct diagnosis more difficult.

What Are the Symptoms of Graves Disease?

People with Graves disease may have common symptoms of hyperthyroidism such as

- nervousness or irritability

- fatigue or muscle weakness

- heat intolerance

- trouble sleeping

- hand tremors

- rapid and irregular heartbeat

- frequent bowel movements or diarrhea

- weight loss

- goiter, which is an enlarged thyroid that may cause the neck to look swollen and can interfere with normal breathing and swallowing

A small number of people with Graves disease also experience thickening and reddening of the skin on their shins. This usually painless problem is called pretibial myxedema or Graves dermopathy.

In addition, the eyes of people with Graves disease may appear enlarged because their eyelids are retracted—seem pulled back into the eye sockets—and their eyes bulge out from the eye sockets. This condition is called Graves ophthalmopathy (GO).

What Is Graves Ophthalmopathy?

Graves ophthalmopathy (GO) is a condition associated with Graves disease that occurs when cells from the immune system attack the muscles and other tissues around the eyes.

The result is inflammation and a buildup of tissue and fat behind the eye socket, causing the eyeballs to bulge out. Rarely, inflammation is severe enough to compress the optic nerve that leads to the eye, causing vision loss.

Other GO symptoms are

- dry, gritty, and irritated eyes

- puffy eyelids

- double vision

- light sensitivity

- pressure or pain in the eyes

- trouble moving the eyes

About 25 to 30 percent of people with Graves disease develop mild GO, and 2 to 5 percent develop severe GO. This eye condition usually lasts 1 to 2 years and often improves on its own.

GO can occur before, at the same time as, or after other symptoms of hyperthyroidism develop and may even occur in people whose thyroid function is normal. Smoking makes GO worse.

Who Is Likely to Develop Graves Disease?

Scientists cannot predict who will develop Graves disease. However, factors such as age, sex, heredity, and emotional and environmental stress are likely involved.

Graves disease usually occurs in people younger than age 40 and is seven to eight times more common in women than men. Women are most often affected between ages 30 and 60. And a person's chance of developing Graves disease increases if other family members have the disease.

Researchers have not been able to find a specific gene that causes the disease to be passed from parent to child. While scientists know some people inherit an immune system that can make antibodies against healthy cells, predicting who will be affected is difficult.

People with other autoimmune diseases have an increased chance of developing Graves disease. Conditions associated with Graves disease include type 1 diabetes, rheumatoid arthritis, and vitiligo—a disorder in which some parts of the skin are not pigmented.

How Is Graves Disease Diagnosed?

Healthcare providers can sometimes diagnose Graves disease based only on a physical examination and a medical history. Blood tests and other diagnostic tests, such as the following, then confirm the diagnosis.

- **TSH test.** The ultrasensitive TSH test is usually the first test performed. This test detects even tiny amounts of TSH in the blood and is the most accurate measure of thyroid activity available.

- **T_3 and T_4 test.** Another blood test used to diagnose Graves disease measures T_3 and T_4 levels. In making a diagnosis, healthcare providers look for below-normal levels of TSH, normal to elevated levels of T_4, and elevated levels of T_3.

Because the combination of low TSH and high T_3 and T_4 can occur with other thyroid problems, healthcare providers may order other tests to finalize the diagnosis. The following two tests use small, safe doses of radioactive iodine because the thyroid uses iodine to make thyroid hormone.

- **Radioactive iodine uptake test.** This test measures the amount of iodine the thyroid collects from the bloodstream. High levels of iodine uptake can indicate Graves disease.

- **Thyroid scan.** This scan shows how and where iodine is distributed in the thyroid. With Graves disease the entire thyroid is involved, so the iodine shows up throughout the gland. Other causes of hyperthyroidism such as nodules—small lumps in the gland—show a different pattern of iodine distribution.

- **TSI test.** Healthcare providers may also recommend the TSI test, although this test usually isn't necessary to diagnose Graves disease. This test, also called a TSH antibody test, measures the level of TSI in the blood. Most people with Graves disease have this antibody, but people whose hyperthyroidism is caused by other conditions do not.

How Is Graves Disease Treated?

People with Graves disease have three treatment options: radioiodine therapy, medications, and thyroid surgery. Radioiodine therapy is the most common treatment for Graves disease in the United States. Graves disease is often diagnosed and treated by an endocrinologist—a doctor who specializes in the body's hormone-secreting glands.

Radioiodine Therapy

In radioiodine therapy, patients take radioactive iodine-131 by mouth. Because the thyroid gland collects iodine to make thyroid hormone, it will collect the radioactive iodine from the bloodstream in the same way. Iodine-131—stronger than the radioactive iodine used in diagnostic tests—gradually destroys the cells that make up the thyroid gland but does not affect other body tissues.

Many healthcare providers use a large enough dose of iodine-131 to shut down the thyroid completely, but some prefer smaller doses to try to bring hormone production into the normal range. More than one round of radioiodine therapy may be needed. Results take time and people undergoing this treatment may not notice improvement in symptoms for several weeks or months.

People with GO should talk with a healthcare provider about any risks associated with radioactive iodine treatments. Several studies suggest radioiodine therapy can worsen GO in some people. Other treatments, such as prescription steroids, may prevent this complication.

Although iodine-131 is not known to cause birth defects or infertility, radioiodine therapy is not used in pregnant women or women who are breastfeeding. Radioactive iodine can be harmful to the fetus' thyroid and can be passed from mother to child in breast milk. Experts recommend that women wait a year after treatment before becoming pregnant.

Almost everyone who receives radioactive iodine treatment eventually develops hypothyroidism, which occurs when the thyroid does not make enough thyroid hormone. People with hypothyroidism must take synthetic thyroid hormone, a medication that replaces their natural thyroid hormone.

Medications

Beta blockers. Healthcare providers may prescribe a medication called a beta blocker to reduce many of the symptoms of hyperthyroidism, such as tremors, rapid heartbeat, and nervousness. But beta blockers do not stop thyroid hormone production.

Anti-thyroid medications. Healthcare providers sometimes prescribe anti-thyroid medications as the only treatment for Graves disease. Anti-thyroid medications interfere with thyroid hormone production but don't usually have permanent results. Use of these medications requires frequent monitoring by a healthcare provider. More often, anti-thyroid medications are used to pretreat patients before surgery or radioiodine therapy, or they are used as supplemental treatment after radioiodine therapy.

Anti-thyroid medications can cause side effects in some people, including

- allergic reactions such as rashes and itching

- a decrease in the number of white blood cells in the body, which can lower a person's resistance to infection

- liver failure, in rare cases

In the United States, healthcare providers prescribe the anti-thyroid medication methimazole (Tapazole, Northyx) for most types of hyperthyroidism.

Anti-thyroid medications and pregnancy. Because pregnant and breastfeeding women cannot receive radioiodine therapy, they are usually treated with an anti-thyroid medication instead. However, experts agree that women in their first trimester of pregnancy should probably not take methimazole due to the rare occurrence of damage to the fetus.

Another anti-thyroid medication, propylthiouracil (PTU), is available for women in this stage of pregnancy or for women who are allergic to or intolerant of methimazole and have no other treatment options. Healthcare providers may prescribe PTU for the first trimester of pregnancy and switch to methimazole for the second and third trimesters.

Some women are able to stop taking anti-thyroid medications in the last 4 to 8 weeks of pregnancy due to the remission of hyperthyroidism that occurs during pregnancy. However, these women should continue to be monitored for recurrence of thyroid problems following delivery.

Studies have shown that mothers taking anti-thyroid medications may safely breastfeed. However, they should take only moderate doses, less than 10–20 milligrams daily, of the anti-thyroid medication methimazole. Doses should be divided and taken after feedings, and the infants should be monitored for side effects.

Women requiring higher doses of the anti-thyroid medication to control hyperthyroidism should not breastfeed.

Stop your anti-thyroid medication and call your healthcare provider right away if you develop any of the following while taking anti-thyroid medications:

- easy bruising

- fatigue

- fever

- loss of appetite

- persistent sore throat

- skin rash or itching

- vague abdominal pain

- weakness

- yellowing of the skin or whites of the eyes, called jaundice

Thyroid Surgery

Surgery is the least-used option for treating Graves disease. Sometimes surgery may be used to treat

- pregnant women who cannot tolerate anti-thyroid medications

- people suspected of having thyroid cancer, though Graves disease does not cause cancer

- people for whom other forms of treatment are not successful

Before surgery, the healthcare provider may prescribe anti-thyroid medications to temporarily bring a patient's thyroid hormone levels into the normal range. This presurgical treatment prevents a condition called thyroid storm—a sudden, severe worsening of symptoms—that can occur when hyperthyroid patients have general anesthesia.

When surgery is used, many healthcare providers recommend the entire thyroid be removed to eliminate the chance that hyperthyroidism will return. If the entire thyroid is removed, lifelong thyroid hormone medication is necessary.

Although uncommon, certain problems can occur in thyroid surgery. The parathyroid glands can be damaged because they are located very close to the thyroid. These glands help control calcium and phosphorous levels in the body. Damage to the laryngeal nerve, also located close to the thyroid, can lead to voice changes or breathing problems.

But when surgery is performed by an experienced surgeon, less than 1 percent of patients have permanent complications.

Eye Care

The eye problems associated with Graves disease may not improve following thyroid treatment, so the two problems are often treated separately.

Eye drops can relieve dry, gritty, irritated eyes—the most common of the milder symptoms. If pain and swelling occur, healthcare providers may prescribe a steroid such as prednisone. Other medications that suppress the immune response may also provide relief.

Special lenses for glasses can help with light sensitivity and double vision. People with eye symptoms may be advised to sleep with their head elevated to reduce eyelid swelling. If the eyelids do not fully close, taping them shut at night can help prevent dry eyes.

In more severe cases, external radiation may be applied to the eyes to reduce inflammation. Like other types of radiation treatment, the benefits are not immediate; most people feel relief from symptoms 1 to 2 months after treatment.

Surgery may be used to improve bulging of the eyes and correct the vision changes caused by pressure on the optic nerve. A procedure called orbital decompression makes the eye socket bigger and gives the eye room to sink back to a more normal position. Eyelid surgery can return retracted eyelids to their normal position.

Can Treatment for Graves Disease Affect Pregnancy?

Treatment for Graves disease can sometimes affect pregnancy. After treatment with surgery or radioactive iodine, TSI antibodies can still be present in the blood, even when thyroid levels are normal. If a pregnant woman has received either of these treatments prior to becoming pregnant, the antibodies she produces may travel across the placenta to the baby's bloodstream and stimulate the fetal thyroid.

A pregnant woman who has been treated with surgery or radioactive iodine should inform her healthcare provider so her baby can be monitored for thyroid-related problems later in the pregnancy. Pregnant women may safely be treated with anti-thyroid medications.

Eating, Diet, and Nutrition

Experts recommend that people eat a balanced diet to obtain most nutrients.

Dietary Supplements

Iodine is an essential mineral for the thyroid. However, people with autoimmune thyroid disease may be sensitive to harmful side effects from iodine. Taking iodine drops or eating foods containing large amounts of iodine—such as seaweed, dulse, or kelp—may cause or worsen hyperthyroidism.

Women need more iodine when they are pregnant—about 250 micrograms a day—because the baby gets iodine from the mother's diet. In the United States, about 7 percent of pregnant women may not get enough iodine in their diet or through prenatal vitamins. Choosing iodized salt—salt supplemented with iodine—over plain salt and prenatal vitamins containing iodine will ensure this need is met.

To help ensure coordinated and safe care, people should discuss their use of dietary supplements, such as iodine, with their healthcare provider.

Section 43.5

Idiopathic Intracranial Hypertension

This section includes text excerpted from "Idiopathic Intracranial Hypertension," National Eye Institute (NEI), April 2014.T

What Is Idiopathic Intracranial Hypertension?

Intracranial hypertension is a condition due to high pressure within the spaces that surround the brain and spinal cord. These spaces are filled with cerebrospinal fluid (CSF), which cushions the brain from mechanical injury, provides nourishment, and carries away waste.

The most common symptoms of intracranial hypertension are headaches and visual loss, including blind spots, poor peripheral (side) vision, double vision, and short temporary episodes of blindness. Many patients experience permanent vision loss. Other common symptoms include pulsatile tinnitus (ringing in the ears) and neck and shoulder pain.

Intracranial hypertension can be either acute or chronic. In chronic intracranial hypertension, the increased CSF pressure can cause swelling and damage to the optic nerve—a condition called papilledema.

Chronic intracranial hypertension can be caused by many conditions including certain drugs such as tetracycline, a blood clot in the brain, excessive intake of vitamin A, or brain tumor. It can also occur without a detectable cause. This is idiopathic intracranial hypertension (IIH).

Because the symptoms of IIH can resemble those of a brain tumor, it is sometimes known by the older name pseudotumor cerebri, which means "false brain tumor."

Who Is at Risk for Idiopathic Intracranial Hypertension?

An estimated 100,000 Americans have IIH, and the number is rising as more people become obese or overweight. The disorder is most common in women between the ages of 20 and 50; about 5 percent of those affected are men. Obesity, defined as a body mass index (BMI) greater than 30, is a major risk factor. BMI is a number based on your weight and height. A recent gain of 5–15 percent of total body weight is also considered a risk factor for this disorder, even for people with a BMI less than 30.

How Is Idiopathic Intracranial Hypertension Diagnosed?

A thorough medical history and physical exam are needed to identify risk factors for IIH and to evaluate for the many potential causes of increased intracranial pressure. A neurological exam will also be performed. In IIH, the exam is normal except for findings related to increased intracranial pressure, including papilledema, visual loss, and possible weakness in the lateral rectus muscles, which are located near your temples and help turn the eyes outward. Weakness in these muscles can cause the eyes to turn inward, toward the nose, producing double vision.

A number of vision tests may also be performed, including a comprehensive dilated eye exam to look for signs of papilledema. Visual field testing is done to evaluate your peripheral vision. This testing measures the area of space you can see at a given instant without moving your head or eyes.

Brain imaging, including computed tomography (CT) and magnetic resonance imaging (MRI) scans, will be performed to look for a brain tumor, injury, or other potential cause for your symptoms. Normal findings on these exams are essential to a diagnosis of IIH.

A lumbar puncture, also known as a spinal tap, will be performed. In this procedure, a needle is inserted into a CSF-filled sac below the spinal cord in the lower back. The CSF pressure will be measured, and a small amount of CSF will be collected for analysis to look for causes of increased intracranial pressure. The procedure may also cause a temporary reduction in CSF pressure and symptoms.

How Is Idiopathic Intracranial Hypertension Treated?

If a diagnosis of IIH is confirmed, regular visual field tests and comprehensive dilated eye exams are recommended to monitor any changes in vision.

Sustainable weight loss through healthy eating, salt restriction, and exercise is a critical part of treatment for people with IIH who are overweight. Studies show that modest weight loss, around 5–10 percent of total body weight, may be sufficient to reduce signs and symptoms. If lifestyle changes are not successful in reducing weight and relieving IIH, weight loss surgery may be recommended for those with a BMI greater than 40.

For many people, weight loss can be difficult to achieve and maintain. And for those who are able to adjust their weight, relief from IIH tends to be gradual. Acetazolamide (Diamox), a drug that decreases CSF production, is therefore often used as an add-on therapy to weight loss. The drug is taken orally. Common side effects include fatigue, nausea, tingling hands and feet, and a metallic taste, usually triggered by carbonated drinks. These can be reversed by lowering the dose or stopping the drug.

It's important to remember that some medications, such as tetracycline, may help trigger IIH, and that stopping them may lead to improvement.

In rapidly progressive cases that do not respond to other treatments, surgery may be needed to relieve pressure on the optic nerve. Therapeutic shunting, which involves surgically inserting a tube to drain CSF from ventricles or inner brain cavities, can be used to remove excess CSF and lower pressure. In a procedure called optic nerve sheath fenestration, pressure on the optic nerve is relieved by making a small window into the covering that surrounds the nerve just behind the eyeball.

What Is the Prognosis?

For most people, IIH usually improves with treatment. For others, it progressively worsens with time, or it can resolve and then recur. About 5–10 percent of women with IIH experience disabling vision loss. Most patients do not need surgical treatment.

Section 43.6

Multiple Sclerosis

This section contains text excerpted from the following sources: Text in this section begins with excerpts from "Multiple Sclerosis," Genetic and Rare Diseases Information Center (GARD), National Center for Advancing Translational Sciences (NCATS), November 21, 2015; Text beginning with the heading "Visual Dysfunction in Multiple Sclerosis" is excerpted from "Visual Dysfunction in Multiple Sclerosis," U.S. Department of Veterans Affairs (VA), September 2009. Reviewed March 2017.

Multiple sclerosis (MS) is a degenerative disorder that affects the central nervous system, specifically the brain and the spinal cord. The disorder is characterized by destruction of the myelin, the fatty tissue that surrounds and protects the nerve fibers and promotes the transmission of nerve impulses, and damage to nerve cells. The symptoms vary widely from person to person, and may include sensory disturbances in the limbs, problems with muscle control, tremors, muscle stiffness (spasticity), exaggerated reflexes (hyperreflexia), weakness, difficulty walking, poor bladder control, and vision problems. Most patients have periods during which they have symptoms (clinical attacks). The clinical attacks are typically followed by periods without any symptoms (remission). After several years, the symptoms worsen continuously. MS is considered an autoimmune disorder but the exact cause is unknown. Risk factors for developing multiple sclerosis include genetic factors like changes in the *HLA-DRB1* gene and in the *IL7R* gene and environmental factors, such as exposure to the Epstein-Barr virus, low levels of vitamin D, and smoking. The goal of treatment of MS is to decrease attacks and the inflammation within the central nervous system.

Visual Dysfunction in Multiple Sclerosis

Patients with multiple sclerosis (MS) can have many different kinds of vision problems, including optic neuritis, diplopia, and nystagmus.

Optic Neuritis

What Is Optic Neuritis?

Optic neuritis is blurry vision or hazy vision affecting one eye. It is usually associated with some eye pain or discomfort, especially with eye movements. Often the center of vision is most affected, making it difficult to see people's faces or creating a "line" in the center of their vision. More than half of all MS patients will experience optic neuritis at one point in their lives. In fact, for 15–20 percent of patients, optic neuritis will be the first presentation of their MS. On examination, a patient with optic neuritis often has an afferent pupillary defect (APD), which is an asymmetry in the two pupils' reaction to light. Initially, the optic nerve head may look normal or mildly swollen. Later on, the optic nerve may develop pallor (paleness).

Can Optic Neuritis Improve?

The good news is that optic neuritis usually gets better, though the vision in the affected eye may not return 100 percent. Vision in the affected eye might not be as clear as before, and colors may seem faded or "washed out." Depth perception is often not as good after an episode of optic neuritis.

What Is the Treatment for Optic Neuritis?

MS patients are often given intravenous methylprednisolone (also known as Solu-Medrol®) for optic neuritis. The steroids do not appear to improve visual outcome in the end, but they do seem to speed up the recovery of vision.

Double Vision (Diplopia)

What Is Double Vision?

Double vision, or diplopia, occurs when the eyes are not moving together so that the brain is getting two slightly different pictures simultaneously. This typically occurs when MS affects the brainstem, where the coordination of eye movements is controlled. One common cause of double vision in MS is an internuclear ophthal-moplegia (also known as an INO). Rarely, MS patients may develop double vision from a sixth nerve palsy or other neuro-ophthalmologic disorder.

Sometimes the patient does not see two completely separate images. MS patients may report a "shadow" or a "blur" instead of frank double vision. An important question to ask is whether the visual problem goes away if either eye is closed. Because diplopia is caused by the brain receiving two different images, one from each eye, as soon as either eye is closed, this type of visual problem will go away. On examination, there may be an obvious problem with the movement of the eyes, but sometimes the misalignment is not easy to see without special equipment.

What Is the Treatment for Double Vision?

Diplopia often resolves on its own. As with optic neuritis, intravenous corticosteroids are often prescribed, in the hopes of speeding up the recovery. Patients may need to wear an eye patch temporarily. The eye patch is guaranteed to "cure" the diplopia, since only one eye will be sending an image to the brain, but some patients may feel self-conscious while wearing the patch. Sometimes, if recovery is incomplete, eyeglasses with prisms can be used to bring the eyes back into alignment. Prism eyeglasses are similar to prescription eyeglasses for reading. The prism prescription and can be added to an already existing eyeglass prescription. In rare cases, strabismus surgery (surgery to correct crossed eye) may be recommended to realign the eyes.

Nystagmus

What Is Nystagmus?

Nystagmus is an involuntary, rhythmic movement of the eyes that can be associated with vertigo (a feeling of "dizziness"), oscillopsia (the illusion that the world is "jumping" or "swinging back and forth"), blurry vision, or diplopia. Nystagmus can occur in the setting of an INO, or due to an MS attack in the vestibular part of the brainstem or cerebellum.

The nystagmus may be visible when the patient is looking straight ahead, but sometimes is only present when the patient is looking off to the side, up, or down. If the nystagmus is very mild, it may only be perceptible while using an ophthalmoscope.

What Are the Treatments for Nystagmus?

Nystagmus can be difficult to treat if it does not resolve on its own. Various medications may help dampen down the nystagmus, including clonazepam (Klonopin®), baclofen (Lioresal®), gabapentin (Neurontin®), and memantine (Namenda®). In rare instances, surgery or botulinum toxin (Botox®) may help.

Summary

In summary, vision can be impaired by MS in many different ways. MS patients with visual problems may benefit from an evaluation by both a neurologist and an ophthalmologist, or a neuro-ophthalmologist if one is available. An accurate analysis of the exact visual problem will help lead to possible treatment options.

Section 43.7

Ocular Rosacea

This section includes text excerpted from "Questions and Answers about Rosacea," National Institute of Arthritis and Musculoskeletal and Skin Diseases (NIAMS), April 2016.

What Is Rosacea?

Rosacea is a chronic (long-term) disease that affects the skin and sometimes the eyes. The disorder is characterized by redness, pimples, and, in advanced stages, thickened skin. Rosacea usually affects the face. Skin on other parts of the upper body is only rarely involved.

Who Gets Rosacea?

Rosacea most often affects middle-age and older adults. It is more common in women (particularly during menopause) than men. Although rosacea can develop in people of any skin color, it tends to occur most frequently and is most apparent in people with fair skin.

What Are the Symptoms of Rosacea?

There are several symptoms and conditions associated with rosacea. These include frequent flushing, vascular rosacea, inflammatory rosacea, and several other conditions involving the skin, eyes, and nose.

Frequent flushing of the center of the face, which may include the forehead, nose, cheeks, and chin, occurs in the earliest stage of rosacea. The flushing often is accompanied by a burning sensation, particularly when creams or cosmetics are applied to the face. Sometimes the face is swollen slightly.

A condition called vascular rosacea causes persistent flushing and redness. Blood vessels under the skin of the face may dilate (enlarge), showing through the skin as small red lines. This is called telangiectasia. The affected skin may be swollen slightly and feel warm.

A condition called inflammatory rosacea causes persistent redness and papules (pink bumps) and pustules (bumps containing pus) on the skin. Eye inflammation and sensitivity as well as telangiectasia also may occur.

In the most advanced stage of rosacea, the skin becomes a deep shade of red and inflammation of the eye is more apparent. Numerous telangiectases are often present, and nodules in the skin may become painful. A condition called rhinophyma also may develop in some men; it is rare in women. Rhinophyma is characterized by an enlarged, bulbous, and red nose resulting from enlargement of the sebaceous (oil-producing) glands beneath the surface of the skin on the nose. People who have rosacea also may develop a thickening of the skin on the forehead, chin, cheeks, or other areas.

In addition to skin problems, many people who have rosacea have eye problems caused by the condition. Typical symptoms include redness, dryness, itching, burning, tearing, and the sensation of having sand in the eye. The eyelids may become inflamed and swollen. Some people say their eyes are sensitive to light and their vision is blurred or otherwise impaired.

What Causes Rosacea?

Doctors do not know the exact cause of rosacea but believe that some people may inherit a tendency to develop the disorder. People who blush frequently may be more likely to develop rosacea. Some researchers believe that rosacea is a disorder where blood vessels dilate too easily, resulting in flushing and redness.

Factors that cause rosacea to flare up in one person may have no effect on another person. Although the following factors have not been well-researched, some people claim that one or more of them have aggravated their rosacea: heat (including hot baths), strenuous exercise, sunlight, wind, very cold temperatures, hot or spicy foods and drinks, alcohol consumption, menopause, emotional stress, long-term use of topical steroids on the face, and bacteria.

How Is Rosacea Treated?

Although there is no cure for rosacea, it can be treated and controlled. A dermatologist (a medical doctor who specializes in diseases of the skin) usually treats rosacea. The goals of treatment are to control the condition and improve the appearance of the patient's skin. It may take several weeks or months of treatment before a person notices an improvement of the skin.

Treatments for rosacea include medicines that are applied directly to the affected skin. Some doctors will prescribe a topical antibiotic, which is applied directly to the affected skin. For people with more severe cases, doctors may prescribe an oral (taken by mouth) antibiotic.

Patients can play an important role in managing rosacea. You can take several steps to keep rosacea under control:

- Keep a written record of when flares occur. This may provide clues about what is irritating the skin.

- Use sunscreen. Most people should use a sunscreen every day that protects against UVA and UVB rays (ultraviolet rays) and has a sun-protecting factor (SPF) of 15 or higher, but sunscreen is particularly important for people whose skin is irritated by exposure to the sun.

- Use a mild lubricant if you find it is helpful, but avoid applying any irritating products to the face. Some people find that a green-tinted makeup effectively conceals skin redness.

Doctors usually treat the eye problems of rosacea with prescription eye medicine. People who develop infections of the eyelids must practice frequent eyelid hygiene. The doctor may recommend scrubbing the eyelids gently with diluted baby shampoo or an over-the-counter eyelid cleaner and applying warm (but not hot) compresses several times a day. Electrosurgery, dermabrasion, and laser surgery may be used if red lines caused by dilated blood vessels appear in the skin or if skin thickening develops.

Ask the doctor about how to manage rosacea and what treatment options are best for you. A combination of treatments may work best. Find out:

- How long the treatment may last.
- How long it will take to see results.
- What the possible side effects are.
- What you should do if the side effects are severe.

Part Seven

Living with Low Vision

Chapter 44

Defining Vision Impairment

Chapter Contents

Section 44.1

What Is Low Vision?

This section includes text excerpted from "Living with
Low Vision: What You Should Know," National Eye
Institute (NEI), September 2016.

What Is Low Vision?

When you have low vision, eyeglasses, contact lenses, medicine,
or surgery may not help. Activities like reading, shopping, cooking,
writing, and watching TV may be hard to do.

In fact, millions of Americans lose some of their sight every year.
While vision loss can affect anyone at any age, low vision is most common for those over age 65.

Low vision is usually caused by eye diseases or health conditions.
Some of these include age-related macular degeneration (AMD),
cataract, diabetes, and glaucoma. Eye injuries and birth defects
are some other causes. Whatever the cause, lost vision cannot be
restored. It can, however, be managed with proper treatment and
vision rehabilitation.

You should visit an eye care professional if you experience any
changes to your eyesight.

How Do I Know If I Have Low Vision?

Below are some signs of low vision. Even when wearing your glasses
or contact lenses, do you still have difficulty with—

- recognizing the faces of family and friends?

- reading, cooking, sewing, or fixing things around the house?

- selecting and matching the color of your clothes?

- seeing clearly with the lights on or feeling like they are dimmer
  than normal?

- reading traffic signs or the names of stores?

These could all be early warning signs of vision loss or eye disease. The sooner vision loss or eye disease is detected by an eye care professional, the greater your chances of keeping your remaining vision.

How Do I Know When to Get an Eye Exam?

Visit your eye care professional regularly for a comprehensive dilated eye exam. However, if you notice changes to your eyes or eyesight, visit your eye care professional right away!

What Can I Do If I Have Low Vision?

To cope with vision loss, you must first **have an excellent support team**. This team should include you, your primary eye care professional, and an optometrist or ophthalmologist specializing in low vision.

Occupational therapists, orientation and mobility specialists, certified low vision therapists, counselors, and social workers are also available to help.

Together, the low vision team can help you make the most of your remaining vision and maintain your independence.

Second, **talk with your eye care professional** about your vision problems. Even though it may be difficult, ask for help. Find out where you can get more information about support services and adaptive devices. Also, find out which services and devices are best for you and which will give you the most independence.

Third, **ask about vision rehabilitation**, even if your eye care professional says that "nothing more can be done for your vision."

Vision rehabilitation programs offer a wide range of services, including training for magnifying and adaptive devices, ways to complete daily living skills safely and independently, guidance on modifying your home, and information on where to locate resources and support to help you cope with your vision loss.

Medicare may cover part or all of a patient's occupational therapy, but the therapy must be ordered by a doctor and provided by a Medicare-approved healthcare provider. To see if you are eligible for Medicare-funded occupational therapy, call 800–MEDICARE or 800–633–4227.

Finally, **be persistent**. Remember that you are your best healthcare advocate. Explore your options, learn as much as you can, and keep asking questions about vision rehabilitation. In fact, write down questions to ask your doctor before your exam, and bring along a notepad to jot down answers.

There are many resources to help people with low vision, and many of these programs, devices, and technologies can help you maintain your normal, everyday way of life.

What Questions Should I Ask My Eye Care Team?

An important part of any doctor–patient relationship is effective communication. Here are some questions to ask your eye care professional or specialist in low vision to jumpstart the discussion about vision loss.

Questions to Ask Your Eye Care Professional

- What changes can I expect in my vision?

- Will my vision loss get worse? How much of my vision will I lose?

- Will regular eyeglasses improve my vision?

- What medical or surgical treatments are available for my condition?

- What can I do to protect or prolong my vision?

- Will diet, exercise, or other lifestyle changes help?

- If my vision can't be corrected, can you refer me to a specialist in low vision?

- Where can I get vision rehabilitation services?

Questions to Ask Your Specialist in Low Vision

- How can I continue my normal, routine activities?

- Are there resources to help me in my job?

- Will any special devices help me with daily activities like reading, sewing, cooking, or fixing things around the house?

- What training and services are available to help me live better and more safely with low vision?

- Where can I find individual or group support to cope with my vision loss?

Section 44.2

What Is Legal Blindness?

Complete or total blindness is the inability to see light, shapes, or anything at all. But legal blindness, as defined by government agencies and statutes, has a different meaning. It refers to a specific level of visual impairment that is required by law for a person to qualify for government-funded disability benefits, or for a person to be disqualified from engaging in certain government-regulated activities (such as driving a car). About 1.3 million people in the United States, or about 0.5 percent of the population, are considered legally blind.

Definition of Legal Blindness

The generally accepted definition of legal blindness includes measurements of two aspects of eyesight: central visual acuity, and field of vision. Having a certain level of visual impairment in either measurement—with corrective eyeglasses or contact lenses—meets the definition of legal blindness. The levels of visual impairment required by the Social Security Administration (SSA) and most other U.S. government agencies are as follows:

- Reduced central visual acuity of 20/200 or less in your better eye with use of the best eyeglass lens or contact lens to correct your eyesight, or

- Limitation of your field of view such that the widest diameter of the visual field in your better eye is no greater than 20°.

Reduced Visual Acuity

Visual acuity is the clarity or sharpness of eyesight. It is measured using a Snellen eye chart, which has rows of letters that gradually decrease in size from top to bottom. The patient typically stands about 20 feet (6 meters) away from the chart, covers one eye, and tries to read the letters on each line. The size of the letters on one of the lines corresponds to normal visual acuity, or what a person with normal eyesight can read from a distance of 20 feet.

Using the Snellen system, a person with normal visual acuity is said to have 20/20 vision. The numerator (top number) of the Snellen fraction refers to the patient's distance from the eye chart, while the denominator (bottom number) refers to the distance at which a person with normal visual acuity can read that line. Therefore, a person with 20/200 vision standing 20 feet away from the eye chart can only read letters that a person with normal visual acuity can read from 200 feet away. In other words, a legally blind person has vision that is 10 times worse than that of a normally sighted person.

To be considered legally blind, a person's visual acuity must be 20/200 or less even while they are using the best possible corrective lenses. If wearing eyeglasses or contact lenses improves their vision beyond that measurement—even in just one eye—they do not meet the definition of legal blindness.

Limited Visual Field

The second aspect of eyesight included in the definition of legal blindness is visual field, also known as peripheral vision. People with a normal field of vision will be able to see almost 180° laterally (directly to either side) and 135° vertically (up and down) without moving their heads. People who are legally blind due to a restricted visual field can see a maximum of 20° in any direction. Their field of vision may be limited in all directions, creating a condition known as tunnel vision, or it may be limited in multiple areas by the presence of blind spots. Peripheral vision is vital to personal safety in many everyday activities, such as driving a car or walking across a street. As a result, people with a severely restricted visual field are considered legally blind even if their central visual acuity is 20/20.

Causes of Legal Blindness

Some people are born with visual disabilities that affect their sight to the point that they are considered legally blind. Some of the conditions that may lead to a diagnosis of legal blindness include congenital cataracts, infantile glaucoma, and retinopathy of prematurity. Many other people become legally blind later in life due to health conditions that affect the eyes, such as age-related macular degeneration (AMD or ARMD), cataracts, diabetic retinopathy, and glaucoma.

Tests for Legal Blindness

Legal blindness must be diagnosed by an eye doctor as part of a comprehensive eye examination. The eye doctor will test the patient's central visual acuity using a Snellen chart while the patient is wearing corrective lenses. If the corrected visual acuity is below 20/200, the patient will be diagnosed as legally blind.

There are several different methods of testing the patient's field of vision. One example is a perimetry test, in which the patient stares at a dot inside a machine. The machine flashes lights at various points around the visual field, and the patient pushes a button each time they see a flash. At the end of the test, the machine prints a report showing gaps or blind spots within the patient's field of vision. If the diameter of the visual field measures less than 20°, the patient will be diagnosed as legally blind.

Upon receiving a diagnosis of legal blindness, a person may become eligible for government-funded disability benefits in the form of financial assistance, tax deductions, educational accommodations, and job training. There are also a number of service organizations that provide training and resources to help people who are legally blind to live independently.

References

1. Hellem, Amy. "What Does 'Legally Blind' Mean?" All About Vision, February 2017.

2. "Legally Blind," Think about Your Eyes, 2016.

3. Wachler, Brian Boxer. "What Does It Mean to Be Legally Blind?" WebMD, 2015.

Chapter 45

Tips for People with Low Vision

Chapter Contents

Section 45.1

Devices to Help Low Vision

This section contains text excerpted from the following sources:
Text in this section begins with excerpts from "Help for People with
Vision Loss," National Eye Institute (NEI), December 22, 2016; Text
beginning with the heading "Magnifying Devices" is excerpted from
"Magnifying Devices," U.S. Library of Congress (LOC), 2014.

Here's eye-opening news: Currently, 4.2 million Americans ages 40
and older are visually impaired. Of these, 3 million have low vision. By
2030, when the last baby boomers turn 65, the number of Americans
who have visual impairments is projected to reach 7.2 million, with 5
million having low vision.

For the millions of people who currently live or will live with low
vision, the good news is there is help.

But first, what is low vision? Low vision is when even with regular
glasses, contact lenses, medicine, or surgery, people have difficulty
seeing, which makes everyday tasks difficult to do. Activities that used
to be simple like reading the mail, shopping, cooking, and writing can
become challenging.

Most people with low vision are age 65 or older. The leading causes
of vision loss in older adults are age-related macular degeneration,
diabetic retinopathy, cataract, and glaucoma. Among younger people,
vision loss is most often caused by inherited eye conditions, infectious
and autoimmune eye diseases, or trauma. For people with low vision,
maximizing their remaining sight is key to helping them continue to
live safe, productive, and rewarding lives.

The first step is to seek help.

"I encourage anyone with low vision to seek guidance about vision
rehabilitation from a low vision specialist," advises Paul A. Sieving,
M.D., Ph.D., director of the National Eye Institute (NEI), one of the
National Institutes of Health (NIH) and the federal government's
principal agency for vision research.

Who is a low vision specialist? A low vision specialist is an ophthalmologist or optometrist who works with people who have low vision.
A low vision specialist can develop a vision rehabilitation plan that

identifies strategies and assistive devices appropriate for the person's particular needs. "A vision rehabilitation plan helps people reach their true visual potential when nothing more can be done from a medical or surgical standpoint," explains Mark Wilkinson, O.D., a low vision specialist at the University of Iowa Hospitals and Clinics and chair of the low vision subcommittee for the National Eye Health Education Program (NEHEP).

Vision rehabilitation can include the following:

- Training to use magnifying and adaptive devices

- Teaching new daily living skills to remain safe and live independently

- Developing strategies to navigate around the home and in public

- Providing resources and support

Magnifying Devices

Magnifying devices assist people with low vision to engage more easily in activities such as reading standard print, enjoying a hobby, or viewing a presentation by increasing the size of text and objects. Magnifiers come in many weights and styles. They may be attached to a handle or a neck cord, on a stand, or as a headset. Prices vary based on factors such as the material and strength of the lens and the type of illumination (if any).

Before buying a magnification device, one should consult a low-vision specialist for evaluation. A local vision-rehabilitation facility may offer information on available resources.

Types of Magnifying Devices

- **Bar magnifiers** provide magnification for one or two lines of type at a time, lie flat on the reading surface, and can be moved down the page as reading progresses. Many have feet to raise the magnifier a few inches above the material.

- **Binocular magnifiers** are worn around the head, either alone or over prescription or safety eyeglasses, for close-up precision use. Some have features such as an adjustable headband or a flip-up frame to move the magnifier out of view.

- **Dome/Globe magnifiers** have a spherical shape that can lay flat on a small reading surface or can be held and used vertically for activities such as threading a needle or reading a thermometer.

- **Fresnel/Page magnifiers** come in a variety of sizes and are useful for viewing an extensive field of text, such as books, puzzles, maps, or a telephone directory. They may be framed or unframed, and may be hand-held or attached to a stand that can sit on a table with an object underneath, or be placed in front of a computer monitor.

- **Hand-held magnifiers** are useful for spot tasks such as reading a label on a medicine bottle, checking a price tag, or consulting a map. Illuminated and non-illuminated models in round or rectangular shapes are available.

- **Magnifying lamps** are available in a variety of models that feature different magnification levels, illumination levels, types of light bulbs, color of light emitted from the magnifier, size of the lens, and weight of the magnifier. A magnifying lamp is usually attached to a flexible arm that can be moved over the reading material.

- **Neck/Pendant magnifiers** rest on the chest and are supported by adjustable cords around the neck. This allows both hands to be free to hold reading material or to work on sewing or other tasks. These come in illuminated and non-illuminated models.

- **Pocket magnifiers** may be housed in hard plastic cases that slide or snap open and shut, or in soft covers that can be used as a handle. They may come with two or more lenses that can be used singly or in combination, and are available in illuminated and non-illuminated models.

- **Screen magnifiers** may be hardware or software. They display the information on a computer or television screen in a variety of magnifications. Some may be used with speech. The software programs are compatible with many computer applications. Some programs offer free trial versions to download.

- **Stand magnifiers** are set in holders that are attached to small legs or other supports. They sit above the page in a frame that is fixed or at a tilt so it automatically maintains a consistent distance from the reading material and remains in focus, even if the user has unsteady hands or tremors. These come in illuminated and non-illuminated models.

- **Video magnifiers** or closed-circuit television (CCTV) systems enlarge print and graphic materials electronically on monitor screens. The screens may be mounted on fixed stands or handheld.

Section 45.2

Everyday Fitness for People with Low Vision

This section includes text excerpted from "Exercise for People with Low Vision," *Go4Life*, National Institutes of Health (NIH), January 24, 2017.

People with low vision can be active in many ways! Before you start an exercise routine, however, talk with your medical doctor and your eye doctor, since bending, lifting, or rapid movement can affect some medical and eye conditions

A fitness instructor at a local gym or community center can help you create an effective exercise program and teach proper form. If you're working out at home:

- Ask a partner to read the exercise descriptions and check your form until you learn the exercises.

- Try the *Go4Life* exercises (www.go4life.nia.nih.gov/exercises). Many can be done sitting down. For others, you can use a sturdy chair, counter, or wall for support.

Walking is great exercise, but play it safe:

- Walk with someone who can point out safety issues along your route, such as objects in your path.

- Take a brisk walk at the mall. Many "mall walking" groups meet before stores open.

Tandem cycling can be highly social, a lot of fun, and good exercise! In addition to providing a great workout, it teaches teamwork.

- A sighted rider sits on the front seat of the "bicycle built for two" and communicates what's ahead to the person sitting on the back seat.

- You may not have to steer, but your partner will appreciate help with pedaling!

Bowling is not only possible, but also highly competitive. You can bowl with sighted guidance or using a guide rail. A sighted assistant aligns the bowler on the approach before the delivery. Lightweight metal rails help guide you straight toward the pins.

Swimming is another excellent endurance activity.

- If you swim laps, count the number of strokes it takes to cover the length of the pool so you can slow down as you approach the end of your lane.

- A pool with ropes separating the lanes helps you stay in your lane and maintain your orientation.

Chapter 46

Home Modifications for People with Low Vision

We've all dealt with a stubbed toe or a bump on the head when our vision isn't cooperating. Here are a few tips and ideas to incorporate into your home environment to reduce trips to the medicine cabinet!

The Bedroom

We spend most of our time in the bedroom when it is dark outside and we rely on lights placed around the room to guide us. Unfortunately, most light projects up toward the ceiling or walls, instead of the floor where we need it most. Use a bed ruffle of a contrasting color to help identify the edge of a bed to prevent bumping into the bed post. Throw rugs of contrasting colors are also helpful if the edges are taped down to avoid tripping or slipping on the edge. Use nightlights to illuminate a pathway from the bedroom to the kitchen or bathroom, so you can move about without turning on the lights.

This chapter contains text excerpted from the following sources: Text in this chapter begins with excerpts from "Home Modifications for Low Vision," © 2017 The Gavin Herbert Eye Institute, UC Irvine. Reprinted with permission; Text beginning with the heading "Lighting Tips for Low Vision Patients" is excerpted from "Helping Your Loved One with Low Vision," U.S. Department of Veterans Affairs (VA), June 21, 2012. Reviewed March 2017.

The Kitchen

Cabinets can be unexpected hazards. By adding lighting under overhead cabinets, the corners and edges of cabinets become more distinct. Applying a strip of LED lights underneath the shelves can help guide you and your eyes to the edge of the shelf.

Stairs

Navigating stairways can be a challenge. Judging the depth when walking downstairs can be difficult, especially if there is poor lighting in the stairwell. Applying a strip of contrasting color or texture to the edge of wooden or metal steps can help guide and assist your step. Also, painting hand rails a contrasting color from the wall can give additional visual guidance.

Occupational or rehabilitation therapists can come to your home and perform an 'audit', giving you specific recommendations for your living space. Ask your optometrist or ophthalmologist for assistance in obtaining a referral to a local agency.

Lighting Tips for Low Vision Patients

- **Increase illumination.** Use floor or table lamps, illuminated magnifiers and flashlights. As we age, we require more light to see well. A visually impaired person may require even more lighting.

- **Decrease glare from lighting.** Glare can reduce vision and cause fatigue. You may be prescribed special tints for indoor and outdoor use.

- **Use goose-neck lamps to provide good illumination.** These lamps are adjustable so they do not increase additional glare.

Low Vision Medication Safety Tips

- Attach a white label with large black print to medication bottles.

- Place your pills on a contrasting color mat so that they will be visible. White pills on a counter top are hard to see.

- Use hand magnifiers to see print.

- Use a talking recorder that is made for medicine bottles such as Script Talk that can record your medicine name and dosage.

- Use a medicine organizer. These are available in large print.

Low Vision Safety Tips for the Home

- Area rugs can be used to define areas but the edges should be tacked down to prevent tripping and falling.

- Floor coverings can be a help or a hindrance some things to remember:

- plain floor covering rather than patterned floor coverings is easier to visualize

- thresholds should not be more than ¼ inch high to prevent tripping

- To increase safety and visibility using stairs localized lighting (like in movie theaters) can be helpful.

- Make sure the handrail to the steps is visible in a contrasting color from the wall.

- Most falls happen on the top stair step so this step should be marked with a different color or illuminated to make contrast. This is also a good idea for the last step as well.

- Use track lighting in hallway or a chair/guide rail to act as a guide.

- Install a runner in a contrasting color down the center of a hallway to serve as guide. **BE SURE TO TACK DOWN THE EDGES TO AVOID TRIPPING.**

- Use different textures in halls and adjacent rooms to provide tactile cues.

- When purchasing tables, consider using ovals or round tables to avoid hitting sharp corners in the event of a fall.

Low Vision Tips for in the Kitchen

Eating

- Use dishes that have dark side and light side to provide contrast to your food.

- Avoid patterns on dinnerware.

- Use placemats or table clothes to increase contrast.
- Do **NOT** use clear glasses or dishes as they appear invisible.
- Use a goose neck lamp directly over your plate.
- Have a system for placing food on the plate, for example, meat at 6:00, potatoes at 9:00 and vegetables at 3:00.
- Eat food inward from the edge to avoid pushing food on the table.

Cooking

- To avoid burns, get in the habit of shutting the burner off before removing food. **Know the off position of the stove knobs.**
- To judge liquid levels, use pots or containers with a white interior to see dark colored liquids and black interiors with white liquids.
- Attach lights to underside of cabinets to improve illumination. Try not to create glare.
- Organize shelves systematically and in alphabetical order.
- Have a system for locating food in the pantry and refrigerator.
- Do not wear loose clothing that could catch on fire.
- Turn pan handles inward from the stove or counter to avoid spills and burns.
- Use Corel or plastic dishes if you are worried about broken glass.
- Set a timer or turn on a light to remind you that the stove or oven is on.
- Mark dials on microwave, stove and refrigerators.
- Use special aids for the kitchen:
  - Large print kitchen timer
  - Cutting board with a black side and a white side to enhance contrast
  - Special measuring cups that enhance contrast
  - Use a knife with an adjustable slicing guide
  - Use an audible liquid level guide when pouring

Low Vision Tips for the Home Workshop

- Use good lighting. Many workshops do not have many windows, and lighting is very important when it comes to making near tasks easier.

- Use a swing arm or gooseneck lamp that can be placed over tools and machines while they are being used.

- Organize tools and mark with larger numbers or bump dots so they are easily located.

- Put contrasting tape on the handles of tools for easy visibility.

- Use a large print measuring tape.

- Make measuring marks with a felt tip pen for heavy black lines that are easier to see.

- Use magnifiers on a gooseneck stand to provide magnification.

- USE SAFETY GOGGLES at all times.

Low Vision Tips for Watching Television

- To see your television more clearly, adjust the rooms lighting to avoid glare that interferes with the images on the television.

- Sit closer to the television. Sitting one foot in front of the TV will **NOT** hurt your eyes.

- Use a large print television remote control or mark your remote control for greater visibility.

- To see your TV more clearly, place it in front of your recliner or buy a larger TV. A high definition television has the most contrast and resolution and may be easier to see.

- Open or close drapes or curtains to adjust for glare. Some people will find that bright illumination is helpful while others find it increases glare problems.

Low Vision Tips for Writing

- To make print easier to see, use a black felt marker (such as a Sharpie) or a gel pen.

- Use special heavy lined paper made specifically for people with vision impairment.

- Place light-colored paper on a dark surface to help define the edges.

- Use writing templates for envelopes, checks and writing paper.

- Use large print checks or checks with tactile lines.

- Use large print address books to keep track of phone numbers.

- Use large print calendars or voice memo recorders to keep track of appointments or important dates.

Chapter 47

Independence and Mobility for People with Low Vision

Experiencing visual impairment or vision loss does not necessarily put an end to independent travel. Orientation and mobility (O&M) is a profession dedicated to helping people with blindness and low vision learn how to move safely from one place to another. Orientation involves figuring out one's current location and then using environmental clues and landmarks to create and follow a mental map to one's desired destination. Mobility involves traveling efficiently and independently by walking or using transportation. O&M training provides children and adults who are blind or visually impaired with the skills and techniques they need to navigate confidently in the home, school, workplace, and community—usually by using a white cane.

Some people with low vision are able to continue driving a car with the help of bioptic lenses, which incorporate miniature telescopes into eyeglasses to magnify distant objects and increase reaction time. A variety of other transportation options are available for people who are no longer able to drive.

Orientation and Mobility

O&M specialists are trained in eye function, blindness, low vision, and the ways in which visual impairments affect people's ability to

"Independence and Mobility for People with Low Vision," © 2017 Omnigraphics. Reviewed March 2017.

perform activities of daily living and travel independently. Although they do not provide physical rehabilitation services, O&M specialists do offer instruction in skills, techniques, and strategies for using a cane, detecting environmental clues, and interpreting sensory information in order to navigate safely and efficiently. They provide services across the lifespan, from infants to elderly adults, through schools, rehabilitation centers, and community programs.

Some of the orientation techniques, travel skills, and mobility instruction offered by O&M specialists include the following:

- Developing and using senses of hearing, smell, and touch to gather information about one's current location;

- Using a cane or other assistive devices to navigate safely and independently;

- Employing human guide techniques to move through various types of indoor and outdoor environments;

- Learning to recognize spatial relationships between objects;

- Following directions, recognizing landmarks, and using navigation apps to locate destinations;

- Developing problem-solving skills for use when disoriented, lost, or forced to alter an established route;

- Learning how to ask for or decline assistance from passersby;

- Employing techniques for crossing streets, walking up and down stairs, and finding dropped objects;

- Using public transportation and transit systems independently.

Driving with Low Vision

For many people with vision impairments, the ability to drive a car is an important component of maintaining independence and freedom. Many states have established legal limits for the minimum visual acuity required to obtain a driver's license. Common standards are 20/40 or 20/60 vision with corrective lenses. People whose visual acuity falls below the limits may still be able to drive with the help of a bioptic lens system.

Bioptic lenses are eyeglasses that incorporate miniature telescopes near the top of the regular prescription lenses (known as carrier lenses), just above the normal line of sight. They enlarge road signs, hazards, and other objects to enable people with visual impairments to see them from a greater distance. Unlike binoculars, however, the user does not look through the bioptic lenses continuously. Instead, they spend 90 to 95 percent of the total driving time looking through the regular lenses and only glance through the bioptic telescopes briefly as needed to magnify distant objects.

The main advantage of bioptic lenses is that they give people with vision impairments additional time to react and make driving decisions and adjustments. The bioptic telescope increases the driver's ability to see distant objects by a factor of the power of the device, so a person using a 4x telescope could see a sign or road hazard from 80 feet away that they could only see from 20 feet away with their normal vision.

One of the main disadvantages of bioptic lenses is that sighting through the telescope obscures part of the normal field of vision, known as the ring scotoma. The missing visual information raises concerns that drivers using the lenses may not notice an obstacle, such as a pedestrian or a bicycle. Proponents of bioptic lenses point out that they provide a similar field of vision to the side and rearview mirrors in cars, and drivers must learn to use them in much the same way. They also argue that normally sighted drivers are equally likely to miss visual information on the road while they change the radio station or check their cell phones.

Bioptic lens systems must be prescribed by an optometrist or ophthalmologist. Most states allow people with low vision to apply for a driver's license while using bioptic lenses, but many states require them to complete formal driver education, including behind-the-wheel instruction, before being permitted to drive.

Arranging Transportation

For people with visual impairments who are not able to drive, finding reliable and affordable transportation can be difficult. Yet managing transportation is an important way to gain independence. People who live in areas without easy access to public transportation must be creative and well-organized to get where they need to go. Some potential transportation options for people with low vision include the following:

Hire a personal driver for a private vehicle that you own and maintain;

- Investigate government-subsidized voucher transportation programs offered through community or senior service centers;

- Check into free, volunteer-driver transportation options provided by local churches or community groups;

- Negotiate discounts with local taxi companies;

- Utilize on-demand ride-share services like Uber and Lyft.

References

1. Demmitt, Audrey. "The Transportation Problem: Finding Rides When You Can't Drive," VisionAware, August 20, 2014.

2. "Driving with Bioptics," Ocutech, 2016.

3. "Driving with Low Vision," VisionAware, 2017.

4. "Mobility: Independent Travel," Second Sense, 2017.

5. "Orientation and Mobility Skills," VisionAware, 2017.

Chapter 48

Low Vision and the Workplace

The Americans with Disabilities Act (ADA), which was amended by the Americans with Disabilities Act Amendments Act of 2008 ("Amendments Act" or "ADAAA"), is a federal law that prohibits discrimination against qualified individuals with disabilities. Individuals with disabilities include those who have impairments that substantially limit a major life activity, have a record (or history) of a substantially limiting impairment, or are regarded as having a disability.

Title I of the ADA covers employment by private employers with 15 or more employees as well as state and local government employers. Section 501 of the Rehabilitation Act provides similar protections related to federal employment. In addition, most states have their own laws prohibiting employment discrimination on the basis of disability. Some of these state laws may apply to smaller employers and may provide protections in addition to those available under the ADA.

This chapter includes text excerpted from "Questions and Answers about Blindness and Vision Impairments in the Workplace and the Americans with Disabilities Act (ADA)," U.S. Equal Employment Opportunity Commission (EEOC), March 6, 2017.

The U.S. Equal Employment Opportunity Commission (EEOC) enforces the employment provisions of the ADA. This chapter explains how the ADA applies to job applicants and employees with vision impairments.

General Information about Vision Impairments

Estimates vary as to the number of Americans who are blind and visually impaired. One reason for the different estimates is that different terminology is used to assess the number of individuals with some degree of vision problems. According to one estimate, approximately 6.6 million people in the United States are blind or visually impaired. Another estimate concluded that there are 10 million blind or visually impaired people in the United States and of these 1.3 million are considered legally blind.

The Centers for Disease Control and Prevention (CDC) define "vision impairment" to mean that a person's eyesight cannot be corrected to a "normal level." Vision impairment may result in a loss of visual acuity, where an individual does not see objects as clearly as the average person, and/or in a loss of visual field, meaning that an individual cannot see as wide an area as the average person without moving the eyes or turning the head. There are varying degrees of vision impairments, and the terms used to describe them are not always consistent. The CDC and the World Health Organization (WHO) define low vision as a visual acuity between 20/70 and 20/400 with the best possible correction, or a visual field of 20 degrees or less. Blindness is described as a visual acuity worse than 20/400 with the best possible correction, or a visual field of 10 degrees or less. In the United States, the term "legally blind," means a visual acuity of 20/200 or worse with the best possible correction, or a visual field of 20 degrees or less. Although there are varying degrees of vision impairments, the visual problems an individual faces cannot be described simply by the numbers; some people can see better than others with the same visual acuity.

There are many possible causes for vision impairment, including damage to the eye and the failure of the brain to interpret messages from the eyes correctly. The most common causes of vision impairment in American adults are: diabetic retinopathy, age-related macular degeneration (AMD), cataracts, and glaucoma. Additionally, many individuals have monocular vision—perfect or nearly perfect vision in one eye, but little or no vision in the other. Vision impairment can occur at any time in life, but adults aged 40 and older are at the greatest risk for eye diseases, such as cataract, diabetic retinopathy, glaucoma, and AMD.

Persons with vision impairments successfully perform a wide range of jobs and can be dependable workers. Yet, many employers still automatically exclude them from certain positions based on generalizations about vision impairments and false assumptions that it would be too expensive, or perhaps even too dangerous, to employ them. Thus, employers may erroneously assume that any accommodation that would allow a person with a vision impairment to do her job would be too costly. Employers also may have liability concerns related to the fear of accidents and/or injuries.

1. When does someone with a vision impairment have a disability within the meaning of the ADA?

As a result of changes made by the ADAAA, people who are blind should easily be found to have a disability within the meaning of the first part of the ADA's definition of disability because they are substantially limited in the major life activity of seeing. Individuals with a vision impairment other than blindness will meet the first part of the ADA's definition of disability if they can show that they are substantially limited in seeing or another major life activity (e.g., the major bodily function of special sense organs). A determination of disability must ignore the positive effects of any mitigating measure that is used. For example, a mitigating measure may include the use of low vision devices that magnify, enhance, or otherwise augment a visual image. Another type of mitigating measure is the use of learned behavioral modifications (for example, a person with monocular vision may turn his head from side to side to compensate for the lack of peripheral vision). A person with monocular vision, regardless of such compensating behaviors, will be substantially limited in seeing compared to most people in the general population.

2. Is everyone who wears glasses a person with a disability?

No, not everyone who wears glasses is a person with a disability under the ADA. Although the ADA generally requires that the positive effects of mitigating measures be ignored in assessing whether someone has a disability, the law requires that one consider the positive effects of the use of ordinary eyeglasses or contact lenses (that is, lenses that are intended to fully correct visual acuity or to eliminate refractive error). If the use of ordinary lenses results in no substantial limitation to a major life activity, then the person's vision impairment does not constitute a disability under the first part of the ADA's definition of disability.

573

Even though individuals who use ordinary eyeglasses or contact lenses that are intended to fully correct their vision will not be covered under the first definition of disability, they are protected from discrimination based on an employer's use of uncorrected vision standards that are not job-related and consistent with business necessity.

Individuals with a history of a vision impairment will be covered under the second part of the definition of disability if they have a record of an impairment that substantially limited a major life activity in the past (for example, where surgery corrected a past substantially limiting vision impairment). Finally, an individual is covered under the third ("regarded as") prong of the definition of disability if an employer takes a prohibited action (for example, refuses to hire or terminates the individual) because of a vision impairment or because the employer believes the individual has a vision impairment, other than an impairment that lasts fewer than six months and is minor.

Obtaining, Using, and Disclosing Medical Information

Title I of the ADA limits an employer's ability to ask questions related to blindness and other disabilities and to conduct medical examinations at three stages: pre-offer, post-offer, and during employment.

Job Applicants

Before an Offer of Employment Is Made

3. May an employer ask a job applicant whether he has or had a vision impairment or about his treatment related to any vision impairment prior to making a job offer?

No. An employer may not ask questions about an applicant's medical condition or require an applicant to have a medical examination before it makes a conditional job offer. This means that an employer cannot legally ask an applicant such questions as:

- whether she has ever had any medical procedures related to her vision (for example, whether the applicant ever had eye surgery);

- whether she uses any prescription medications, including medications for conditions related to the eye; or

- whether she has any condition that may have caused a vision impairment (for example, whether the applicant has diabetes).

Of course, an employer may ask questions pertaining to the applicant's ability to perform the essential functions of the position, with or without reasonable accommodation, such as:

- whether the applicant can read labels on packages that need to be stocked

- whether the applicant can work the night shift

- whether the applicant can inspect small electronic components to determine if they have been damaged.

4. Does the ADA require an applicant to disclose that she has or had a vision impairment or some other disability before accepting a job offer?

No. The ADA does not require applicants to disclose that they have or had a vision impairment or another disability unless they will need a reasonable accommodation for the application process (for example, written application materials to be printed in a larger font). Some individuals with a vision impairment, however, choose to disclose or discuss their condition to dispel myths about vision loss or to ensure that employers do not assume that the impairment means the person is unable to do the job.

Sometimes, the decision to disclose depends on whether an individual will need a reasonable accommodation to perform the job (for example, specialized equipment, removal of a marginal function, or another type of job restructuring). A person with a vision impairment, however, may request an accommodation after becoming an employee even if she did not do so when applying for the job or after receiving the job offer.

5. May an employer ask questions about an obvious vision impairment, or follow-up questions if an applicant discloses a non-obvious vision impairment?

No. An employer generally may not ask an applicant about obvious impairments. Nor may an employer ask an applicant who has voluntarily disclosed that he has a vision impairment any questions about the nature of the impairment, when it began, or how the individual copes with the impairment. However, if an applicant has an obvious impairment or has voluntarily disclosed the existence of a vision impairment and the employer reasonably believes that he will require an accommodation to perform the job because of the impairment, the employer may ask whether the applicant will need an accommodation and what type. The employer must keep any information an applicant discloses about his medical condition confidential.

After an Offer of Employment Is Made

After making a job offer, an employer may ask questions about the applicant's health (including questions about the applicant's disability) and may require a medical examination, as long as all applicants for the same type of job are treated equally (that is, all applicants are asked the same questions and are required to take the same examination). After an employer has obtained basic medical information from all individuals who have received job offers, it may ask specific individuals for more medical information if the request is medically related to the previously obtained medical information. For example, if an employer asks all applicants post-offer about their general physical and mental health, it can ask individuals who disclose a particular illness, disease, or impairment for medical information or require them to have a medical examination related to the condition disclosed.

6. What may an employer do when it learns that an applicant has or had a vision impairment after she has been offered a job but before she starts working?

When an applicant discloses after receiving a conditional job offer that she has or had a vision impairment, an employer may ask the applicant additional questions, such as how long she has had the vision impairment; what, if any, vision the applicant has; what specific visual limitations the individual experiences; and what, if any, reasonable accommodations the applicant may need to perform the job. The employer also may send the applicant for a follow-up vision or medical examination or ask her to submit documentation from her doctor answering questions specifically designed to assess her ability to perform the job's functions safely. Permissible follow-up questions at this stage differ from those at the pre-offer stage when an employer only may ask an applicant who voluntarily discloses a disability whether she needs an accommodation to perform the job and what type.

An employer may not withdraw an offer from an applicant with a vision impairment if the applicant is able to perform the essential functions of the job, with or without reasonable accommodation, without posing a direct threat (that is, a significant risk of substantial harm) to the health or safety of himself or others that cannot be eliminated or reduced through reasonable accommodation.

Employees

The ADA strictly limits the circumstances under which an employer may ask questions about an employee's medical condition or require the employee to have a medical examination. Once an employee is on the job, his actual performance is the best measure of ability to do the job.

7. When may an employer ask an employee if a vision impairment, or some other medical condition, may be causing her performance problems?

Generally, an employer may ask disability-related questions or require an employee to have a medical examination when it knows about a particular employee's medical condition, has observed performance problems, and reasonably believes that the problems are related to a medical condition. At other times, an employer may ask for medical information when it has observed symptoms, such as difficulties visually focusing, or has received reliable information from someone else (for example, a family member or co-worker) indicating that the employee may have a medical condition that is causing performance problems. Often, however, poor job performance is unrelated to a medical condition and generally should be handled in accordance with an employer's existing policies concerning performance.

8. Are there any other instances when an employer may ask an employee with a vision impairment about her condition?

Yes. An employer also may ask an employee about a vision impairment when it has a reasonable belief that the employee will be unable to safely perform the essential functions of her job because of the vision impairment. In addition, an employer may ask an employee about her vision impairment to the extent the information is necessary:

- to support the employee's request for a reasonable accommodation needed because of her vision impairment;

- to verify the employee's use of sick leave related to her vision impairment if the employer requires all employees to submit a doctor's note to justify their use of sick leave; or

- to enable the employee to participate in a voluntary wellness program.

Keeping Medical Information Confidential

With limited exceptions, an employer must keep confidential any medical information it learns about an applicant or employee. Under the following circumstances, however, an employer may disclose that an employee has a vision impairment:

- to supervisors and managers, if necessary to provide a reasonable accommodation or meet an employee's work restrictions;

- to first aid and safety personnel if an employee may need emergency treatment or require some other assistance at work;

- to individuals investigating compliance with the ADA and similar state and local laws; and

- where needed for workers' compensation or insurance purposes (for example, to process a claim).

9. May an employer tell employees who ask why their co-worker is allowed to do something that generally is not permitted (such as working at home or working a modified schedule) that she is receiving a reasonable accommodation?

No. Telling co-workers that an employee is receiving a reasonable accommodation amounts to a disclosure that the employee has a disability. Rather than disclosing that the employee is receiving a reasonable accommodation, the employer should focus on the importance of maintaining the privacy of all employees and emphasize that its policy is to refrain from discussing the work situation of any employee with co-workers. Employers may be able to avoid many of these kinds of questions by training all employees on the requirements of equal employment laws, including the ADA.

Additionally, an employer will benefit from providing information about reasonable accommodation to all of its employees. This can be done in a number of ways, such as through written reasonable accommodation procedures, employee handbooks, staff meetings, and periodic training. This kind of proactive approach may lead to fewer questions from employees who misperceive co-worker accommodations as "special treatment."

Accommodating Employees with Visual Disabilities

The ADA requires employers to provide adjustments or modifications—called reasonable accommodations—to enable applicants and employees with disabilities to enjoy equal employment opportunities unless doing so would be an undue hardship (that is, a significant difficulty or expense). Accommodations vary depending on the needs of the individual with a disability. Not all employees with a visual disability will need an accommodation or require the same accommodations.

10. What types of reasonable accommodations may employees with visual disabilities need?

Some employees may need one or more of the following accommodations:

assistive technology, including:

- a closed circuit television system (CCTV) for reading printed materials

- an external computer screen magnifier

- digital recorders

- software that will read information on the computer screen

- an optical scanner that can create documents in electronic form from printed ones

- a refreshable Braille display

- a Braille embosser

- written materials in an accessible format, such as in large print, Braille, in a recorded format, or on a computer disk

- modification of employer policies to allow use of a guide dog in the workplace

- modification of an employment test

- a person to read printed materials

- a driver or payment for the cost of transportation to enable performance of essential functions

- an accessible website

- permission to work at home

- modified training or training in the use of assistive technology.

- a modified work schedule

- time off, in the form of accrued paid leave or unpaid leave if paid leave has been exhausted or is unavailable

- reassignment to a vacant position

Although these are some examples of the types of accommodations commonly requested by employees with visual disabilities, other employees may need different changes or adjustments. Employers should ask the particular employee requesting an accommodation what he needs that will help him do his job. There also are extensive public and private resources to help employers identify reasonable accommodations. For example, the website for the Job Accommodation Network (JAN) (askjan.org) provides information about many types of accommodations for employees with visual disabilities.

11. How does an employee with a visual disability request a reasonable accommodation?

There are no "magic words" that a person has to use when requesting a reasonable accommodation. A person simply has to tell the employer that she needs an adjustment or change at work because of her visual impairment. A request for reasonable accommodation also can come from a family member, friend, health professional, or other representative on behalf of a person with a visual disability. If an employer requires more information about the disability and why an accommodation is needed, it should engage in an "interactive process"—a dialogue with the employee—to obtain information that will help the employer in handling the request.

12. May an employer request documentation when an employee who has a visual disability requests a reasonable accommodation?

Sometimes. When a person's vision impairment is not obvious, the employer may ask the person to provide reasonable documentation about how the condition limits major life activities (that is, whether the person has a disability) and why a reasonable accommodation is needed. An employer, however, is entitled only to documentation sufficient to establish that the employee has a visual disability and to explain why an accommodation is needed. A request for an employee's entire medical record, for example, would be inappropriate, as it likely would include information about conditions other than the employee's visual disability.

13. Does an employer have to grant every request for a reasonable accommodation?

No. An employer does not have to provide an accommodation if doing so would be an undue hardship. Undue hardship means that providing the reasonable accommodation will result in significant difficulty or expense. An employer also does not have to eliminate an essential function of a job as a reasonable accommodation, tolerate performance that does not meet its standards, or excuse violations of conduct rules that are job-related and consistent with business necessity and that the employer applies consistently to all employees (such as rules prohibiting violence, threatening behavior, theft, or destruction of property). Nor do employers have to provide employees with personal use items, such as eyeglasses or other devices that are used both on and off the job.

If more than one accommodation would be effective, the employee's preference should be given primary consideration, although the employer is not required to provide the employee's first choice of reasonable accommodation. If a requested accommodation is too difficult or expensive, an employer may choose to provide an easier or less costly accommodation as long as it is effective in meeting the employee's needs.

14. May an employer be required to provide more than one accommodation for the same employee with a visual disability?

Yes. The duty to provide a reasonable accommodation is an ongoing one. Although some employees with visual disabilities may require only one reasonable accommodation, others may need more than one. An employer must consider each request for a reasonable accommodation and determine whether it would be effective and whether providing it would pose an undue hardship.

15. What kinds of reasonable accommodations are related to the benefits and privileges of employment?

Reasonable accommodations related to the benefits and privileges of employment include accommodations that are necessary to provide individuals with disabilities access to facilities or portions of facilities to which all employees are granted access (for example, employee break rooms and cafeterias), access to information communicated in the workplace, and the opportunity to participate in employer-sponsored training and social events.

An employer will not be excused from providing an employee with a visual disability with a necessary accommodation because the employer has contracted with another entity to conduct the event.

Concerns about Safety

When it comes to safety concerns, an employer should be careful not to act on the basis of myths, fears, or stereotypes about vision impairments. Instead, the employer should evaluate each individual on her skills, knowledge, experience, and how the visual disability affects her.

16. When may an employer refuse to hire, terminate, or temporarily restrict the duties of a person who has or had a vision impairment because of safety concerns?

An employer only may exclude an individual with a vision impairment from a job for safety reasons when the individual poses a direct threat. A "direct threat" is a significant risk of substantial harm to the individual or others that cannot be eliminated or reduced through reasonable accommodation. This determination must be based on objective, factual evidence, including the best recent medical evidence.

In making a direct threat assessment, the employer must evaluate the individual's present ability to safely perform the job. The employer also must consider:

- the duration of the risk;
- the nature and severity of the potential harm;
- the likelihood that the potential harm will occur; and
- the imminence of the potential harm.

The harm must be serious and likely to occur, not remote or speculative. Finally, the employer must determine whether any reasonable accommodation would reduce or eliminate the risk.

17. What should an employer do when another federal law prohibits it from hiring anyone with a vision impairment?

If a federal law prohibits an employer from hiring a person with a vision impairment, the employer would not be liable under the ADA.

The employer should be certain, however, that compliance with the law actually is required, not voluntary. The employer also should be sure that the law does not contain any exceptions or waivers.

Harassment

The ADA prohibits harassment, or offensive conduct, based on disability just as other federal laws prohibit harassment based on race, sex, color, national origin, religion, age, and genetic information. Offensive conduct may include, but is not limited to, offensive jokes, slurs, epithets or name calling, physical assaults or threats, intimidation, ridicule or mockery, insults or put-downs, offensive objects or pictures, and interference with work performance. Although the law does not prohibit simple teasing, offhand comments, or isolated incidents that are not very serious, harassment is illegal when it is so frequent or severe that it creates a hostile or offensive work environment or when it results in an adverse employment decision (such as the victim being fired or demoted).

18. What should employers do to prevent and correct harassment?

Employers should make clear that they will not tolerate harassment based on disability or on any other basis. This can be done in a number of ways, such as through a written policy, employee handbooks, staff meetings, and periodic training. The employer should emphasize that harassment is prohibited and that employees should promptly report such conduct to a manager. Finally, the employer should immediately conduct a thorough investigation of any report of harassment and take swift and appropriate corrective action. For more information on the standards governing harassment under all of the EEO laws, see www.eeoc.gov/policy/docs/harassment.html.

Retaliation

The ADA prohibits retaliation by an employer against someone who opposes discriminatory employment practices, files a charge of employment discrimination, or testifies or participates in any way in an investigation, proceeding, or litigation related to a charge of employment discrimination. It is also unlawful for an employer to retaliate against someone for requesting a reasonable accommodation. Persons who believe that they have been retaliated against may file a charge of retaliation as described below.

19. How does an employee file a charge of employment discrimination?

Against Private Employers and State/Local Governments

Any person who believes that his or her employment rights have been violated on the basis of disability and wants to make a claim against an employer must file a charge of discrimination with the EEOC. A third party may also file a charge on behalf of another person who believes he or she experienced discrimination. For example, a family member, social worker, or other representative can file a charge on behalf of someone with a vision impairment. The charge must be filed by mail or in person with the local EEOC office within 180 days from the date of the alleged violation. The 180-day filing deadline is extended to 300 days if a state or local anti-discrimination agency has the authority to grant or seek relief as to the challenged unlawful employment practice.

The EEOC will send the parties a copy of the charge and may ask for responses and supporting information. Before formal investigation, the EEOC may select the charge for EEOC's mediation program. Both parties have to agree to mediation, which may prevent a time consuming investigation of the charge. Participation in mediation is free, voluntary, and confidential. For a detailed description of the process, you can visit their website at www.eeoc.gov/employees/charge.cfm.

Against the Federal Government

If you are a federal employee or job applicant and you believe that a federal agency has discriminated against you, you have a right to file a complaint. Each agency is required to post information about how to contact the agency's EEO Office. You can contact an EEO Counselor by calling the office responsible for the agency's EEO complaints program. Generally, you must contact the EEO Counselor within 45 days from the day the discrimination occurred. In most cases the EEO Counselor will give you the choice of participating either in EEO counseling or in an alternative dispute resolution (ADR) program, such as a mediation program.

If you do not settle the dispute during counseling or through ADR, you can file a formal discrimination complaint against the agency with the agency's EEO Office. You must file within 15 days from the day you receive notice from your EEO Counselor about how to file. For a detailed description of the process, you can visit their website at www.eeoc.gov/eeoc/publications/fs-fed.cfm.

Chapter 49

Social Security If You're Blind or Have Low Vision

If You're Blind or Have Low Vision

If you're blind, U.S. Social Security Administration (SSA) has special rules that allow you to receive benefits when you are unable to work.

SSA pays benefits to people who are blind under two programs: the Social Security Disability Insurance program and the Supplemental Security Income (SSI) program. The medical rules they use to decide whether you are blind are the same for each program. Other rules are different.

You Can Get Disability Benefits If You're Blind

You may qualify for Social Security or SSI disability benefits if you're blind. SSA considers you to be blind if your vision can't be corrected to better than 20/200 in your better eye or if your visual field is 20 degrees or less in your better eye for a period that lasted or is expected to last at least 12 months.

You Can Get Disability Benefits Even If You're Not Blind

If your vision doesn't meet Social Security's definition of blindness, you may still qualify for disability benefits if your vision problems

---

This chapter includes text excerpted from "If You're Blind or Have Low Vision—How We Can Help," U.S. Social Security Administration (SSA), January 2017.

alone, or combined with other health problems, prevent you from working. For Social Security disability benefits, you must also have worked long enough in a job where you paid Social Security taxes. For SSI payments based on disability and blindness, you need not have worked, but your income and resources must be under certain dollar limits.

How You Qualify for Social Security Disability Benefits

When you work and pay Social Security taxes, you earn credits that count toward future Social Security benefits.

If you're blind, you can earn credits anytime during your working years. Credits for your work after you become blind can be used to qualify you for benefits if you don't have enough credits at the time you become blind.

Also, if you don't have enough credits to get Social Security disability benefits based on your own earnings, you may be able to get benefits based on the earnings of one of your parents or your spouse.

Disability Freeze

There is a special rule that may help you get higher retirement or disability benefits someday. You can use this rule if you are blind but aren't getting disability benefits now because you are still working. If your earnings are lower because of your blindness, SSA can exclude those years when they calculate your Social Security retirement or disability benefit in the future. Because Social Security benefits are based on your average lifetime earnings, your benefit will be higher if they don't count those years. SSA calls this rule a "disability freeze."

You Can Get SSI Disability Payments

SSI payments are based on need. Your income and resources must be less than certain dollar limits. The income limits vary from one state to another. You need not have worked under Social Security to qualify for SSI. Ask your local Social Security office about the income limits in your state.

You Can Work While Receiving Benefits

Rules, called "work incentives," make it easier for people receiving disability benefits to work.

People getting Social Security disability benefits can continue to receive their benefits when they work as long as their earnings are not more than an amount set by law.

If you're receiving Social Security disability benefits and you're blind, you can earn as much as $1,950 a month in 2017. This is higher than the earnings limit of $1,170 a month that applies to disabled workers who aren't blind. The earnings limits usually change each year.

Additionally, if you're blind and self-employed, SSA doesn't evaluate the time you spend working in your business as they do for people who aren't blind. This means you can be doing a lot of work for your business, but still receive disability benefits, as long as your net profit averages $1,950 or less a month in 2017.

Work Figured Differently after Age 55

If you are age 55 or older, and blind, SSA uses determination rules about work for you that are different from the rules they use for people who aren't blind. After age 55, even if your earnings exceed $1,950 a month in 2017, benefits are only suspended, not terminated, if the work you're doing requires a lower level of skill and ability than what you did before you reached 55. They'll pay you disability benefits for any month your earnings fall below this limit.

Different work incentives apply to people getting SSI.

Part Eight

Additional Help and Information

Chapter 50

Vision Health Initiative (VHI)

The Centers for Disease Control and Prevention's (CDC) Vision Health Initiative (VHI) has joined with others committed to vision health to create a more effective multilevel network for vision loss prevention and eye health promotion. VHI has the unique role of collaborating with state and national partners, to strengthen science and develop interventions to improve eye health, reduce vision loss and blindness, and promote the health of people with vision loss.

VHI Mission

The CDC/VHI, a group in the Division of Diabetes Translation, is designed to promote vision health and quality of life for all populations, throughout all life stages, by preventing and controlling eye disease, eye injury, and vision loss resulting in disability.

VHI Goals

- Promote eye health and prevent vision loss.

- Improve the health and lives of people with vision loss by preventing complications, disabilities, and burden.

This chapter contains text excerpted from the following sources: Text in this chapter begins with excerpts from "Vision Health Initiative (VHI)," Centers for Disease Control and Prevention (CDC), December 12, 2013. Reviewed March 2017; Text under the heading "VHI: The Numbers" is excerpted from "Vision Health Initiative: Improving the Nation's Vision Health," Centers for Disease Control and Prevention (CDC), January 18, 2016.

593

- Reduce vision and eye health related disparities.

- Integrate vision health with other public health strategies.

VHI Objectives

1. To assess and monitor the burden of vision impairment and blindness. The VHI develops and refines vision surveillance at the state and national level and helps states develop their capacity to implement effective state-based surveillance systems.

2. To build capacity for conducting epidemiologic, behavioral, and health services research related to vision loss at all life stages and translate scientific evidence into public health practice, health policy, and health promotion strategies.

3. To identify, prioritize, and disseminate evidence-based, efficient, and cost-effective public health interventions to improve quality of life, increase access to needed eye care, and reduce health disparities among people with or at high risk for vision loss.

4. To leverage resources, facilitate strategic partnerships and provide technical assistance to national, state and community-based partners to preserve, protect, and enhance vision health.

5. To integrate appropriate and effective vision health activities into existing state and community public health programs.

Future Directions

Future vision and eye health initiatives must incorporate innovative, comprehensive and multidisciplinary approaches that ensure positioning eye health within any healthy lifestyle intervention.

Working with its partners, CDC aims to expand surveillance activities, programs and interventions nationwide to improve the care for people with or at risk for vision loss. CDC is also working to develop an integration model at the state level to address vision and eye disease problems.

Healthy People 2010

Healthy People 2010 (HP 2010) for the first time included a chapter on vision as well as hearing. *HP 2010* is sponsored by the U.S. Department of Health and Human Services (HHS). It identifies the most significant threats to health and establishes national goals to reduce those threats.

Chapter 28 of *HP 2010* assert the national goal to "improve the visual and hearing health of the nation through prevention, early detection, treatment, and rehabilitation." Vision objectives include increasing the proportion of people who have regular dilated eye examinations and increasing the proportion of children aged 5 years and younger who have vision screenings. *HP 2010* also proposes to reduce visual impairment as a result of refractive errors and to reduce blindness and vision impairment among children aged 17 years and younger. The chapter calls visual impairment "one of the 10 most frequent causes of disability in America," discusses the importance of vision rehabilitation, and addresses visual impairment due to diabetic retinopathy, age-related macular degeneration, glaucoma, cataract, and refractive error, saying that "visual impairment is associated with loss of personal independence, decreased quality of life, and difficulty maintaining employment. For older adults, visual problems have a pronounced negative impact on quality of life, equivalent to that of life-threatening conditions such as heart disease and cancer.

Healthy People 2020

In *Healthy People 2020*, National Eye Institute (NEI) serves as the lead agency for the vision objectives. CDC/VHI serves on the *Healthy People 2020* Vision Work Group to assist in setting up the direction for eye health and safety for the next decade. The work will continue building on the success of *HP 2010* and continue the efforts to make vision and eye health a health priority.

VHI: The Numbers

- 14 million individuals in the United States aged 12 years and older have visual impairment; 80 percent could have their vision improved through refractive correction.

- Glaucoma is 4–5 times higher in African Americans than whites.

- 89 percent of the U.S. adult population are NOT aware that eye complications caused by diabetes usually have no early warning symptoms.

- 14 percent of adults in poor families reported vision trouble compared to 7 percent of adults in families that are not poor.

- State data show that more than 50 percent of adults who did not seek eye care reported lack of awareness or costs as the main reasons.

- $139 billion is the total economic burden of eye disorders and vision impairment in the United States.

Chapter 51

Glossary of Terms Related to Eyes and Eye Disorders

ablation zone: The area of tissue that is removed during laser surgery.

accommodation: The ability of the eye to increase its focusing power. As an object is viewed closer up, greater focusing power is needed to continue to see it clearly.

acuity: Clearness, or sharpness of vision.

adaptive and assistive devices: Prescription and nonprescription devices that help people with low vision enhance their remaining vision.

age-related macular degeneration: An eye disease that results in a loss of central, "straight-ahead" vision.

anterior chamber: The space in the front portion of the eye between the cornea and the iris. The space is filled with a clear fluid.

astigmatism: A distortion of the image on the retina caused by irregularities in the cornea or lens.

blood vessels: Arteries, veins, and capillaries that carry blood through the body.

cataract: A clouding of the lens. People with a cataract see through a haze.

This glossary contains terms excerpted from documents produced by several sources deemed reliable.

conjunctivitis: Eye infection, pink eye, swelling and redness around your eyes.

cornea: clear outer part of the focusing system that is located at the front of the eye.

corneal edema: Abnormal fluid build-up in the cornea that can cause haziness and swelling of the cornea and resulting blurred vision.

corneal transplant: Surgical treatment where the patient's cloudy cornea is cut away and a clear cornea, donated by someone who has died, is sewn into its place.

diabetes: A chronic disease related to high blood sugar that may lead to vision loss (diabetic retinopathy).

diabetic eye disease: A group of eye problems that people with diabetes may get. All of these eye problems can lead to vision loss or blindness.

diabetic retinopathy: Damage to the blood vessels in the retina due to diabetes.

dilate: Widening or enlargement of the pupil so that the retina is more visible.

dilated eye exam: An eye examination where drops are placed in your eyes to widen, or dilate, the pupils. The eye care professional uses a special magnifying lens to examine the retina and optic nerve for signs of damage and other eye problems.

dominant optic nerve atrophy: Hereditary damage to the optic nerve, resulting in a loss of vision.

double vision: Seeing two images of a single object instead of one.

dry eye syndrome: A common condition that occurs when the eyes do not produce enough tears to keep the eye moist and comfortable.

endothelial cells: The cells that line the inner surface of the cornea in a single layer (endothelium). They are responsible for pumping fluid out of the cornea to keep it clear.

endothelium: The innermost layer of cells lining the inner surface of the cornea.

epithelium: The outermost layer of cells of the cornea and the eye's first defense against infection.

excimer laser: An ultraviolet laser used in refractive surgery to remove corneal tissue.

eyelash: The fringe of hair edging the eyelid; they close to keep particles, like dust, out of your eyes.

eyelid: The skin-covered structure that protects the front of the eye. It limits light entering the eye and spreads tears over the cornea.

focal laser treatment: A laser surgery treatment where an ophthalmologist places up to several hundred small laser burns in the areas of retinal leakage surrounding the macula.

fovea: The center of the macula, which gives the sharpest vision.

glare: Scatter from bright light that causes discomfort and can decrease vision and the ability to perform tasks like driving.

glaucoma: A group of eye diseases in which the normal fluid pressure inside the eyes slowly rises, leading to vision loss or even blindness.

hyperopia/farsightedness : The inability to see near objects as clearly as distant objects, and the need for accommodation to see distant objects clearly.

hyperopia/ farsightedness: The inability to see near objects as clearly as distant objects.

intraocular lens: A lens that is surgically implanted inside the eye.

intraocular pressure: The pressure of fluid inside the eye.

iridotomy: Incision of the iris.

iris: The colored part of the eye; it regulates the amount of light entering the eye.

iritis: Inflammation of the front portion of the eye that can lead to scarring inside the eye and glaucoma.

keratectomy: The surgical removal of corneal tissue.

keratitis: Inflammation of the cornea.

keratoconus: A disorder characterized by an irregular corneal surface (cone-shaped) resulting in blurred and distorted images.

keratomileusis: Carving of the cornea to reshape it.

keratotomy: A surgical incision (cut) of the cornea.

laser trabeculoplasty: A surgical procedure that helps open up the drainage angle to allow more fluid to pass out of the eye.

lens: The clear part of the eye behind the iris that helps to focus light on the retina. It allows the eye to focus on both far and near objects.

low vision: A visual impairment, not corrected by standard eyeglasses, contact lenses, medication, or surgery, which interferes with the ability to perform everyday activities.

low vision therapist: A vision rehabilitation professional who trains people with low vision to use optical and nonoptical devices and adaptive techniques to make the most of their remaining vision.

macula: The small, sensitive area of the retina that gives central vision.

macular edema: When fluid leaks into the center of the macula, the part of the eye where sharp, straight-ahead vision occurs. The fluid makes the macula swell, blurring vision.

microkeratome: A mechanical surgical device that is affixed to the eye by use of a vacuum ring. When secured, a very sharp blade cuts a layer of the cornea at a predetermined depth.

microvascular disease: Disease of the smallest blood vessels, such as those found in the eyes, nerves, and kidneys.

mild nonproliferative retinopathy: The first stage of diabetic retinopathy where small areas of balloon-like swelling (microaneurysms) occur in the tiny blood vessels of the retina.

moderate nonproliferative retinopathy: The second stage of diabetic retinopathy where blood vessels that nourish the retina are blocked.

monovision: The purposeful adjustment of one eye for near vision and the other eye for distance vision.

myopia/nearsightedness: The inability to see distant objects as clearly as near objects, because the focusing power of the eye is too strong.

occupational therapist: A rehabilitation professional who works with persons with disabilities, including low vision, to complete the everyday activities that they need for independence and quality of life.

ophthalmologist: A medical doctor who diagnoses and treats all diseases and disorders of the eye and prescribes glasses and contact lenses.

optic nerve: Bundle of more than 1 million nerve fibers that carry visual messages from the retina to the brain.

orientation and mobility specialist: A vision rehabilitation professional who trains people with low vision to move about safely in the home and travel by themselves.

over correction: The refractive error of the eye is corrected too much causing someone who is nearsighted to become farsighted or someone who is farsighted to become nearsighted.

peripheral iridectomy: Surgical removal of part of the iris near its outer edge.

posterior chamber: The space in the eye between the back of the iris and the front of the vitreous (the jelly-like substance that fills the space in the back central portion of the eyeball).

presbyopia: The inability to maintain a clear image (focus) as objects are moved closer.

pseudoexfoliation: Abnormal deposits of white, flaky material seen on the structures in the front part of the eye that may be associated with cataracts and high pressure in the eye or glaucoma.

pupil: The opening at the center of the iris. The iris adjusts the size of the pupil and controls the amount of light that can enter the eye.

pupillary block: Blockage of the flow of fluid from the posterior chamber to the anterior chamber of the eye through the pupil. This can cause the pressure to build up inside the eye and can result in glaucoma.

refraction: A test to determine the refractive power of the eye; also, the bending of light as it passes from one medium into another.

refractive errors: Imperfections in the focusing power of the eye, for example, hyperopia, myopia, and astigmatism.

refractive power: The ability of an object, such as the eye, to bend light as light passes through it.

refractive surgery: General term referring to many different procedures to correct the refractive error of the eye.

retina: Light-sensitive tissue lining the back of the eyeball. It sends electrical impulses to the brain.

retinal detachment: Separation of the retina from its attachments to the back of the eyeball often resulting in loss of vision. Flashing lights, floating spots, and blank spots in vision can be symptoms of a retinal detachment.

scatter laser surgery: A laser surgery treatment where an ophthalmologist places 1,000 to 2,000 laser burns in the areas of the retina away from the macula, causing the abnormal blood vessels to shrink.

sclera: The tough, white, outer layer (coat) of the eyeball that, along with the cornea, protects the eyeball.

Sjogren syndrome: Dry eyes and mouth.

specialist in low vision: An ophthalmologist or optometrist who specializes in the evaluation of low vision. This professional prescribes magnifying devices.

stroma: The middle, thickest layer of tissue in the cornea.

tonometry: An instrument that measures the pressure inside your eye. Numbing drops may be applied to your eye during this test.

under correction: The refractive error of the eye is not corrected enough leaving someone who is nearsighted still nearsighted or someone who is farsighted still farsighted to a certain degree.

uveitis: Inflammation of the inner eye that includes the iris, the tissue that holds the lens of the eye, and a network of blood vessels surrounding the eyeball called the choroid plexus.

vision rehabilitation therapists: Professionals who teach adaptive independentliving skills, enabling adults who are blind or have low vision to confidently perform a range of daily activities.

visual acuity: The sharpness of vision; the measurement of the eye's ability to distinguish object details and shape.

visual acuity test: An eye chart test that measures how well you see at various distances.

vitrectomy: A surgical treatment where an ophthalmologist removes the vitreous gel and replaces it with a salt solution.

vitreous gel: Transparent, colorless mass that fills the rear two-thirds of the eyeball, between the lens and the retina.

vitreous humor: The clear gel that fills the inside of the eye.

wavefront: A measure of the total refractive errors of the eye, including nearsightedness, farsightedness, astigmatism, and other refractive errors that cannot be corrected with glasses or contacts.

Chapter 52

Directory of Resources Related to Eye Disorders and Vision Loss

General

All About Vision (AAV)
1010 Turquoise St.
Ste. 275
San Diego, CA 92109
Phone: 858-454-2145
Website: www.allaboutvision.com

American Academy of Ophthalmology (AAO)
655 Beach St.
San Francisco, CA 94109
Phone: 415-561-8500
Fax: 415-561-8533
Website: www.aao.org
E-mail: eyesmart@aao.org

American Association for Pediatric Ophthalmology and Strabismus (AAPOS)
655 Beach St.
San Francisco, CA 94109-1336
Phone: 415-561-8505
Fax: 415-561-8531
Website: www.aapos.org
E-mail: aapos@aao.org

Resources in this chapter were compiled from several sources deemed reliable; all contact information was verified and updated in March 2017.

American Foundation for the Blind (AFB)
Two Penn Plaza
Ste. 1102
New York, NY 10121
Toll-Free: 800-AFB-LINE
(800-232-5463)
Phone: 212-502-7600
Fax: 888-545-8331
Website: www.afb.org
E-mail: afbinfo@afb.net

American Optometric Association (AOA)
243 N. Lindbergh Blvd.
First Fl.
St. Louis, MO 63141-7881
Toll-Free: 800-365-2219
Phone: 314-991-4100
Fax: 314-991-4101
Website: www.aoa.org

Boston Children's Hospital
300 Longwood Ave.
Boston, MA 02115
Toll-Free: 800-355-7944
Phone: 617-355-6000
Website: www.childrenshospital.org

eMedicineHealth
WebMD LLC
1201 Peachtree St., N.E.
400 Colony Sq.
Ste. 2100
Atlanta, GA 30361
Toll-Free: 866-788-3097
Website: www.emedicinehealth.com

EyeCare America
The Foundation of the American Academy of Ophthalmology (AAO)
P.O. Box 429098
San Francisco, CA 94142-9098
Toll-Free: 877-887-6327
Fax: 415-561-8567
Website: www.eyecareamerica.org
E-mail: pubserv@aao.org

Eye Surgery Education Council (ESEC)
American Society of Cataract and Refractive Surgery (ASCRS) Foundation
4000 Legato Rd.
Ste. 700
Fairfax, VA 22033-4003
Phone: 703-591-2220
Fax: 703-591-0614
Website: www.eyeworld.org
E-mail: ascrs@ascrs.org

Foundation Fighting Blindness
7168 Columbia Gateway Dr.
Ste. 100
Columbia, MD 21046
Toll-Free: 800-683-5555
Phone: 410-423-0600
TDD: 410-363-7139
Website: www.blindness.org
E-mail: info@FightBlindness.org

Junior Blind of America (JBA)
5300 Angeles Vista Blvd.
Los Angeles, CA 90043
Toll-Free: 800-352-2290
Phone: 323-295-4555
Fax: 323-296-0424
Website: www.juniorblind.org
E-mail: info@juniorblind.org

Lighthouse Guild International
15 W. 65th St.
New York, NY 10023
Toll-Free: 800-284-4422
Phone: 212-769-6200
Website: www.lighthouseguild.org

National Eye Institute (NEI)
National Institutes of Health (NIH)
31 Center Dr. MSC 2510
Bethesda, MD 20892-2510
Phone: 301-496-5248
Website: nei.nih.gov
E-mail: 2020@nei.nih.gov

National Stroke Association (NSA)
9707 E. Easter Ln.
Ste. B
Centennial, CO 80112
Toll-Free: 800-STROKES (800-787-6537)
Website: www.stroke.org
E-mail: info@stroke.org

North American Neuro-Ophthalmology Society (NANOS)
5841 Cedar Lake Rd.
Ste. 204
Minneapolis, MN 55416
Phone: 952-646-2037
Fax: 952-545-6073
Website: www.nanosweb.org
E-mail: info@nanosweb.org

Optometric Physicians of Washington (OPW)
14450 N.E. 29th Pl.
Ste. 115
Bellevue, WA 98007-3697
Phone: 425-455-0874
Fax: 425-646-9646
Website: www.eyes.org
E-mail: opw@eyes.org

Prevent Blindness America (PBA)
211 W. Wacker Dr.
Ste. 1700
Chicago, IL 60606
Toll-Free: 800-331-2020
Website: www.preventblindness.org
E-mail: info@preventblindness.org

St. Luke's Cataract and Laser Institute
43309 U.S. Hwy 19 N
Tarpon Springs, FL 34689
Toll-Free: 888-904-0000
Phone: 727-938-2020
Fax: 727-938-5606
Website: www.stlukeseye.com

*University of Illinois Eye
and Ear Infirmary (IEEI)*
Department of Ophthalmology
and Visual Sciences (DOVS)
1855 W. Taylor St. m/c 648
Rm. 3.138
Chicago, IL 60612
Phone: 312-996-6591
Fax: 312-996-7770
Website: eyecare.uic.edu
E-mail: eyeweb@uic.edu

Your-Eye-Sight.org
Website: www.your-eye-sight.org

Achromatopsia

Achromatopsia.info
The Low Vision Centers of
Indiana
9002 N. Meridian St.
Ste. 109
Indianapolis, IN 46260
Phone: 317-844-0919
Website: www.achromatopsia.
info

Anophthalmia

*International Children's
Anophthalmia Network
(ICAN)*
c/o Center for Developmental
Medicine and Genetics
5501 Old York Rd.
Genetics, Levy 2 West
Philadelphia, PA 19141
Toll-Free: 800-580-ICAN
(800-580-4226)
Website: www.anophthalmia.org
E-mail: ican@anophthalmia.org

Choroideremia

*Choroideremia Research
Foundation, Inc. (CRF)*
23 E. Brundreth St.
Springfield, MA 01109-2110
Toll-Free: 800-210-0233
Phone: 413-781-2274
Website: www.curechm.org

Disorders of Cornea

*Cornea Research Foundation
of America (CRFA)*
9002 N. Meridian St.
Ste. 212
Indianapolis, IN 46260
Phone: 317-814-2993
Fax: 317-814-2806
Website: www.cornea.org

*Sjögren's Syndrome
Foundation (SSF)*
6706 Democracy Blvd.
Ste. 325
Bethesda, MD 20817
Toll-Free: 800-475-6473
Phone: 301-530-4420
Fax: 301-530-4415
Website: www.sjogrens.org

*Stevens Johnson Syndrome
Foundation (SJS)*
P.O. Box 350333
Westminster, CO 80035
Phone: 303-635-1241
Fax: 303-648-6686
Website: www.sjsupport.org
E-mail: sjsupport@gmail.com

Diabetic Eye Disorders

American Diabetes Association (ADA)
2451 Crystal Dr.
Ste. 900
Arlington, VA 22202
Toll-Free: 800-DIABETES
(800-342-2383)
Website: www.diabetes.org
E-mail: askada@diabetes.org

Glaucoma

Children's Glaucoma Foundation (CGF)
2 Longfellow Pl.
Ste. 201
Boston, MA 02114
Phone: 617-227-3011
Fax: 617-227-9538
Website: www.
childrensglaucomafoundation.
org
E-mail: info@
childrensglaucomafoundation.
org

The Glaucoma Foundation (TGF)
80 Maiden Ln.
Ste. 700
New York, NY 10038
Phone: 212-285-0080
Website: www.
glaucomafoundation.org
E-mail: info@
glaucomafoundation.org

Glaucoma Research Foundation (GRF)
251 Post St.
Ste. 600
San Francisco, CA 94108
Toll-Free: 800-826-6693
Phone: 415-986-3162
Website: www.glaucoma.org
E-mail: question@glaucoma.org

Keratoconus

National Keratoconus Foundation (NKCF)
850 Health Sciences Rd.
Irvine, CA 92697
Toll-Free: 800-521-2524
Phone: 310-623-4466
Fax: 310-623-1837
Website: www.nkcf.org
E-mail: info@nkcf.org

Macular Degeneration

AMD Alliance International
111 E. 59th St.
New York, NY 10022
Toll-Free: 800-829-0500
Phone: 212-821-9200
Website: www.amdalliance.org
E-mail: info@amdalliance.org

Macular Degeneration Partnership (AMD)
850 Health Sciences Rd.
Irvine, CA 92697
Toll-Free: 888-430-9898
Phone: 310-623-4466
Website: www.amd.org
E-mail: ContactUs@AMD.org

607

Optic Nerve Disease

International Foundation for Optic Nerve Disease (IFOND)
P. O. Box 777
Cornwall, NY 12518
Phone: 6572067250
Website: www.ifond.org
E-mail: ifond@aol.com

Retinoblastoma

National Cancer Institute (NCI)
National Institutes of Health (NIH)
9609 Medical Center Dr.
Rockville, MD 20850
Toll-Free: 800-4-CANCER
(800-422-6237)
Phone: 301-435-3848
Toll-Free TTY: 800-332-8615
Website: www.cancer.gov

Uveitis

American Uveitis Society (AUS)
700 18th St. S.
Ste. 601
Birmingham, AL 35233
Phone: 205-325-8507
Fax: 205-325-8200
Website: www.uveitissociety.org

Ocular Immunology and Uveitis Foundation (OIUF)
1440 Main St.
Ste. 201
Waltham, MA 02451
Phone: 781-647-1431
Fax: 617-621-2953
Website: www.uveitis.org

Index

Index

National Cancer Institute (NCI)
   contact 608
   publications
      retinoblastoma treatment 287n
      uveal melanoma
         treatment 321n
National Eye Institute (NEI)
   contact 605
   publications
      Age-Related Eye Disease Study
         (AREDS) 12n
      age-related macular
         degeneration (AMD) 239n
      amblyopia 94n
      astigmatism 79n
      blepharitis 388n
      brain and eye70n
      cataract 203n
      color blindness 442n
      common vision problems 54n
      comprehensive dilated eye
         exam 38n
      cornea and corneal disease
         189n
      diabetes and blindness 505n
      diabetic eye disease 508n
      dry eye 226n
      eye disease statistics 24n
      eye health 10n, 117n
      eyewear 361n
      floaters 308n
      glaucoma 259n
      healthy eyes 117n
      helping older adults 60n
      hyperopia 82n
      idiopathic intracranial
         hypertension 535n
      macular hole 252n
      macular pucker 256n
      myopia 84n
      presbyopia 90n
      refractive errors 76n
      retinal detachment 280n
      retinitis pigmentosa 282n
      retinopathy of prematurity
         (ROP) 299n
      sports and eye safety 361n
      talking to eye doctor 45n
      uveal coloboma 314n

National Eye Institute (NEI)
   publications, *continued*
      uveitis 328n
      vision loss help 556n
      workplace eye safety 341n
National Human Genome Research
   Institute (NHGRI)
   publication
      Duane syndrome 453n
National Institute of Arthritis and
   Musculoskeletal and Skin Diseases
   (NIAMS)
   publications
      Behçet disease 520n
      rosacea 541n
National Institute of Diabetes and
   Digestive and Kidney Diseases
   (NIDDK)
   publications
      diabetic eye disease 500n, 505n
      Graves disease 526n
National Institute of Neurological
   Disorders and Stroke (NINDS)
   publication
      neuromyelitis optica 270n
National Institutes of Health (NIH)
   publications
      blindness 68n
      longitudinal study of ocular
         complications of AIDS
         (LSOCA) 516n
      studies of ocular complications
         of AIDS (SOCA)—ganciclovir-
         cidofovir CMV retinitis trial
         (GCCRT) 516n
National Institute on Aging (NIA)
   publications
      aging and eyes 56n
      eye doctor visit 45n
National Keratoconus Foundation
   (NKCF), contact 607
National Stroke Association (NSA)
   contact 605
   publication
      stroke and vision loss 489n
NCT *see* non-contact tonometry
neovascular age-related macular
   degeneration (neovascular AMD),
   described 243

O

vitrectomy
  defined 602
  described 513
  floaters 309
  fungal eye infection 487
  macular hole 254
  macular pucker 257
  retinal detachment 281
  retinopathy of prematurity 303
vitreous
  described 253
  see also floaters; vitreous humor
vitreous detachment, macular
  pucker 257
vitreous gel
  defined 500, 602
  anti-VEGF injection therapy 512
  see also vitreous humor
vitreous humor
  defined 4, 602
  depicted *330*
  disorders 307
  endophthalmitis 484
  hemorrhage 494
  macular hole 253
  uveitis 329
  Wagner syndrome 433
  see also aqueous humor;
    vitrectomy
VRT *see* vision restoration therapy

W

Wagner syndrome, overview 432–4
"Wagner Syndrome" (GARD) 432n
"Wagner Syndrome" (GHR) 432n
"WAGR syndrome" (GHR) 460n
wavefront, defined 602
wavefront LASIK, described 161
wear schedule, contact lenses 122
WebMD LLC (eMedicineHealth)
  contact 604
  publications
      chemical eye burns 374n
      foreign body and eye 381n
welding helmet, personal protective
  eyewear 342

welding protector, welding
  protection 355
wet AMD
  described 243
  risks 18
  see also age-related macular
      degeneration; neovascular age-
      related macular degeneration
"What Is a Comprehensive Dilated
  Eye Exam?" (NEI) 38n
"What Is LASIK?" (FDA) 144n
"What Is Legal Blindness?"
  (Omnigraphics) 551n
"What to Know If Your Child Wants
  Contact Lenses" (FDA) 139n
"When Is LASIK Not for Me?" (FDA)
  144n
"Why Is Vision Loss a Public Health
  Problem?" (CDC) 28n
Wildervanck syndrome, Duane
  syndrome 454
Wilms tumor, WAGR syndrome, 460
workplace
  eye injury 348
  hazard assessment 342
  low vision 571
"Workplace Safety and Health Topics:
  Eye Safety" (NIOSH) 341n

X

X-linked juvenile retinoschisis,
  overview 304–5
"X-Linked Juvenile Retinoschisis"
  (GHR) 304n
X-ray, eye exams 290

Y

Your-Eye-Sight.org, website
  address 606

Z

zeaxanthin, age-related macular
  degeneration (AMD) 12
zinc, Age-Related Eye Disease
  Study 12, 244